BASIC AND CLINICAL ASPECTS OF NUTRITION AND BRAIN DEVELOPMENT

Editors

David K. Rassin
Department of Pediatrics
Division of Developmental Nutrition and Metabolism
University of Texas Medical Branch
Galveston, Texas

Bernard Haber
Marine Biomedical Institute
University of Texas Medical Branch
Galveston, Texas

Boris Drujan
Instituto Venezolano de Investigaciones Cientificas
Caracas, Venezuela

Alan R. Liss, Inc., New York

Library of Congress Cataloging-in-Publication Data

Basic and clinical aspects of nutrition and brain
  development.

  (Current topics in nutrition and disease ; v. 16)
  Presentations from a symposium sponsored by
El Centro Latinoamericano de Biológica–United
Nations Educational, Scientific, and Cultural
Organization (CLAB-UNESCO), held in Caracas,
Venezuela, Dec. 1985.
  Includes bibliographies and index.
  1. Brain—Diseases—Nutritional aspects—Congresses.
2. Brain—Growth—Congresses. 3. Infants—Nutrition—
Congresses. 4. Pediatric neurology—Congresses.
I. Rassin, David K. II. Haber, Bernard. III. Drujan,
Boris. IV. Centro Latino Americano de Ciencias
Biológicas. V. Series. [DNLM: 1. Brain—growth &
development—congresses. 2. Brain Diseases—etiology—
congresses. 3. Infant Nutrition—congresses.
4. Models, Biological—congresses. 5. Nutrition
Disorders—complications—congresses.
W1 CU82R v.16 / WL 300 B3107 1985]
RC386.2.B38   1987   616.8'04   87-16871
ISBN 0-8451-1615-0

Contents

Contributors

Miriam Banay-Schwartz, N.S. Kline Institute for Psychiatric Research, New York, NY 10035 **[43]**

A. Barbeau, Clinical Research Institute of Montréal, Department of Neurobiology, Montréal, Québec H2W 1R7, Canada **[271]**

F. Bélanger, Clinical Research Institute of Montréal, Department of Neurobiology, Montréal, Québec H2W 1R7, Canada **[271]**

N.F. Butte, Children's Nutrition Center and Department of Pediatrics, Baylor University, Houston, TX 77030 **[3]**

Roger F. Butterworth, Laboratory of Neurochemistry, André-Viallet Clinical Research Centre, Hôpital Saint-Luc, University of Montréal, Montréal, Québec H2X 3J4, Canada **[287]**

Rosemary E.A. Craig, Department of Nutritional Sciences, Faculty of Medicine, University of Toronto, Toronto, Ontario, Canada M5S 1A8 **[159]**

Janina R. Galler, Center for Behavioral Development and Mental Retardation, Boston University School of Medicine, Boston, MA 02118 **[57]**

C. Garza, Children's Nutrition Center and Department of Pediatrics, Baylor University, Houston, TX 77030 **[3]**

Giorgio Gombos, Centre de Neurochimie du CNRS, 67000 Strasbourg, France **[99]**

Carol E. Greenwood, Department of Nutritional Sciences, Faculty of Medicine, University of Toronto, Toronto, Ontario, Canada M5S 1A8 **[159]**

D. Hachey, Children's Nutrition Center and Department of Pediatrics, Baylor University, Houston, TX 77030 **[3]**

A.V. Juorio, Psychiatric Research Division, University of Saskatchewan, Saskatoon, Saskatchewan S7N 0W0, Canada **[305]**

Karla B. Kanis, Center for Behavioral Development and Mental Retardation, Boston University School of Medicine, Boston, MA 02118 **[57]**

Barry B. Kaplan, Molecular Neurobiology Program, Department of Psychiatry, Western Psychiatric Institute and Clinic, University of Pittsburgh School of Medicine, Pittsburgh, PA 15213 **[131]**

Kinya Kuriyama, Department of Pharmacology, Kyoto Prefectural University of Medicine, Kawaramachi-Hirokoji, Kamikyo-Ku, Kyoto 602, Japan **[255]**

The numbers in brackets are the opening page numbers of the contributors' articles.

Abel Lajtha, N.S. Kline Institute for Psychiatric Research, New York, NY 10035 **[43]**

Ricardo López-Escalera, Instituto de Fisiología Celular, Universidad Nacional Autónoma de México, 04510 México, D.F., México **[217]**

Dimitra Mangoura, Departments of Psychiatry and Pharmacology, University of Colorado School of Medicine, Denver, CO 80262 **[75]**

Julio Morán, Instituto de Fisiología Celular, Universidad Nacional Autónoma de México, 04510 México, D.F., México **[217]**

Seitaro Ohkuma, Department of Pharmacology, Kyoto Prefectural University of Medicine, Kawaramachi-Hirokoji, Kamikyo-Ku, Kyoto 602, Japan **[255]**

S. Paris, Clinical Research Institute of Montréal, Department of Neurobiology, Montréal, Québec H2W 1R7, Canada **[271]**

Herminia Pasantes-Morales, Instituto de Fisiología Celular, Universidad Nacional Autónoma de México, 04510 México, D.F., México **[217]**

David K. Rassin, Department of Pediatrics, University of Texas Medical Branch at Galveston, Galveston, TX 77550 **[ix, 19]**

Pedro Rosso, Escuela de Medicina, Pontificia Universidad Católica de Chile, Santiago, Chile **[339]**

M. Roy, Clinical Research Institute of Montréal, Department of Neurobiology, Montréal, Québec H2W 1R7, Canada **[271]**

Nikos Sakellaridis, Departments of Psychiatry and Pharmacology, University of Colorado School of Medicine, Denver, CO 80262 **[75]**

R.J. Schanler, Children's Nutrition Center and Department of Pediatrics, Baylor University, Houston, TX 77030 **[3]**

Zena Stein, Gertrude H. Sergievsky Center, Columbia University and New York Psychiatric Institute, New York, NY 10032 **[323]**

Anna Maria Giuffrida Stella, Instituto di Chimica Biologica, Dell'Universita di Catania, 95125 Catania, Italy **[43]**

J.A. Sturman, Department of Developmental Biochemistry, Institute for Basic Research in Developmental Disabilities, Staten Island, NY 10314 **[245]**

Mervyn Susser, Gertrude H. Sergievsky Center, Columbia University and New York Psychiatric Institute, New York, NY 10032 **[317,323]**

N.M. van Gelder, Clinical Research Institute of Montréal, Department of Neurobiology, Montréal, Québec H2W 1R7, Canada **[271]**

Antonia Vernadakis, Departments of Psychiatry and Pharmacology, University of Colorado School of Medicine, Denver, CO 80262 **[75]**

Francesco Vitiello, Istituto di Fisiologia Umana, Facoltà di Medicina e Chirurgia, Bari, Italy **[99]**

W.W. Wong, Children's Nutrition Center and Department of Pediatrics, Baylor University, Houston, TX 77030 **[3]**

Preface

In recent years there has been an increasing interest in the mechanisms by which nutrition may influence brain function. It has become apparent that the concept of protection of the brain from variations in plasma concentrations of nutrients responding to dietary intake does not hold true and so indeed some behaviors may reflect the latest meal. Of special interest are the effects that variations in the diet of the pregnant mother and the neonate may have upon the critical development of the central nervous system during fetal and early neonatal life. The disciplines of nutrition and the neurosciences have been developing separately at an extremely rapid pace during the last two decades but with few attempts to bridge the gap between the two. This volume is an attempt to bridge this gap with special reference to the nutrition and neurochemistry of the developing brain.

The overall concept has been to present some aspects of basic infant nutrition and then progress into a number of specific areas of neurochemistry and brain development that often reflect nutritional manipulations and/or developmental changes. The last section is then a return to an analysis of how nutrition may have influenced outcome in the infant and child. Hopefully, those readers interested in nutrition will be persuaded to delve into the neurochemical sections and those interested in neurochemistry will take the opportunity to learn about some of the unsolved problems in nutrition.

The conception of this volume came about as the result of a meeting held in Caracas, Venezuela in December of 1985 on "Nutrition, Neurochemistry, and Brain Development." Although the body of the book reflects presentations at that symposium, several solicited chapters were added to better address the topic. Most of the contributed material was received in the fall of 1986.

This work would not have come to fruition without the support of the Instituto Venezolano de Investigaciones Cientificas (IVIC) which hosted the symposium. The program was sponsored by El Centro Latinoamericano de Biológica—United Nations Educational, Scientific and Cultural Organization (CLAB-UNESCO). We are grateful for additional support that was received from the International Society for Neurochemistry, the National Science Foundation (U.S.A.), Ross Laboratories, and Mead Johnson Laboratories.

David K. Rassin
Bernard Haber
Boris Drujan

SECTION I: BIOCHEMICAL BASIS OF EARLY NUTRITION

Current Topics in Nutrition and Disease, Volume 16
Basic and Clinical Aspects of Nutrition and Brain Development,
pages 3–18
© 1987 Alan R. Liss, Inc.

Current Approaches for Assessing Nutritional Status of Infants

C. Garza, R.J. Schanler, N.F. Butte, W.W. Wong, and D. Hachey
Children's Nutrition Center and Department of Pediatrics,
Baylor University, Houston, Texas 77030

INTRODUCTION

The nutritional status of infants is usually assessed from measurements of growth performance, biochemical indices, and/or dietary intake. Standards are derived from reference populations and carry the implicit assumption that the achievement of "normative" values results in functional benefits. Indeed, applications of anthropometric, biochemical, or dietary standards carry implied warranties of sensitive relationships between the standard and a related function. The sensitivity of conventional standards as proxy indicators for specific functional competences, however, is not well established (Solomons and Allen, 1983). Assessments of putative relationships are complicated by interactive effects among complex environmental factors and genetic diversity. The major challenges in pediatric nutrition include the scrutiny of alleged relationships between standards and functional competences, the comprehension of adaptive mechanisms to varying levels of specific nutrient intakes, and the discernment of how the environment and genetic endowment influence those relationships. This chapter will present recent data from the Children's Nutrition Research Center, Houston, that illustrate these challenges and will identify potential approaches that functionally assess the nutritional status of infants, with emphasis on the utilization of energy and protein because of the pervasive roles they play in metabolism.

ASSESSMENT OF ENERGY AND PROTEIN INTAKE

Energy requirements of infants have been estimated by the measurement of ad libitum intakes in "reference" populations and the factorial method, the summation of energy expended for basal metabolism (including the cost of synthetic processes associated with growth), activity, the thermic response to food, and the energy retained in tissues accumulated as a result of growth

(Butte et al., 1985). A series of studies have been conducted by our group to assess the energy needs of infants (Butte et al., 1984; Stuff et al., 1986, 1987; Montandon et al., 1986).

The reference population consisted of breast-fed infants from upper-middle-class households. In the first study, 45 infants were followed longitudinally (Butte et al., 1984). A support staff trained to assist mothers in the successful management of lactation was available throughout the study. The attrition rate was less than 10%. Subjects who left the study did so for reasons unrelated to their breastfeeding. Milk intakes plateaued at 733 g/day over the 4 months of observation. Nutrient intakes were based on the analysis of milk samples from each participant. Twenty-four-hour samples of milk were collected monthly. Energy intakes on a body weight basis fell from 110 kcal/kg at month 1 to 71 kcal/kg at month 4. Therefore, by the fourth month, these infants consumed less than 65% of the energy recommended by the National Research Council (NRC) for infants of this age (Committee on Dietary Allowances, 1980).

These data raised questions regarding estimates of the protein needs of infants. For infants 6 months of age or younger, the NRC set the allowance at 2.2 g protein/kg body weight (Committee on Dietary Allowances, 1980). This estimate was based on the ''amount of protein provided by the quantity of milk required to ensure a satisfactory rate of growth.'' Allowances were estimated to fall gradually from 2.4 g/kg/day during the first month of life to approximately 1.5 g/kg/day by the sixth month. A 75% adjustment was made in the allowance for older children to account for the decreased efficiency of protein utilization from a mixed diet.

The mean plus two standard deviations of protein intakes observed in our study of 45 exclusively breast-fed infants agrees well with protein allowances recommended by the NRC, but the mean value is substantially below factorially derived estimates of protein requirements (Table I). The factorial method of protein requirement determination sums the amounts of nitrogen needed for maintenance and growth. That sum represents the minimal amount of protein required for normal growth and development. The corresponding estimates are summarized in Table I. Estimates of mean requirements derived by the factorial method are 17, 33, 29, and 30% above the intakes of protein N measured at 1, 2, 3, and 4, respectively. If we assume that both protein and non-protein nitrogen in human milk are nutritionally available to the infant, mean intakes match well the factorially derived estimates of requirement.

Both the energy recommendation and the estimated protein allowance refer to amounts of energy and protein that provide for ''normal growth.'' The mean weight-for-age, length-for-age, and weight-for-length percentiles of the study subjects remained at or above the 50th NCHS percentile for the

TABLE I. Estimated Energy and Protein Requirements

Age (mo)	Energy requirements (kcal/kg/day)[a]	Observed energy intake (kcal/kg/day)[b]	Nitrogen requirements (mg/kg/day)	Observed protein nitrogen intake (mg/kg/day)	Observed total nitrogen intake (mg/kg/day)
0–1	93–115	110	310	260	345
1–2	88–110	83	270	180	250
2–3	82–103	74	220	160	215
3–4	79–101	71	200	140	200

[a]Adapted from Butte et al., 1985.
[b]Gross energy.

4 months of study (Butte et al., 1984). Nevertheless, a statistically significant decrease in the weight-for-age percentile occurred after the first month at an average rate of 2.6 percentiles/month and in the weight-for-length percentile at a rate of 3.9 percentiles/month. No change in length-for-age percentiles was detected. These observations raise several questions. Is lactation performance among these women inadequate to maintain the growth rates of their infants projected by body size in very early infancy; are present growth standards inappropriate for exclusively breast-fed infants; or do these growth patterns reflect a regression toward the mean?

These questions were addressed in subsequent studies (Stuff et al., 1986, 1987). A pilot study was designed to assess the feasibility of extending estimates of intake obtained over 24 hours to estimates obtained over 120 consecutive hours (Stuff et al., 1986). That study was semilongitudinal in design. Seventeen infants were studied: nine at months 5 and 6 and eight at months 6 and 7. All were exclusively breast-fed for 5 months. Solid foods were introduced at 6 months. Infants were studied before and 30 and 60 days after solid foods were added to an exclusively human milk diet. Growth was measured monthly, and intakes of milk and other foods were measured for 5 consecutive days. We anticipated that if lactation performance were limiting intake, the addition of ad libitum quantities of solid foods after nursing would result in a significant increase in energy intake and possibly a growth spurt. Neither was observed. Intake in the second group of infants was approximately 70 kcal/kg during the period of exclusive breastfeeding and remained at that level after solid foods were added to the diet. Relative weight gain demonstrated a negative trend similar to that observed in the initial study.

A more comprehensive, longitudinal study is in progress (Stuff et al., 1987). Approximately 45 of a projected 60 subjects have been recruited. Only women who plan to breast-feed their infants exclusively for 4 to 6 months are eligible, and all subjects are recruited in the last trimester of pregnancy. Infants are studied longitudinally from birth to at least 3 months after the introduction of solid foods. The decision to introduce solid foods is made by each mother in consultation with her infant's pediatrician. Intakes are measured monthly from 16 weeks of age until 3 months after the introduction of solid foods. Data collected thus far are consistent with results obtained in previous studies; intakes were approximately 70 to 80 kcal/kg before and after solid foods were added to the diets of the infants, and their pattern of growth differed significantly from NCHS standards.

If the adequacy of growth is assessed on the basis of single cross-sectional observations, the results are compatible with adequate intakes; the group's mean weight-for-age, length-for-age, and weight-for-length remained above the 50th percentile in all cases but one weight-for-length in the pilot study. The large size of these infants at birth probably reflects the relatively high socio-economic status of the households from which subjects have been drawn. If growth is evaluated on the basis of the longitudinal observations, the breast-fed infants followed for approximately 8 months grew less rapidly than anticipated from the growth trajectory projected by their body weights in early infancy. This pattern is consistent with results obtained in our first longitudinal study.

MEASUREMENT OF INTAKE

Questions raised in the preceding section assumed that milk intakes were measured accurately. Several methodologic approaches are available to measure the volume of milk consumed. The current method of choice is the test-weighing procedure, i.e., weighing the infant before and after each nursing (Woolridge et al., 1985). We have used three approaches: Test-weighing, and dosing the infant, or the mother, with ^2H_2O. In the past, measurement difficulties that resulted from the infant's movements and the relatively inadequate sensitivity of available balances made test-weighing highly unreliable. The integrating function of recently developed electronic scales minimizes the interference of the infant's movements during weighing, and the sensitivity of the scales usually allows for a precision of $\pm$ 1 or 2 g and an overall accuracy of approximately $\pm$ 5 g in the estimation of differences in weights.

Coward et al. have described two alternate methods that use ^2H_2O for the determination of human milk intakes (Coward et al., 1979, 1982). These methods are particularly promising for field applications and are attractive because they do not interfere with usual feeding routines. In the first, the tracer was administered to the infant. The decay of deuterium enrichment in the infant's body water was followed to estimate milk intake. The method overestimated milk intake when results obtained were compared with those from the conventional test-weighing procedure (Butte et al., 1983). In a subsequent study we compared the second approach described by Coward with the test-weighing approach (Butte et al., 1987). The ^2H_2O was administered orally to the mother, and the decay in isotopic enrichment in the infant's body water was followed for 14 days. We modified the method originally described by Coward (1979). $H_2^{18}O$ was administered to the infant for the determination of total body water, deuterium enrichment was measured in the infant's urine rather than in saliva, the frequency of sampling was increased, and the compartmental model used to calculate milk intake was altered slightly. The mean difference between estimates of 24-hr intakes obtained by the isotopic and test-weighing methods was $\pm$ 32 g/day. This difference was not statistically different from zero.

The new electronic scales provide a means of assessing intakes during single feedings or over several days of feedings. The isotopic approach provides a means for assessing usual intake over a longer period. Both methods represent significant advances in estimating intakes, and the similarity in results increases confidence in both approaches.

FUNCTIONAL SIGNIFICANCE OF RECENT OBSERVATIONS OF MILK INTAKE

The functional significance of energy intakes below recommended levels is of obvious interest. Reports that the energy intakes of bottle-fed infants, compared with those of breast-fed infants, coincide more closely with accepted estimates of energy requirements intensify that interest (Montandon et al., 1986), as do data suggesting that the growth patterns of breast-fed infants may differ from those of the NCHS reference population (Garza, 1987c). Various methods may be used to assess the functional implications of these differences. One approach is to examine the partitioning of energy expenditure. The most promising method appears to be a combination of a relatively old technology, indirect calorimetry (Davidsen et al., 1982), and a more recent one, mass spectrometry (Klein and Klein, 1984). Total energy expenditure can be measured by the use of ^2H_2O and $H_2^{18}O$ (Lifson et al., 1955). The method is considered in more detail below. Indirect calorimetry can aid in partitioning total energy expenditure.

Total energy expenditure can be subdivided into energy expended for basal metabolic needs (BMR), in response to food (dietary-induced thermogenesis, DIT), and for all other purposes, i.e., activity. The synthetic costs associated with growth processes are likely subsumed in estimates of an infant's basal metabolic rate. Adjustments to low levels of intake, i.e., uncomplicated partial starvation, include reductions in BMR and activity (Keys et al., 1950). These adjustments have been described in malnourished children

(Rutishauser and Whitehead, 1972; Parra et al., 1973) and in adults partially starved under metabolically controlled conditions (Keys et al., 1950). Reductions in BMR under conditions of partial starvation in adults have been associated with functional deficits in multiple organ systems (Keys et al., 1950).

An alternative approach is to examine the composition of tissues gained during growth. The accumulation of fat and lean tissue during early growth is known to be partially dependent on the quality and quantity of intake (Blaxter, 1975). The functional outcomes associated with the accumulation of various proportions of fat and lean tissue have been difficult to assess largely because of technological problems in the accurate measurement of the body composition of infants. A number of new techniques appear to overcome previous obstacles (Sheng et al., 1986; Dell et al., 1986; Fiorotto et al., 1986) and are discussed below.

Another approach is to explore possible mechanisms that affect the efficiency with which nutrients are metabolized, e.g., examination of amino acid metabolism and protein utilization. Technological advances in gas chromatography/mass spectrometry may permit the expanded use of tracer methodologies in young infants (Hachey et al., 1987). Examples of this application will be discussed.

Energy Utilization

The amount and proportion of energy expended for BMR, DIT, and activity provide measures of the functional consequences of various levels of energy intake. Of most interest is the quantitation of energy expended for activity. Adjustments in activity may precede other functional compromises that result in reduction in BMR (Ferro-Luzzi, 1985). Ideally, energy expended for activity should be measured throughout the day, and the behaviors comprising discreet activities should be characterized simultaneously. To determine energy expenditure rates on a time scale sufficient to accomplish this objective, however, is not possible in infants using conventional portable techniques. Total energy expenditure under field conditions traditionally has been measured by portable indirect calorimetric techniques that permit the measurement of gas exchange while the subject works. This approach requires significant subject cooperation and is not applicable to studies of infants. The accuracy of these methods is questionable because the equipment may augment the workload and decrease work efficiency. The alternative is to obtain values of energy expenditure over longer times. If measurement errors are not unacceptably large, the energy expended for total activity in infants may be estimated indirectly from the difference between total energy expenditure and the sum of BMR and DIT. This approach also may permit one to measure expenditure for limited ranges of activities characteristic of infancy.

The approach developed by Lifson may be used to estimate total energy expenditure (Lifson et al., 1955). The method requires the ability to approximate the water space measured by desiccation, the proportion of total water output accounted for by insensible water losses, and the decay (over 10 to 14 days) in ^2H and ^{18}O enrichment of body water after an orally administered bolus of both labels. The rate of CO_2 production is calculated from the differences between the turnover rates of ^2H and ^{18}O. Deuterium in labeled water equilibrates with the total body water pool (the exchange of deuterium with organic hydrogen is ignored), and ^{18}O in the administered tracer exchanges with total body water and carbon dioxide. The amount of oxygen consumed and its energy equivalent are estimated from the average respiratory quotient and the experimentally determined rate of CO_2 production. The method has been compared recently in adults and infants against conventional indirect and direct calorimetry and with measurements of dietary energy intake (Klein et al., 1984; Roberts et al., 1986; Schoeller and Webb, 1984). The method currently is undergoing study in our laboratory (Wong et al., 1987). We are investigating the energy expenditure of 1- and 4-month-old breast- and bottle-fed infants. Preliminary results indicate that total energy expenditure is below measurements of energy intake obtained by test-weighing and ^2H_2O dilution techniques. BMR and DIT also have been estimated in the study infants. If the accuracy of methods permit, combining measurements of total energy expenditure with measures of BMR and DIT, as described above, permits the estimation of energy expended for activity. Very preliminary estimates indicate that breast-fed 4-month-old infants expend approximately 20 kcal/kg for activity and that the ratio of total energy expenditure to BMR is approximately 1.4.

Body Composition

Theoretically, measurements of total energy intake and total energy expenditure permit one to indirectly calculate the energy density of tissues accumulated during growth. This calculation is possible if metabolizable energy is determined either from direct observations or approximated from literature values. Weight gain can be determined easily; the contribution of mineral accretion is ignored. The ratio of the difference between metabolizable energy and total energy expenditure to weight gain represents the energy density of accumulated tissue.

The resurgence of interest in body composition, however, has also recently led to the development of alternative methods for measurements of body composition: total body electrical conductivity (TOBEC) (Fiorotto et al., 1986), air displacement (Dell et al., 1986), and acoustic plethysmography

(Sheng et al., 1986). Although these methods assess body composition indirectly, possible cross-checking between methods that focus on anthropometric types of measurements and those that emphasize the balance between energy intake and expenditure is an attractive approach to validation. The estimated gains of water, protein, and fat during longitudinal studies permit an approximation of the energy density of accumulated tissues.

Acoustic plethysmography. Body composition is often deduced from determinations of body density. This approach requires one to estimate total body volume. The use of body volumes to measure body composition is based on the Archimedian principle (Keys and Grande, 1976). Densitometry is applied appropriately to estimate total body fat and lean body mass (total body weight − total body fat) of adults. The relative size of these compartments is estimated from the assumed densities of fat, lean body mass, and the experimental determination of total body density. With cooperative subjects, body density is determined from body weights obtained under water, an approach that is not feasible with infants.

A new approach for obtaining body volume is acoustic plethysmography (Sheng et al., 1984, 1987). The acoustic plethysmography is based on the principle of the Helmoltz resonator, i.e., the resonant frequency of a resonating chamber is inversely proportional to the square root of the chamber volume. A complete description of the prototype has been published (Deskins et al., 1985). The model has been tested in minipigs and very low birthweight infants (Sheng et al., 1986).

The use of densitometry in infants has led to an expansion of the two-compartment model of body composition (fat and lean body mass) to a four-compartment model: total body water (TBW), total body fat (TBF), total body protein (TBP), and total body minerals (TBM). Expansion to four compartments permits the estimation of total body fat and protein without requiring any assumptions about the density of the lean body mass compartment. The four-compartment model is especially important in studies of infants because of their chemical immaturity (Sheng et al., 1984). The water content of the lean body mass compartment decreases with age. The decrease is non-linear, and the water content of lean tissue may not reach stability until late childhood. Changes in the water content of the lean body mass of children are most significant in studies of the body composition of very low birthweight infants and are progressively less important in chemically more mature children.

Expansion to the four compartment model is based on the following questions: total body mass = TBF + TBP + TBW + TBM; total body volume = TBF/FD + TBP/PD + TBW/WD + TBM/MD. FD, PD, WD, and MD represent the densities of fat, protein, water, and mineral, respectively. The respective densities are obtained from the physical constants measured in various animal studies. Total body mass is determined by weighing the subject, water may be measured by tracer methodologies or the TOBEC instrument; TBM is estimated from literature values for the reference fetus or infant, and total body volume is measured by acoustic plethysmography. The two equations are solved simultaneously for the two unknowns, TBF and TBP.

Comparisons of total body protein and fat estimated by the four-compartment model with values determined by direct chemical analysis are favorable (Sheng et al., 1984). These initial results support the feasibility of the method.

Air displacement. The principal of air displacement also has been used to determine the body volume of infants. Dell and colleagues recently described the body density of infants provided one of six diets comprised of diverse proportions of energy and protein (Dell et al., 1986). The body volumes used to compute body density were determined by an "air displacement" approach. The instrument used to obtain this measurement consisted of two identical Plexiglas cylinders enclosed in a larger thermostatically controlled enclosure. The unit includes a manometer for determining pressure differences between the two cylinders. Pressure differences are a function of the volume occupied by an infant placed in one of the two cylinders.

Total body electrical conductivity. TOBEC appears to be the most promising new development for measuring body composition, and the instrument used has been evaluated most recently by Fiorotto et al. (1987). The signal generated by the TOBEC instrument is a function of the conductive and dielectric properties of the index body's FFM. Additionally, Fiorotto and her colleagues stress the need to account for the length of the subject. Two conductors of equal volume and composition but unequal lengths generate unequal TOBEC signals. These investigators used infant miniature pigs that ranged from 10 to 33 days of age to assess the accuracy of the TOBEC measurements of body composition. Measurements of TBW and FFM obtained by direct chemical analysis of carcasses were compared with the square root of the product of the TOBEC signal and the animal's recumbent length. The calibration of the transformed signal against the results of the chemical analysis yielded the following two relationships (body weight in g and body length in cm):

FFM (kg) = $- 1.35 + 0.036$ (TOBEC signal $*$ length)$^{1/2}$ $+ 0.82$ (body weight/L^2); r = 0.999, SEE = 0.042.

TBW (kg) = $- 0.96 + 0.028$ (TOBEC signal $*$ length)$^{1/2}$ $+ 0.58$ (body weight/L^2); r = 0.999, SEE = 0.033.

The 95% prediction intervals appear sufficiently narrow to be of potential use in longitudinal studies of energy utilization. The body composition of young term infants and young miniature pigs is sufficiently similar to use the calibration to predict the FFM and TBW of infants. These equations require more detailed evaluations in infants. Use of the method with young infants will further evaluate the TOBEC instrument's potential. TBF may be estimated from the difference between total body weight and the FFM.

FUNCTIONAL SIGNIFICANCE OF RECENT OBSERVATIONS OF PROTEIN INTAKES

Protein intakes of exclusively breast-fed infants are lower than those predicted by factorially derived estimates of protein requirement for normal growth and development (Table I). Nonetheless, clinical protein deficiency is seldom, if ever, encountered in exclusively breast-fed infants whose mothers successfully manage their lactation. Although failure to thrive is documented in breast-fed infants, abnormal milk composition has rarely been implicated without evidence of concomitant mammary gland involution (Lawrence, 1980). Low milk volumes due to mismanagement usually have been the cause of inadequate energy and protein intakes (Lawrence, 1980). The specific properties of human milk that promote the highly efficient utilization of its nitrogen contents are not known, nor have the mechanisms been definitely identified that are used by the infant to achieve a high level of efficiency (Garza et al., 1987a).

To improve our understanding of protein utilization in infancy our laboratory has conducted studies in very low birthweight infants (Schanler et al., 1986; Schanler and Garza, 1987). Although these studies are not directly applicable to term infants, they have provided direction for the design of future studies. Thirty-one VLBW infants were enrolled in a longitudinal study during the first week of life, after which they were assigned to a human milk or formula feeding group based on parental choice, and enteral feeding was instituted. Infants were fed either their mother's milk fortified with lyophilized fractions of skim and cream derived from pasteurized (72°C, 15 sec) mature human milk or a whey-dominant cow-milk formula (Goldblum et al., 1984). Infants were maintained on a single feeding regimen throughout the study. All infants received a continuous enteral infusion of isonitrogenous, isocaloric preparations of either human milk fortified with pasteurized lyophilized fractions of mature milk or the whey-dominant cow-milk formula. A 96-hr nutrient balance was performed at 2 to 3 weeks of life to estimate metabolizable energy intake and the absorption and retention of nitrogen and minerals. The amounts of lactoferrin, lysozyme, and secretory IgA (sIgA) in the milk and in the infant's feces and urine also were determined (Schanler et al., 1986; Goldblum et al., 1984). Plasma amino acids, total protein, albumin, prealbumin, BUN, and whole blood hemoglobin were measured during the balance study.

Serum total protein, albumin, and prealbumin, blood urea nitrogen, and hemoglobin values fell with increases in postnatal age (Schanler et al., 1985). No differences, however, were noted between the groups. The decline in serum protein concentrations has been observed previously and is usually ascribed to the rapid growth of VLBW infants and to the immaturity of their livers (Hillman and Haddad, 1983). Some investigators have suggested that these changes are normal and reflect extrauterine conditions (Gaull et al., 1977). This explanation is not wholly satisfactory in view of the fetal ability to increase the concentration of serum proteins in utero when the fetus has a greater relative rate of growth, a more expanded extracellular space, and a comparably mature liver than the extrauterine infant of similar postconceptional age. Alternatively, falling levels of serum proteins may signal stress, unrecognized redistribution of serum protein within extravascular compartments, or unmet nutritional needs.

We have speculated that if amino acid or protein intakes were optimal, positive or negative relationships would be unlikely between plasma amino acid levels and other measures of protein status (Garza et al., 1987b). We anticipate that amino acid plasma levels should not be correlated to other functional indices when protein or amino acid intakes are neither excessive nor deficient. In studies of very low birthweight infants, plasma amino acid levels were not associated with other indices of protein status in infants fed fortified human milk, but not in those fed a cow milk-based formula (Schanler et al., 1987). A single positive correlation was observed in the fortified human milk group: plasma lysine and serum total protein ($r = 0.66$, $p < 0.01$). Many more relationships were noted in the formula group (r values ranged from 0.71 to 0.74, $p < 0.01$): nitrogen retention was related to plasma alanine, tryptophan, and glycine; N retention/N intake was related to plasma isoleucine and phenylalanine. Plasma alanine, tryptophan, and glycine levels together accounted for 82% of the variability in nitrogen retention in the formula group. Negative correlations ($r = -0.71$ to -0.81) were noted between whole blood hemoglobin and the plasma levels of isoleucine, glycine, alanine, proline, and leucine, and total and essential amino acids. The five plasma amino acid levels accounted for 89% of the variability of whole blood hemogloblin levels in the formula group. The relationships between plasma amino acid levels and serum total protein and whole blood hemoglobin in infants fed fortified human milk and whey-dominant formula, respectively, suggest that the synthesis of specific functional proteins should be examined more closely than has been done in previous studies seeking to establish optimal intakes and function.

Hachey and his colleagues recently described the analyses of small quantities of serum proteins enriched with ^{13}C and ^{15}N amino acids (Hachey et al., 1987). These techniques may be pivotal in the elucidation of associations such as those observed in our feeding study. Under favorable analytical conditions, modern mass spectrometers are sufficiently sensitive to quantitate less than 0.01 mole percent excess isotope in 1–2 ng of analyzable material. The isotopic analyses of protein-bound amino acids isolated from small plasma samples (< 200 μl) have been demonstrated. The incorporation of deuterium-labeled lysine into albumin, prealbumin and α_1-antitrypsin after a single bolus dose of labeled lysine has been described. These proteins were isolated in pure form by immunochemical and electrophoretic techniques, hydrolyzed, and the isotopic enrichment of specific amino acids determined by gas chromatography/mass spectrometry.

These technological advances may be used to assess another aspect of nutritional status unique to infancy. As alluded to above, nitrogen absorption was similar between the groups fed fortified human milk and cow-milk-based formula. This observation is of particular interest because of the expected resistance to digestion of key functional components in human milk. The quantities of lactoferrin, sIgA, and lysozyme measured in the stool were approximately 3, 9, and 0.1% of the respective amounts of each component that was fed (Schanler et al., 1986). Measurements of urinary nitrogen support the conclusion that the biological value of absorbed nitrogen is similar for fortified human milk and the commercial formula studied (Schanler et al., 1985). Seventeen to twenty percent of absorbed nitrogen was excreted in urine. This finding suggests that obligatory nitrogen was similar in both feeding groups. Balance data do not allow an evaluation of this assumption.

The underlying premise in studies assessing the utilization of specific proteins by infants fed human milk is that the index proteins in the feces of these infants originate primarily from human milk. Recent results have led us to question this predominant view (Schanler et al., 1986; Goldblum et al., 1985). An alternate consideration is that such fecal constituents are synthesized partially by the infant. Feces of infants fed fortified human milk had significantly greater quantities of lactoferrin, lysozyme, and sIgA than those of infants fed the cow-milk-based formula. Specific sIgA antibodies to *Escherichia coli* were detected in the feces of 90% of the human-milk-fed infants, but in none of the infants fed the cow-milk-based formula. Other than a significant correlation between the fecal concentrations of specific sIgA antibodies to *E. coli* O somatic antigens and the concentration of these antibodies in the fortified human milk, no other significant relationships were detected between the milk concentrations or the infants' intakes of the other selection immune factors and the excretion of these factors in their feces. In contrast to these findings, significant relationships were noted among the immune factors in the feces of the group fed fortified human milk. The increased quantity of selected immune factors in the feces of this group, therefore, may have resulted from the passive ingestion and persistence of these factors through the gastrointestinal tract and/or from endogenous synthesis induced by unidentified factors in the milk. The detection of increased quantities of lactoferrin and sIgA in the urine of the fortified human-milk-fed group supports the latter possibility. Gas chromatography/ mass spectrometry techniques capable of quantitating relative enrichments of very small quantities of proteins with specially labeled amino acids may help to resolve these issues.

SUMMARY

Studies of term and very low birthweight infants fed human milk or commercial formula have raised a number of questions which have prompted the development of new approaches for assessing nutritional status. The capability of measuring total energy expenditure and body composition permits an integrated approach for assessing the relationships among energy intake, growth performance, and protein and amino acid utilization. These improved techniques for assessing nutritional status may provide the long-awaited means to assess relationships between diet and the metabolic responses to specific stresses and such functional outcomes as motor and cognitive development.

ACKNOWLEDGMENTS

This project has been funded in part with federal funds from the U.S. Department of Agriculture, Agricultural Research Service under Cooperative Agreement 58-7MN1-6-100. The contents of this publication do not necessarily reflect the views or policies of the U.S. Department of Agriculture. Mention of trade names, commercial products, or organizations does not imply endorsement by the U.S. Government. This work is a publication of the U.S. Department of Agriculture, Agricultural Research Service, Children's Nutrition Research Center, Department of Pediatrics, Baylor College of Medicine, and Texas Children's Hospital, Houston, Texas.

REFERENCES

Blaxter KL (1975): Energy utilization and obesity in domesticated animals. In Bray GA (ed): "Obesity in Perspective." DHEW Publication no. (NIH) 75–708. Washington, D.C.: U.S. Government Printing Office.

Butte NF, Garza C (1985): Energy and protein intakes of exclusively breastfed infants during the first four months of life. In Gracey M, Falkner F (eds): "Nutritional Needs and Assessment of Normal Growth." New York: Nestle Nutrition, Vevey/Raven Press.

Butte NF, Garza C, Smith EO, Nichols BL (1983): Evaluation of the deuterium dilution technique against the test-weighing procedure for the determination of breast milk intake. Am J Clin Nutr 37:996–1003.

Butte NF, Garza C, Smith EO, Nichols BL (1984): Human milk intake and growth in exclusively breast-fed infants. J Pediatr 104:187–195.

Butte NF, Wong W, Patterson B, Garza C, Klein PD (1987): Human milk intake measured by administration of deuterium oxide to the mother: A comparison with test-weighing. Fed Proc, 46:571.

Committee on Dietary Allowances, Food and Nutrition Board (1980): "Recommended Dietary Allowances." Washington, D.C.: National Academy of Sciences.

Coward WA, Cole TJ, Sawyer MB, Prentice AM (1982): Breast-milk intake measurement in mixed-fed infants by administration of deuterium oxide to their mothers. Hum Nutr Clin Nutr 36C:141–148.

Coward WA, Sawyer MB, Whitehead RG, Prentice AM, Evans J (1979): New method for measuring milk intakes in breast-fed babies. Lancet 7:13–14.

Dell RB, Aksoy Y, Kashyap S, Forsythe M, Ramakrishnan R, Zucker C, Heird WC (1987): Relationship between density and body weight in prematurely born infants receiving different diets. In Ellis KJ (ed): "In Vivo Body Composition Studies," Institute of Physical Sciences in Medicine. London, in press.

Deskins WG, Winter DC, Sheng H-P, Garza C (1985): Use of resonating cavity to measure body volume. J Acoust Soc Am 77:756–758.

Ferro-Luzzi A (1985): Work capacity and productivity in long-term adaptation to low energy intakes. In Blaxter K, Waterlow JC (eds): "Nutritional Adaptation in Man." London: John Libbey & Company.

Fiorotto ML, Cochran WJ, Funk RC, Sheng H-P, Klish WJ (1987): Analysis of body composition using total body electrical conductivity (TOBEC) measurements: Effects of body geometry and composition. Am J Physiol, 252:R794–R800.

Fiorotto M, Cochran W, Sheng H-P, Klish W (1987): An evaluation of total body electrical conductivity (TOBEC) measurements for the determination of body composition in the human infant. In Ellis KJ (ed): "In Vivo Body Composition Studies," Institute of Physical Sciences in Medicine. London, in press.

Garza C, Schanler RJ, Butte NF, Motil KJ (1987a): Special properties of human milk. In Conover (ed): "Clinics in Perinatology." New York: W. B. Saunders, 14(1):11–32.

Garza C, Schanler RJ, Goldblum R, Goldman AS (1987b): Fortified human milk feeding in the premature infant. In Lindblad B (ed): "Perinatal Nutrition." New York: Academic Press, in press.

Garza C, Stuff JS, Butte NF (1987c): Growth of the breast-fed infant. In Goldman AS (ed): "The Effects of Human Milk Upon The Recipient Infant." New York: Plenum Press, in press.

Gaull GE, Rassin DK, Raiha NCR (1977): Protein intake of premature infants: A reply. J Pediatr 90:507.

Goldblum RM, Dill CW, Albrecht TB, Alford ES, Garza C, Goldman AS (1984): Rapid high temperature treatment of human milk. J Pediatr 104:380–385.

Goldblum RM, Schanler RJ, Garza C, Goldman AS (1985): Enhanced urinary lactoferrin excretion in premature infants fed human milk. Pediatr Res 19:342A.

Hachey D, Patterson B, Marks L, Booth L, Boriack J, Klein P (1987): Albumin, prealbumin, and $_1$-antitrypsin turnover studies by GC/MS after an IV bolus dose of L-lysine-[4,4,5,5,-^{2}H$_4$]. Fed Proc, 46:879.

Hillman LS, Haddad JG (1983): Serial analyses of serum vitamin D-binding protein in preterm infants from birth to postconceptual maturity. J Clin Edocrinol Metab 56:189.

Keys A, Brozek J, Henschel A, Mickelsen O, Taylor HL (1950): "The Biology of Human Starvation, Volume 1." Minneapolis: The University of Minnesota Press.

Keys A, Grande F (1976): Body weight, body composition and calorie status. In Goodhart RS, Shils ME (eds): "Modern Nutrition in Health and Disease Dietotherapy." London: Henry Kimpton Publishers.

Klein PD, James WPT, Wong WW, Irving CS, Murgatroyd P, Cabrera M, Dallasso H, Klein ER, Nichols BL (1984): Calorimetric validation of the doubly labeled water method for determination of energy expenditure in man. Hum Nutr Clin Nutr 38C:95–106.

Klein PD, Klein ER (1984): Stable isotopes and mass spectrometry in nutrition science. In Grigerio A, Milon H (eds): "Proceedings of the International Symposium on Chromatography and Mass Spectrometry in Nutrition Science and Food Safety." Amsterdam: Elsevier, pp 155–166.

Lavoisier AL (1982): Letter to Joseph Black (1790). In Davidsen S, Passmore R, Brock JF (eds) (1982): "Human Nutrition and Dietetics," 5th ed. Baltimore: Williams and Wilkins, pp 25–26.

Lawrence RA (1980): "Breastfeeding: A Guide for the Medical Profession." St. Louis: C.V. Mosby.

Lifson N. Gordon GB, McClintock R (1955): Measurement of total carbon dioxide production by means of D_2O^{18}. J Appl Physiol 7:704–710.

Montandon CM, Wills CA, Garza C, Smith EO, Nichols BL (1986): Formula intake of one- and four-month-old infants. J Pediatr Gastroenterol Nutr 5:434–438.

Parra A, Garza C, Garza Y, Saravia L, Hazlewood C, Nichols BL (1973): Changes in growth hormone, insulin, and thyroxine values, and in energy metabolism of marasmic infants. J Pediatr 83:144.

Roberts SB, Coward WA, Schlingenseipen KH, Nohria V, Lucas A (1986): Comparison of the doubly labeled water ($^2H_2^{18}O$) method with indirect calorimetry and a nutrient-balance study for simultaneous determination of energy expenditure, water intake, and metabolizable energy intake in preterm infants. Am J Clin Nutr 44:315–322.

Rutishauser IHE, Whitehead RG (1982): Energy intake and expenditure in 1–3-year-old Ugandan children living in a rural environment. Br J Nutr 28:145–152.

Schanler RJ, Garza C (1987): Plasma amino acid differences in very low birthweight infants fed either human milk or whey-dominant cow milk formula. Pediatr Res 21:301–305.

Schanler RJ, Garza C, Nichols BL (1985): Fortified mother's milk for very low birth weight infants: Results of growth and nutrient balance studies. J Pediatr 107:437–445.

Schanler RJ, Goldblum RM, Garza C, Goldman AS (1986): Enhanced fecal excretion of selected immune factors in very low birth weight infants fed fortified human milk. Pediatr Res 20:711–715.

Schoeller DA, Webb P (1984): Five-day comparison of the doubly labeled water method with respiratory gas exchange. Am J Clin Nutr 40:153–158.

Sheng H-P, Huggins RA (1979): A review of body composition studies with emphasis on total body water and fat. Am J Clin Nutr 32:630–647.

Sheng H-P, Dang T, Schanler R, Garza C (1987): Infant body volume measurement by acoustic plethysmography. In Ellis KJ (ed): "In Vivo Body Composition Studies." Institute of Physical Sciences in Medicine. London, in press.

Sheng H-P, Deskins W, Winter D, Garza C (1984): Estimation of total body fat and protein by densitometry. Pediatr Res 18:212A.

Solomons NW, Allen LH (1983): The functional assessment of nutritional status: Principles, practice and potential. Nutr Rev 41:33–50.

Stuff J, Garza C, Boutte C, Fraley JK, Smith EO, Klein ER, Nichols BL (1986): Sources of variation in milk and caloric intakes in breast-fed infants: Implications for lactation study design and interpretation. Am J Clin Nutr 43:361–366.

Stuff J, Garza C, Nichols BL (1987): Solid food supplementation in older breast-fed infants: Feeding pattern, energy intake, and growth patterns. Fed Proc 46:1194.

Wong WW, Butte NF, Garza C, Klein PD (1987): Energy expenditures of term infants determined by the doubly labeled water ($^2H_2^{18}O$) method, indirect calorimetry, and test-weighing. Pediatr Res 21:282A.

Woolridge MW, Butte NF, Dewey KG, Ferris AM, Garza C, Keller RP (1985): Methods for the measurement of milk volume intake of the breast-fed infant. In Neville M, Jensen R (eds): "Human Lactation: Methodologies." New York: Plenum Press, pp. 5–22.

Current Topics in Nutrition and Disease, Volume 16
Basic and Clinical Aspects of Nutrition and Brain Development,
pages 19–39
© 1987 Alan R. Liss, Inc.

Protein Nutrition in the Neonate: Assessment and Implications for Brain Development

David K. Rassin

Department of Pediatrics, University of Texas Medical Branch at
Galveston, Galveston, Texas 77550

INTRODUCTION

Nutrition is the single greatest environmental influence on the human neonate. An appropriate supply of essential nutrients is required for the maintenance of growth as well as the normal development of physiological functions. Early concerns of those involved in the nutrition of neonates primarily revolved around support of growth, as this measure was easy to determine. However, with the continued development of improved support for breastfeeding, improved infant formulas, and more sophisticated measures of nutritional status, growth has become too insensitive a determination of nutritional status (Rassin, 1987). Obviously it is important to maintain growth, but, with few exceptions, most feeding regimens used in neonates support adequate growth. It is now of more importance to assess some of the finer consequences of less than optimal nutrition, such as ability to resist infection, immunological status, renal and hepatic function, biochemical status, and neurologic outcome.

The intent of this volume is to integrate some of our knowledge regarding nutrition and brain development, and in this chapter the potential for protein nutrition to influence the central nervous system will be assessed. Optimal neurologic outcome is certainly a major goal to most investigators involved in the refinement of nutrition for the neonate. All nutrients would be expected to have some influence on brain development, but protein appears to be the component most likely allied with neurologic function. Many amino acids are precursors of neurotransmitters or are neurotransmitters themselves. Thus, variations in protein intake that affect plasma amino acid patterns would be expected to influence a variety of central nervous system neurotransmitter functions. The influence of such changes in protein nutrition could occur both at the level of the blood brain barrier, where competition for transport into the brain occurs, and within the brain, where lack of saturation of neurotransmitter synthetic enzymes may result in changes in the amount of synthesis as precursor pools change.

In general several different areas must be assessed in addressing the consequences of neonatal nutrition. There are the problems of understanding the different requirements of the preterm versus the term infant. It may be assumed that the breast fed normal term infant represents a standard against which other nutrient regimens in term infants may be contrasted. However, such an assumption cannot be made for the preterm infant who is in a developmental stage intermediate between that which exists in utero and that which usually exists ex utero. Thus, considerable controversy exists regarding the true nutritional requirements of preterm infants and how they should be assessed because of the lack of an obvious control.

Further complicating the assessment of neonatal nutrition is the question concerning the influence of enteral versus parenteral feeding. Total parenteral nutrition (TPN) is commonly used in the sick neonate who cannot be fed orally. This regimen is not utilized as frequently in the term infant. Within each of these modes of feeding the problems of both amount of protein and the quality of protein (amino acid composition) have to be considered.

This review will briefly discuss the functions of amino acids, the essentiality of amino acids, enteral feeding, parenteral feeding, and the potential for the various feeding regimens used in neonates to influence the central nervous system during its development.

AMINO ACID FUNCTION

Amino acids are primarily thought of by those involved in nutrition support as precursors of the structural proteins that are essential for growth. However, they serve a vast variety of other functions that are important in the maintenance of normal body homeostasis, growth, and development. Amino acids are direct precursors of enzymes, peptide hormones, and peptide transmitters in addition to structural proteins. The amino acid glycine is a precursor for porphyrin and purine synthesis. Glycine and taurine are precursors for bile salt synthesis. Tyrosine is a precursor for thyroxin and melanin synthesis. Most of the amino acids serve as precursors for gluconeogenesis, with leucine being the only major exception.

Many of the amino acids function either as neurotransmitters themselves or as precursors to neurotransmitters (Table I). The evidence for these functions has been thoroughly reviewed and continues to accumulate (Fonnum, 1978; DeFeudis and Mandel, 1981). Such evidence includes presence at the synapse, synthesis in the neuron, mechanism for inactivation at the synapse, identity of action with endogenous transmitter mechanisms, and responses to pharmacologic agents similar to endogenous neurotransmitters (Werman, 1966; Dudel, 1968). The amino acid gamma-aminobutyric acid (GABA), synthesized from glutamic acid, is not a constituent of proteins but may be

TABLE I. Amino Acid Neurotransmitters or Neurotransmitter Precursors

Neuroactive amino acids	
Gamma-aminobutyrate	Cysteic acid
Glutamate	Cysteinesulfinic acid
Aspartate	Proline
Taurine	Glycine
β-Alanine	Cystathionine
Neurotransmitter precursors	Neurotransmitters
Phenylalanine, tyrosine	Dopamine, norepinephrine
Tryptophan	Serotonin
Glutamate	GABA
Methionine, cysteine	Cysteineusulfinic acid, taurine
Histidine	Histamine
Histidine	Carnosine
Serine	Glycine

responsible for fulfilling a neurotransmitter function at more sites than any other compound in the central nervous system, including acetylcholine, norepinephrine, and dopamine (Snyder et al., 1973). Other amino acids which have been strong neurotransmitter candidates, such as glycine and glutamate, are more difficult to characterize because of their ubiquitous distribution and close association with intermediary metabolism.

The amino acids that are intimately involved with neurotransmission appear to fall into several categories. There are those compounds like GABA, β-alanine, taurine, and cystathionine that are amino acids but are not precursors of proteins. There are those amino acids such as glutamate, aspartate, and glycine which are intimately involved in intermediary metabolism, are protein precursors, and may be neurotransmitters. Lastly, there are amino acids that serve as precursors to other neurotransmitters, such as phenylalanine and tyrosine (dopamine, norepinephrine), tryptophan (serotonin), and histidine (histamine).

Thus, the broad involvement of amino acids in the function of the central nervous system goes far beyond just simple support of protein synthetic function.

AMINO ACID ESSENTIALITY

Amino acids fall into three categories with respect to whether they are indispensable (essential) or not. There are those amino acids which are clearly needed in the diet to support growth and positive nitrogen balance (such as leucine and threonine). There are those amino acids that may be synthesized sufficiently in vivo (such as alanine and serine), and there are

TABLE II. Nutritionally Essential and Non-essential Amino Acids

Essential	Semiessential	Nonessential
Valine	Tyrosine	Glycine
Isoleucine	Cysteine	Alanine
Leucine	Taurine	Aspartate
Phenylalanine	Histidine	Glutamate
Methionine		Serine
Threonine		Arginine
Tryptophan		Proline
Lysine		

those amino acids for which the evidence for essentiality is either equivocal or which may be essential depending upon the developmental or health status of the individual (such as histidine and arginine). Irwin and Hegsted (1971) have reviewed the data regarding the essentiality of amino acids based upon studies of growth and nitrogen balance. These studies have resulted in each of the amino acids being placed into one of the above three categories (Table II). More recently it has been suggested that essentiality should be defined on the basis of synthetic capacity and should be subcategorized based upon the ability of the organism to synthesize the carbon skeleton of the amino acid, to aminate the carbon skeleton, to do neither of these functions, or to do both of these functions (Jackson, 1983). Thus, amino acids such as alanine or glutamate would be *non-essential* because their carbon skeleton can be synthesized and they can be aminated. Amino acids such as leucine and valine have *essential carbon skeletons*, their keto-analogs can be aminated, but the carbon skeleton cannot be synthesized. Amino acids such as glycine and serine may be *semiessential* because their carbon skeletons can be synthesized, but amination may not take place. Lysine would be *essential* because the carbon skeleton can be neither synthesized nor aminated.

Growth data in small numbers of infants fed diets lacking histidine (Snyderman et al., 1963) and in one infant fed a diet lacking cysteine (Snyderman, 1971) led to the suggestion that these amino acids might be essential during early development. One example of the way in which estimates of requirements have been refined in more recent years has been the evaluation of cysteine. That this latter amino acid may be essential or semiessential (Pohlandt, 1974) in the infant has been further supported by the lack of activity of the hepatic enzyme responsible for its synthesis, cystathionase, in the fetus and the reduced hepatic activity of this enzyme in the neonate (Gaull et al., 1972; Pascal et al., 1972). Other investigators have found this enzyme to be active in other fetal tissues (such as the kidney) and suggested sufficient enzymatic capacity may exist. However, supplementation with cysteine did appear to enhance sulfur and nitrogen retention (Zlotkin and Anderson, 1982; Malloy et al., 1984).

Tyrosine also may be essential to the neonate based upon growth data (Snyderman, 1971). However, in the case of this amino acid, the very low activity of its catabolic enzymes in fetal development (Kretchmer et al., 1956, 1957) would appear to make the neonate particularly susceptible to excess amounts of this potentially toxic amino acid (Rassin et al., 1977b; Menkes et al., 1972). The application of stable isotope turnover studies to infants has resulted in the suggestion that glycine might be essential in infants (Jackson et al., 1981). These investigators did not observe an enrichment of urinary [^{15}N]urea from systemically administered [^{15}N]glycine, a finding that would be compatible with an essential amino acid. Other investigators (Pencharz et al., 1983) failed to duplicate this finding and suggested that the inconsistency in the data reflected the dosages of [^{15}N]glycine used rather than a limited dietary supply of the amino acid. The lack of agreement in these studies and the variation in data obtained from stable isotope studies depending upon the amino acid used as a precursor and the urinary compound used as a product (Stein et al., 1986) illustrate the difficulties in interpreting data from this newer technique.

Other amino acids have been suggested to be essential based upon evidence derived from special nutritional situations (arginine) or animal studies (taurine). When low amounts of arginine were fed in TPN solutions, a depletion in the body was followed by hyperammonemia and orotic aciduria (Anderson et al., 1977). These metabolic abnormalities could be avoided by supplementing arginine in the TPN solution. It was suggested that the additional anabolic need of the infant relative to the adult for arginine might result in depletion of this amino acid if fed in only marginal amounts. Based upon animal studies, arginine would appear to be important for maintenance of ammonia homeostasis (Czarncki and Baker, 1984). However, excess supplementation might also be hazardous to the pancreas (Mizunuma et al., 1984).

Taurine, on the other hand, while it has been shown to decrease in the plasma and urine of infants fed low taurine-containing formulas (Gaull et al., 1977b; Jarvenpaa et al., 1982; Rassin et al., 1983), has not yet been proved to be required by man. However, the dramatic findings of retinal degeneration in the cat (Hayes et al., 1975) and the rhesus monkey (Sturman et al., 1984), and the failure of cerebellar development in taurine-deficient cats (Sturman et al., 1985) have led to the widespread supplementation of taurine to formulas prepared for human infants.

The data briefly presented above indicate the evolution of the concept of amino acid essentiality. Further refinements will certainly occur as definitions improve; certainly growth and nitrogen balance alone are no longer sufficient indicators of adequacy in the diet. At the present, proper evaluation of essentiality would appear to require a spectrum of assessment from growth to nitrogen balance to protein status and plasma amino acid patterns to physiologic functions to, ultimately, long-term outcome.

ENTERAL NEONATAL AMINO ACID NUTRITION

The major modes of feeding neonates enterally are breastfeeding and formula-feeding. In general, term infants are fed either human milk or a formula which consists of either bovine-casein-predominant proteins (in a ratio of 18:82, whey:casein) or bovine-whey-predominant proteins (in a ratio of 60:40, whey:casein). The formulas for term infants usually contain about 1.5 g/dl of their respective protein mixes. By contrast human milk usually contains from 0.9 to 1.1 g/dl protein and is whey-protein-predominant with a ratio of approximately 70:30, whey: casein (Macy, 1949; Macy et al., 1953; Hambraeus et al., 1978; Hambraeus, 1977). Human milk casein proteins are different than bovine milk casein proteins. Human milk contains primarily β-casein, while bovine milk contains primarily α-s_1 casein (Jenness, 1974a,b). Human whey proteins are primarily made up of α-lactalbumin, while bovine whey proteins are primarily β-lactoglobulin, a protein that does not appear in human milk (Hambraeus, 1977).

The consequence of these differences in type of protein is that even when bovine proteins are adapted to present the neonate with a ratio of whey to casein proteins similar to that observed in human milk, different amounts of amino acids are fed. For example bovine whey proteins contain considerably more threonine than human whey proteins (Rassin et al., 1977a). Casein proteins also have different amounts of amino acids than whey proteins so that when a whey-protein-predominant formula is compared to a casein-protein-predominant formula at equal amounts of total protein, different amino acids are fed. For example casein proteins have more of the aromatic amino acids tyrosine and phenylalanine than do whey proteins (Rassin et al., 1977b). Thus, the three common feeding regimens for term neonates (human milk, 1.5 g% casein-protein-predominant formula, and 1.5 g% whey-protein-predominant formula) each supply the infant with different amino acid intakes reflecting both differences in the quantity of proteins (human milk is low) and the quality (type) of protein (Table III). Occasionally, other oral preparations are also used in these infants for a variety of clinical indications, for example formulas based on soy proteins, formulas based on casein hydrolysates, and so-called elemental formulas (containing individual amino acids). All of these preparations would also give different amino acid intakes to the infant. It is generally accepted that the healthy breastfed term infant

**TABLE III. Plasma Amino Acid Concentrations (μM)
in Term Infants at 4 Weeks of Age[a]**

	Human milk	Whey-predominant formula (1.5 g/dl)	Casein-predominant formula (1.5 g/dl)
Taurine[b]	97	64	42
Aspartate[b]	24	21	18
Threonine[b]	168	275	217
Serine[b]	210	215	193
Glutamate[b]	254	286	265
Glutamine[b]	732	801	819
Glycine[b]	257	272	295
Alanine[b]	404	389	459
Citrulline[b]	18	27	36
Valine[b]	202	255	321
Cystine[b]	112	102	118
Methionine[b]	42	51	49
Isoleucine[b]	79	102	95
Leucine[b]	156	172	175
Tyrosine[b]	109	98	142
Phenylalanine[b]	59	67	80
Lysine[c]	196	238	194
Histidine[c]	89	95	104
Arginine[c]	99	93	81
Valine/glycine[d]	0.83	0.96	1.10

[a]Variances are not given for simplicity of presentation but are included in the original publications.
[b]Adapted from Jarvenpaa et al., 1982.
[c]Adapted from Janas et al., 1985.
[d]The valine/glycine ratio is given as a general index of protein nutritional status. When this ratio reaches a number less than 0.3 it is usually indicative of protein malnutrition (see column 1, Table V) unless glycine is increased as a result of unusual feeding (see column 3, Table V).

should serve as a standard against which all these various formulas should be measured (Committee on Nutrition, American Academy of Pediatrics, 1976, 1978).

In contrast, it is difficult to determine the protein requirement of the preterm infant. Protein has been fed to these infants in amounts ranging from 1.7–9 g/kg/d. In general, infants fed less than 2.25 g protein/kg/d have not gained weight as well as infants who have been fed larger amounts of protein (Davidson et al., 1967; Babson and Bramhall, 1969). However, feeding these infants larger amounts of protein (4.5 g/kg/day) has resulted in a variety of abnormal metabolic responses (aminoacidemia, metabolic acidosis, azotemia, hyperammonemia), as well as unacceptable clinical responses (Menkes et al., 1966; Goldman et al., 1969; Snyderman et al., 1969; Raiha et al., 1976; Rassin and Gaull, 1977). Thus, in feeding the preterm neonate, a balance must be reached between the metabolic cost of the high protein and the growth disadvantages of low protein.

Further compounding the problem of feeding the preterm infant is the question of the role of human milk. The low protein content of this milk (1.0 g protein/dl or approximately 1.8 g/kg/day) is less than the minimum recommendation (2.25–5 g/kg/d) of some professional groups for these infants (Committee on Nutrition, American Academy of Pediatrics, 1977) and is less than that found in currently available commercial formulas. There is evidence that mothers who give birth to preterm infants have slightly more protein in their milk than those mothers who have term infants (Atkinson et al., 1978; Gross et al., 1981; Lemons et al., 1982). However, the appropriateness of such milk for feeding these infants remains to be demonstrated. The growth of preterm infants fed various volumes of pooled human milk (Jarvenpaa et al., 1983) or their own mother's milk (Gross, 1983) appears to be appropriate, but some concerns remain regarding the adequacy of such feeding (Fomon and Ziegler, 1977, Gaull et al., 1977a).

Most significant in the preterm infant have been the dramatic biochemical responses to different amounts and quality of protein (Raiha et al., 1976; Gaull et al., 1977b; Rassin et al., 1977a,b), especially with respect to the amino acid responses of these infants. Infants fed high protein (3.0 g/dl) casein-protein-predominant formulas had especially high plasma concentrations of tyrosine and phenylalanine (Levine et al., 1941; Mathews and Partington, 1964; Partington, 1968; Rassin et al., 1977b), a finding associated with subsequent poor neurologic outcome (Menkes et al., 1972; Mamunes et al., 1976). In contrast, whey-protein-predominant formulas resulted in especially high concentrations of plasma threonine. A comparison of some of the amino acids observed in these infants after 4 weeks of feeding illustrates some of the differences observed (Table IV).

Thus, enteral feeding in both the term and the preterm infant results in a plasma amino acid pattern that is characteristic of the type of feeding. The plasma amino acid pattern reflects the substrate milieu in which the brain is expected to develop. This milieu may represent one factor in the reduced intellectual (Rodgers, 1978) and health outcome of formula-fed infants when compared to breast-fed infants (Report of the Task Force on the Assessment of the Scientific Evidence Relating to Infant Feeding Practices and Infant Health, 1984).

PARENTERAL NEONATAL AMINO ACID NUTRITION

TPN has been an invaluable aid in the nutritional support of sick infants, often preterm infants, who cannot be fed enterally. Current TPN solutions

TABLE IV. Plasma Amino Acid Concentrations (μM) in Preterm Infants at 4 Weeks of Age[a]

	Pooled human milk			Whey-predominant formula		Casein-predominant formula	
				1.5 g/dl	3.0 g/dl	1.5 g/dl	3.0 g/dl
Volume (ml/kg/d)	170	185	200	150	150	150	150
Taurine	70	80	96	61	50	50	55
Aspartate	10	18	23	14	20	16	22
Threonine	170	127	163	286	348	218	291
Serine	135	177	200	159	224	194	224
Glutamate	157	141	164	172	181	199	205
Glutamine	400	448	479	531	611	635	609
Proline	178	N.M.	N.M.	193	227	186	323
Glycine	197	229	274	229	227	284	263
Alanine	279	294	316	323	360	376	363
Citrulline	16	31	12	23	46	27	48
α-NH₂-butyrate	2	N.M.	N.M.	8	33	7	34
Valine	125	118	121	156	264	219	326
Cystine	80	106	157	89	85	102	106
Methionine	16	32	26	35	49	43	53
Isoleucine	57	41	46	73	113	90	122
Leucine	102	84	91	100	170	125	189
Tyrosine	71	54	60	97	164	167	496
Phenylalanine	47	39	44	52	74	74	161
Orthithine	65	N.M.	N.M.	92	118	101	132
Lysine	70	N.M.	N.M.	161	252	157	254
Histidine	68	N.M.	N.M.	68	85	76	89
Arginine	48	N.M.	N.M.	81	89	78	100
Valine/glycine	0.63	0.52	0.44	0.68	1.16	0.77	1.24

[a]Adapted from Rassin et al., 1977a,b; Gaull et al., 1977b; Jarvenpaa et al., 1983; and unpublished data.

[b]NM = not measured.

consist of mixtures of carbohydrate (usually glucose), electrolytes, vitamins, lipids, and crystalline amino acids which can be infused into the infant either by a central or a peripheral vein (depending upon the length of time of infusion or amount of TPN to be infused). The composition of the amino acid component of the TPN solutions has evolved from casein hydrolysates to crystalline amino acid mixtures that supported growth to current crystalline amino acid mixtures which are closer in composition to physiologic (human milk protein) amino acid intakes (Table V) (Stegink, 1983). Determining the requirements for amino acids in sick preterm infants is confounded by the problem of delineating a "normal" preterm infant, as discussed above, but is also confounded by the fact that the infant is usually ill (changing nutrient requirements); the direct infusion of nutrients into the circulatory system,

TABLE V. Plasma Amino Acid Concentrations (μM) in Preterm Infants
Fed 6 Days of Total Parenteral Nutrition[a]

	Day 0	Day 6	Day 6
Protein	0	1.5 g/kg/day	2.5 g/kg/day
Taurine	71	36	95
Aspartate	15	8	6
Threonine	132	165	320
Serine	100	105	249
Glutamate	48	30	61
Glutamine	322	250	361
Proline	89	86	176
Glycine	215	294	653
Alanine	114	119	204
Valine	56	109	172
Cystine	58	66	62
Methionine	18	26	43
Isoleucine	5	32	51
Leucine	47	55	88
Tyrosine	129	29	23
Phenylalanine	65	57	53
Ornithine	40	50	91
Lysine	122	124	171
Histidine	62	49	66
Arginine	14	36	81
Valine/glycine	0.26	0.37	0.26

[a]Adapted from Malloy et al., 1984.

bypassing regulatory mechanisms of the gut; and the potential interactions of nutrients in the bottle.

The composition of amino acid solutions used for TPN partly reflects attempts to modify early solutions based upon recommendations derived from current understanding of infant amino acid requirements (Winters, 1975). The present composition of these mixtures also represents some practical considerations. Amino acids that are poorly soluble (tyrosine and cystine) are included in minimal amounts. Unstable amino acids are not included (cysteine). Inexpensive amino acids are used to make up much of the nitrogen load that is given (glycine and alanine). Some amino acids may be neurotoxic (glutamate and aspartate) and so have been included in minimal quantities at best (Olney et al., 1972a,b; Olney, 1986), even though these amino acids represent a major proportion of human milk proteins. Unfortunately these practical considerations have resulted in nutrient intakes that may be less than optimum for the preterm neonate. As mentioned above, tyrosine and cysteine may be essential yet cannot be easily delivered by this route of nutrition. Glycine has the potential to be neurotoxic, is a neuroinhibitory compound (Aprison and Daly, 1978), and when present in large amounts, such as in non-ketotic hyperglycinemia, has serious clinical consequences (Nyhan, 1983). Yet glycine, because it is an inexpensive nitrogen source, is often infused in fairly large concentrations (Table V). Some efforts are being made to deal with these problems, for example N-acetyltyrosine may be a practical soluble analog of tyrosine (Stegink et al., 1982).

Infusion of TPN solutions has been associated with a number of untoward responses in infants: azotemia, hyperammonemia, cholestasis, and abnormal plasma amino acid patterns (Heird, 1981). Modifications of the TPN solution may ameliorate some of these problems; for example addition of taurine may aid in preventing cholestasis (Dorvil et al., 1983; Cook et al., 1984), but the effect of the abnormal amino acid patterns on the developing brain is less easy to assess. The plasma amino acid concentrations of infants fed by TPN tend to reflect the composition of the solutions used. Generally plasma tyrosine, cystine, taurine, valine, isoleucine, and leucine are present in reduced concentrations. In contrast threonine, glycine, alanine, methionine, and phenylalanine are frequently present in high concentrations (Winters et al., 1977; Zlotkin et al., 1981; Bell et al., 1983; Malloy et al., 1984). Patterns of amino acids in these infants are difficult to evaluate because they often are preceded by a period of fasting (low or no protein intake of several days) due to the clinical state of the infant. The amino acid profiles of such infants are quite different from those of infants fed enterally.

Thus, parenteral nutrition, while being a life-saving nutritional regimen, may result in the brain developing in a less than optimal nutritional milieu. In beagle puppies, similar feeding results in abnormal plasma amino acid profiles as well as abnormal tissue (brain and liver) free amino acid profiles (Malloy et al., 1981a,b; Malloy and Rassin, 1984). The brains of these puppies also contained considerably less protein (but not less DNA) than control puppies, indicating a selective effect of this type of feeding on brain cell size (Heird and Malloy, 1979; Malloy and Rassin, 1984). The potential for such a nutritional regimen to influence the development of an infant's brain seems very real under these circumstances.

AMINO ACID NUTRITION AND BRAIN DEVELOPMENT

In the preceding discussion the role of amino acids as neurotransmitters or neurotransmitter precursors has been discussed, their potential essentiality as nutrients has been presented, and the differential effect of various modes of protein nutrition on the plasma-free amino acid pools of preterm and term infants, has been documented. The potential for these changes in plasma-free amino acid pools to influence the brain are inferred from the properties at two steps in the progression of an amino acid from plasma to central nervous system neurotransmitter. The first step is its transport across the blood brain barrier, a transport that is competitive and unsaturated and so is open to modification by changes in the precursor pool. The second step is its metabolism; once inside the central nervous system, the capacity for neurotransmitter synthetic systems to respond to changes in the precursor pool exists (Cohen and Wurtman, 1979).

Information regarding the second step is primarily limited to evidence that has been gathered in in vitro animal studies. Generally it is presumed that if the in vitro K_m for an enzyme is greater than the brain concentration of the precursor for that enzyme, then the enzyme is not saturated. If the enzyme is not saturated with precursor then increases in the precursor pool will result in increased synthesis of the neurotransmitter up to the point that the enzyme is saturated. Several neurotransmitter systems have been demonstrated to have these properties and, thus, be open to regulation by changes in the precursor pool. These metabolic systems include the synthetic mechanisms for serotonin, dopamine, norepinephrine, S-adenosylmethionine (important for neurotransmitter degradation), and acetylcholine.

Tryptophan hydroxylase (which catalyzes the conversion of tryptophan to 5-hydroxytryptophan) appears to be the rate limiting step in serotonin (5-hydroxytryptamine) synthesis. The K_m for this enzyme has been found to be approximately 3×10^{-4} M in vitro (Lovenberg et al., 1968), while the brain concentration of tryptophan is about $4-8 \times 10^{-5}$ M (McKean et al., 1968; Fernstrom and Wurtman, 1974). In a similar manner the K_m for tyrosine hydroxylase (which catalyzes the conversion of tyrosine to DOPA) appears to be the rate limiting step in the synthesis of dopamine and norepinephrine. The apparent K_m of this enzyme is 1×10^{-4} M, while the brain concentration of tyrosine is in the range of $6-18 \times 10^{-5}$ M (Gibson and Wurtman, 1978). The apparent K_m for methionine adenosyltransferase (which catalyzes the conversion of methionine to S-adenosylmethionine) appears to be the rate limiting step in the synthesis of S-adenosylmethionine, a compound essential to the catabolism of many neurotransmitters via methylation reactions. The apparent K_m for this enzyme is 90 μM (Matthysse et al., 1972), while brain concentrations of methionine are about 80–150 μM (Lombardini et al., 1971; Rubin et al., 1974). Thus, steps in both the synthesis and catabolism of several important transmitter systems are unsaturated and may respond to variations in precursor availability with increased or decreased synthesis potentially changing the neuronal activity of the central nervous system.

It is interesting to note that the amino acids involved in the above reactions all belong to a single transport group, the large neutral amino acids that compete for transport at the blood brain barrier (Pardridge, 1977). The "brain uptake index" technique developed by Oldendorf (1971) has been used to define a group of amino acids that compete for similar transport sites that corresponds closely to the System L described by Christensen (1979) in his more general treatment of membrane amino acid transport. This group of nine amino acids includes phenylalanine, tyrosine, valine, isoleucine, leucine, threonine, methionine, histidine, and tryptophan.

These interactions have been studied (Wurtman and Fernstrom, 1976; Cohen and Wurtman, 1979) using the ratio of any one large neutral amino acid to the sum of all the large neutral amino acids, and this approach give some insights into the regulation of entry into the brain. However, in an approach that takes into account more of the individual properties of the amino acids, Pardridge and his coworkers have developed kinetic constants in the rat and the rabbit using the brain uptake index technique to describe the brain influx of this group of amino acids in the presence of various plasma concentrations (Pardridge, 1977, 1986; Pardridge and Mietus, 1982; Miller et al., 1985; Pardridge et al., 1985). These investigators developed a K_m and a V_{max} for each amino acid and then developed a mathematical approach first to derive a K_m apparent based upon plasma amino acid concentrations and then to calculate a brain influx of the amino acid (Pardridge, 1977). While several different sets of kinetic parameters have been developed for the rat reflecting such differences as the presence or absence of anesthetic agents or the use of linear transformation versus non-linear regression treatments, these differences will cancel out when the apparent K_m values are derived to calculate influxes (Pardridge et al., 1985; Pardridge, personal communication).

These derived kinetic measures have been used to calculate amino acid influxes in rats fed various amounts of protein and made diabetic by administration of streptozotocin (Glanville and Anderson, 1985). In general, these latter authors found a good correlation for the calculated influx and brain amino acid concentrations for threonine, methionine, tryptophan, and tyrosine in diabetic and for threonine and tyrosine in control rats (Glanville and Anderson, 1985). Thus, even though a direct correlation might not be expected between calculated influx and brain amino acid concentration because of further metabolism once the compounds were inside the central nervous system, there was evidence of some predictive ability of the calculated influx rates.

Assuming that the derived kinetic parameters for the rat give some representation for the human situation, brain influx rates were calculated for the various dietary situations described in Tables III and V. These influx rates were calculated using the kinetic parameters and the following formulas described by Pardridge (1977):

$$K_{mapp}^{aa} = K_m^{aa} \left(1 + \sum \frac{[AA]}{K_m^{aa}} \right)$$

$$v = \frac{V_{max}^{aa}\,[AA]}{K_{mapp}^{aa} + [AA],}$$

K_m = affinity constant (μM),
K_{mapp} = apparent affinity constant (μM),
[AA] = plasma amino acid concentration (μM),
V_{max} = velocity constant (μmol·min^{-1} · g^{-1}), and
v = amino acid influx (μmol·min^{-1} · g^{-1}).
aa = amino acid of interest

First the K_{mapp} is calculated for each amino acid in a given environment of plasma-free amino acid concentrations. Then the influx velocity for each of these amino acids may be calculated.

The formula-fed term infant, as reflected by the moderate changes in plasma amino acid concentrations, only had a few modifications of the predicted amino acid influx. Those infants fed a whey-protein-predominant formula (1.5 g, 60:40) had a reduction in the predicted influx of tyrosine and an increase in the predicted influx of threonine (Table VI). In contrast, those infants fed a casein-protein-predominant formula (1.5 g, 18:82) had an increase in phenylalanine and valine predicted brain influxes (Table VI). Thus, while mild, there is certainly a potential for differences in dietary protein to influence the milieu of the developing term infant's brain.

The preterm infant is much more liable to influences of changes in dietary protein quantity and quality. Feeding different volumes of human milk resulted in several changes in the predicted influxes, especially with respect to methionine (reduced) and threonine (increased) (Table VII). The formulas had a much more dramatic effect, with those infants fed the whey-protein-predominant formulas having especially large increases in tyrosine, isoleucine, and threonine and decreases in methionine and histidine predicted influxes (Table VII) The casein-protein-predominant formulas resulted in increases in tyrosine, phenylalanine, and isoleucine and decreases in methionine and histidine predicted influxes (Table VII). In the high protein intake group of the casein-protein-predominant formula, the large increases in tyrosine and phenylalanine predicted influxes reflect the particularly large changes in the plasma concentrations of these two amino acids.

The preterm infant fed parenterally also had noticeable changes in predicted amino acid influxes. At the time of initiating TPN, most infants had not been fed protein for some time (often several days) due to their

TABLE VI. Predicted Brain Influx of Large Neutral Amino Acids in Term Infants[a]

Human-milk-fed (μmol · min^{-1}g^{-1})		Formula-fed (% human milk-fed)	
		1.5 g (60:40)	1.5 g (18:82)
Phenylalanine	2.77	103	113
Tyrosine	5.68	84	109
Valine	3.05	114	131
Isoleucine	2.69	117	101
Leucine	5.85	100	94
Threonine	1.68	146	109
Methionine	1.44	110	99
Histidine	2.35	97	99

[a]Calculated from the data presented in Table III and the formulas in the text. The kinetic constants used were as presented by Pardridge (1977).

clinical condition. The predicted influxes at day 0 reflected a situation similar to that seen in protein malnutrition with very low branch chain amino acids (valine, isoleucine, and leucine). However, these infants tended to have high plasma tyrosine and phenylalanine concentrations, possibly due to immature liver function, resulting in high predicted influxes (Table VII). The initiation of TPN resulted in several changes in the predicted influxes, with an especially dramatic decrease in tyrosine, and increase in valine and threonine predicted influxes (Table VII).

Unfortunately, only minimal data are available for tryptophan in all of these various nutritional paradigms, reflecting the analytical difficulty associated with measurement of this amino acid by standard amino acid analysis techniques. The data that are available indicate that tryptophan does not vary as much as many of the other amino acids. These data, when used in the calculations described above, indicate that, generally, tryptophan predicted influxes would decrease in the formula-fed groups, primarily reflecting the large increases in the aromatic amino acids.

Thus, in general, one might predict that formula-fed infants have higher brain concentrations of catecholamines and lower concentrations of serotonin and histamine than human-milk-fed infants. In contrast, TPN-supported infants may have decreased brain catecholamine concentrations. While these data and calculations do not prove that changes in feeding regimens in the human neonate can cause changes in the neurotransmitter composition of the brain, the evidence from animal studies would certainly support this conclusion. It is clear that new techniques are needed to define the characteristics of brain amino acid influx in the human neonate, but for the moment it would appear prudent to modify protein nutrient composition and amount with caution because of the potential effects on brain neurotransmitter systems.

TABLE VII. Predicted Brain Influx of Large Neutral Amino Acids in Preterm Infants[a]

	Human milk			Formulas (% of human milk-185 g group)[b]	
	185 ml/kg/d	170 ml/kg/d $(\mu mol \cdot min^{-1} g^{-1})$	200 ml/kg/d	1.5 g (60:40)	3.0 g (60:40)
Phenylalanine	2.61 (94)	109	107	106	109
Tyrosine	4.14 (73)	118	106	138	165
Valine	2.55 (84)	97	98	105	128
Isoleucine	2.00 (74)	126	107	140	157
Leucine	4.66 (80)	109	103	95	115
Threonine	1.80 (107)	121	121	172	154
Methionine	1.55 (108)	47	79	88	90
Histidine	2.53 (108)	92	96	81	74

	Formulas		Total parenteral nutrition (% of human milk-185 g group)			
	1.5 g (18:82)	3.0 g (18:82)	No protein (0 d)	1.25 g Protein (6 d)	1.5 g Protein (6 d)	2.5 g Protein (6 d)
Phenylalanine	122	151	152	152		120
Tyrosine	186	288	206	61		41
Valine	120	106	47	101		129
Isoleucine	142	114	12	86		112
Leucine	98	88	58	74		95
Threonine	112	88	99	139		213
Methionine	89	65	55	90		120
Histidine	75	52	88	80		88

[a]These predicted influxes have been calculated from the data presented in Tables IV and V and the formulas in the text. The kinetic constants used were as presented by Pardridge (1977).

[b]The numbers in parentheses are the influxes of the 185 ml/kg/d human-milk-fed group expressed as a percentage of the data from the term breast-fed infants (Table VI).

SUMMARY

Amino acids serve as neurotransmitter precursors and as neurotransmitters in the brain. Classic approaches to determining the essentiality of nutrients based upon growth and nitrogen balance studies tend to ignore these important functions. The various types of protein nutrition used in the neonate, different quality and quantity of protein or enteral versus parenteral feeding, results in different plasma amino acid patterns. These plasma amino acid patterns probably influence the influx of amino acids into the brain resulting in changes in both neurotransmitter precursor and neurotransmitter pools. Considerable refinement in techniques of evaluation will be necessary before it will be possible to determine whether or not the brain is subject to functional differences as a result of developing in different pools of neurotransmitter substrate.

REFERENCES

Anderson TL, Heird WC, Winters RW (1977): Clinical and physiological consequences of total parenteral nutrition in the pediatric patient. In Greep JM, Soeterz PB, Wesdorp RIC, Phaf CWC, Fischer JE (eds): "Current Concepts in Parenteral Nutrition." The Hague: Marinus Nijhoff, pp 117–127.

Aprison MH, Daly EC (1978): Biochemical aspects of transmission at inhibitory synapses: The role of glycine. Adv Neurochem 3:203–294.

Atkinson SA, Bryan MH, Anderson GH (1978): Human milk: Difference in nitrogen concentration in milk from mothers of term and premature infants. J Pediatr 93:67–69.

Babson SG, Bramhall JL (1969): Diet and growth in the premature infant: The effect of different dietary intakes of ash-electrolyte and protein on weight gain and linear growth. J Pediatr 74:890–900.

Bell EF, Filer LJ, Jr, Wong AP, Stegink LD (1983): Effects of a parenteral nutrition regimen containing dicarboxylic amino acids on plasma, erythrocyte and urinary amino acid concentrations of young infants. Am J Clin Nutr 37:99–107.

Christensen HN (1979): Exploiting amino acid structure to learn about membrance transport. Adv Enzymol 49:41–101.

Cohen EL, Wurtman RJ (1979): Nutrition and brain neurotransmitters. In Winick M (ed): "Human Nutrition: A Comprehensive Treatise." Vol. 1, "Nutrition: Pre- and Postnatal Development." New York: Plenum Press, pp 103–132.

Committee on Nutrition, American Academy of Pediatrics (1976): Commentary on breast-feeding and infant formulas including proposed standards for formulas. Pediatric 57:278–285.

Committee on Nutrition, American Academy of Pediatrics (1977): Nutritional needs of low-birth-weight infants. Pediatrics 60:519–530.

Committee on Nutrition, American Academy of Pediatrics (1978): Breastfeeding. Pediatrics 62:591–601.

Cooke RJ, Whitington RF, Kelts D (1984): Effects of taurine supplementation on hepatic function during short-term parenteral nutrition in the premature infant. J Pediatr Gastroenterol Nutr 3:234–238.

Czarncki GL, Baker DJ (1984): Urea cycle function in the dog with emphasis on the role of arginine. J Nutr 114:581–590.

Davidson M, Levine SZ, Bauer CH, Dann M (1967): Feeding studies in low-birth-weight infants: Relationships of dietary protein, fat and elctrolyte to rates of weight-gain, clinical courses and serum chemical concentrations. J Pediatr 70:695–713.

DeFeudis FV, Mandel P (eds) (1981): "Amino Acid Neurotransmitters." New York: Raven Press.

Dorvil NP, Yousef IM, Tuchweber B, Roy CC (1983): Taurine prevents cholestasis induced by lithocholic acid sulfate in guinea pigs. Am J Clin Nutr 37:221–232.

Dudel J (1986): Criteria for identification of transmitter substances, In von Euler C, Skoglund S, V Soderburg (eds): "Structure and Function of Inhibitory Neuronal Mechanisms." Oxford: Pergamon Press, pp 523–525.

Fernstrom JD, Wurtman RJ (1974): Control of brain serotonin levels by the diet. In Costa E, Sandler M (eds): "Serotonin—New Vistas," Advances in Psychopharmacology, vol. 11. New York: Raven Press, pp 133–142.

Fomon SJ, Ziegler EE (1977): Protein intake of premature infants: Interpretation of data. J Pediatr 90:504–506.

Fonnum F (ed) (1978): "Amino Acids as Chemical transmitters." New York: Plenum Press.

Gaull GA, Rassin DK, Raiha NCR (1977a): Protein intake of premature infants: A reply. J Pediatr 90:507–510.

Gaull GE, Rassin DK, Raiha NCR, Heinonen K (1977b): Milk protein quantity and quality in low-birth-weight infants III. Effects on sulfur-containing amino acids in plasma and urine. J Pediatr 90:348–355.

Gaull GE, Sturman JA, Raiha NCR (1972): Development of mammalian sulfur metabolism: Absence of cystathionase in human fetal tissues. Pediatr Res 6:538–547.

Gibson CJ, Wurtman RJ (1987): Psysiological control of brain norepinephrine synthesis by brain tyrosine concentration. Life Sci 22:1399–1406.

Glanville NT, Anderson GH (1985): The effect of insulin deficiency, dietary protein intake and plasma amino acid concentrations on brain amino acid levels in rats. Can J Physiol Pharmacol 63:487–494.

Goldman HI, Freudenthal R, Holland B, Karelitz S (1969): Clinical effects of two different levels of protein intake on low-birth-weight infants. J Pediatr 74:881–889.

Gross SJ (1983): Growth and biochemical response of preterm infants fed human milk or modified infant formula. N Engl J Med 308:237–241.

Gross SJ, Geller J, Tomarelli RM (1981): Composition of breast milk from mothers of preterm infants. Pediatrics 68:490–493.

Hambraeus L (1977); Proprietary milk versus human breast milk in infant feeding: A critical appraisal from the nutritional point of view. Pediatr Clin North Am 24:17–36.

Hambraeus L, Lonnderdal B, Forsum E, Gebre-Medhin M (1978): Nitrogen and protein components of human milk. Acta Paediatr Scand 67:561–565.

Hayes KC, Carey RE, Schmidt SY (1975): Retinal degeneration associated with taurine deficiency in the cat. Science 188:949–951.

Heird WC (1981): Total parenteral nutrition. In Lebenthal E (ed): "Textbook of Gastroenterology and Nutrition in Infancy." New York: Raven Press, pp 659–670.

Heird WC, Malloy MH (1979): Brain composition of beagle puppies receiving total parenteral nutrition. In Visser HKA (ed): "Nutrition and Metabolism of the Fetus and Infant." The Hague: Martinus Nijhof, pp 365–375.

Irwin MI, Hegsted DM (1971): A conspectus of research on amino acid requirments of man. J Nutr 101:539–556.

Jackson AA (1983): Amino acids: Essential and non-essential? Lancet 1:1034–1036.

Jackson AA, Shaw JCL, Barber A, Golden MHN (1981): Nitrogen metabolism in preterm infants fed donor breast milk: The possible essentiality of glycine. Pediatr Res 15:1454–1461.

Janas LM, Picciano MF, Hatch TF (1985): Indicies of protein metabolism in term infants fed human milk, whey-predominant formula, or cow's milk formula. Pediatric 75:775–784.

Jarvenpaa A-L, Raiha NCR, Rassin DK, Gaull GE (1983): Preterm infants fed human milk attain intrauterine weight-gain. Acta Paediatr Scand 72:239–243.

Jarvenpaa A-L, Rassin DK, Raiha NCR, Gaull GE (1982): Milk protein quantity and quality in the term infant. II. Effects on acidic and neutral amino acids. Pediatrics 70:221–230.

Jenness R (1974a): The composition of milk. In Larson BL, Smith VR (eds): "Lactation: A Comprehensive Treatise," vol. 3. New York: Academic Press, pp 3–107.

Jenness R (1974b): Biosynthesis and composition of milk. J Invest Dermatol 63:109–118.

Kretchmer N, Levine SZ, McNamara H (1957): The in vitro metabolism of tyrosine and its intermediates in the liver of the premature infant. AMA J Dis Child 93:19–20.

Kretchmer N, Levine SZ, McNamare H, Barrett HL (1956): Certain aspects of tyrosine metabilism in the young. I. The development of the tyrosine oxidizing system in human liver. J Clin Invest 35:235–244.

Lemons JA, Moy L, Hall D, Simmons M (1982): Differences in the composition of preterm and term human milk during early lactation. Pediatr Res 16:113–117.

Levine S, Maples E, Gordon H (1941): A defect in the metabilism of tyrosine and phenylalanine in premature infant. I. Identification and assay of intermediary products. J Clin Invest 20:199–207.

Lombardini JB, Burch MK, Talalay P (1971): An enzymatic derivative double isotope assay for L-methionine. J Biol Chem 246:4465–4470.

Lovenberg W, Jequier E, Sjoerdsma A (1968): A trytophan hydroxylation in mammalian systems. Adv Pharmacol 6A:21–36.

Macy IG (1949): Composition of human colostrum and milk. Am J Dis Child 78:589–603.

Macy IG, Kelly HG, Sloan RE (1953): The composition of milks. Nat Acad Sci, Washington, D.C., Nat Res Council Public. 254.

Malloy MH, Rassin DK (1984): Cysteine supplementation of total parenteral nutrition: The effect in beagle pups. Pediatr Res 18:747–751.

Malloy MH, Rassin DK, Gaull GE, Heird WC (1981a): Development of taurine metabolism in beagle pups: Effects of taurine free total parenteral nutrition. Biol Neonate 40:1–8.

Malloy MH, Rassin DK, Heird WC, Gaull GE (1981b): Transsulfuration in parenterally nourished beagle pups. Am J Clin Nutr 34:1520–1525.

Malloy MH, Rassin DK, Richardson CJ (1984): Total parenteral nutrition in sick preterm infants: Effects of cysteine supplementation with nitrogen intakes of 240 and 400 mg/kg/day. J Pediatr Gastroenterol Nutr 3:239–244.

Mamunes P, Prince PE, Thornton NH, Hunt PA, Hitchcock ES (1976): Intellectual deficits after transient tyrosinemia in the term neonate. Pediatrics 57:675–680.

Mathews J, Partington MW (1964): The plasma tyrosine levels of premature babies. Arch Dis Child 39:371–378.

Matthysse S, Baldessarini RJ, Vogt M (1972): Methionine advenosyltransferase: A double-isotope derivative enzymatic assay. Anal Biochem 48:410–421

McKean CM, Boggs DE, Peterson NA (1968): The influence of high phenylalanine and tyrosine on the concentrations of essential amino acids in brain. J Neurochem 15:235–241.

Menkes JH, Chernick V, Ringel B (1966): Effect of elevated blood tyrosine on subsequent intellectual development of premature infants. J Pediatr 69:583–588.

Menkes JH, Welcher DW, Levi HS (1972): Relationship of elevated blood tyrosine to the ultimate intellectual performance of premature infants. Pediatrics 49:218–224.

Miller LP, Pardridge WM, Braun LD, Oldendorf WH (1985): Kinetic constants for blood-brain barrier amino acid transport in conscious rats. J Neurochem 45:1427–1432.

Mizunuma T, Kawamura S, Kishino Y (1984): Effects of ingesting excess arginine on rat pancreas. J Nutr 114:467–471.

Nyhan WL (1983): Nonketotic hyperglycinemia. In Stanbury JB, Wyngaarden JB, Frederickson DS, Goldstein JL, Brown MS (eds): "The Metabolic Basis of Inherited Disease." 5th Ed. New York: McGraw Hill, pp 561–569.

Oldendorf WH (1971): Brain uptake of radiolabelled amino acids, amines, and hexoses after arterial injection. Am J Physiol 221:1629–1639.

Olney JW (1986): Excitotoxic amino acids. News in Physiological Sciences 1:19–25.

Olney JW, Ho OL, Rhee V (1972a): Cytotoxic effects of acidic and sulphur containing amino acids on the infant mouse central nervous system. Exp Brain Res 14:61–76.

Olney JW, Sharpe LG, Feigin RD (1972b): Glutamate-induced brain damage in infant primates. J Neuropathol Exp Neurol 31:464–488.

Pardridge WM (1977): Regulation of amino acid availability to the brain. In Wurtman RJ, Wurtman JJ (eds): "Nutrition and the Brain," vol. 1. New York: Raven Press, pp 141–204.

Pardridge WM (1986): Effects of the dipeptide sweetener aspartame on the brain. In Wurtman RJ, Wurtmann JJ (eds): "Nutrition and the Brain," vol. 7. New York: Raven Press, pp 199–241.

Pardridge WM, Landew EM, Miller LP, Braun LD, Oldernof WH (1985): Carotid artery injection technique: Bounds for bolus mixing by plasma and by brain. J Cereb Blood Flow Metab 5:576–583.

Pardridge WM, Mietus LJ (1982): Kinetics of neutral amino acid transport through the blood-brain barrier of the newborn rabbit. J Neurochem 38:955–962.

Partington MW (1968): Neonatal tyrosinemia. Biol Neonate 12:316–330.

Pascal TA, Gillam BM, Gaull GE (1972): Cystathionase: Immunochemical evidence for absence from human fetal liver. Pediatr Res 6:773–778.

Pencharz PB, Farri L, Papageorgiou A (1983): The effects of human milk and low-protein formulae on the rates of total body protein turnover and urinary 3-methylhistidine excretion of preterm infants. Clin Sci 64:611–616.

Pohlandt F (1974): Cysteine: A semiessential amino acid in the newborn infant. Acta Paediatr Scand 63:801–804.

Raiha NCR, Heinonen K, Rassin DK, Gaull GE (1976): Milk protein quantity and quality in low-birth-weight-infants I. Metabolic responses and effects on growth. Pediatrics 57:659–674.

Rassin DK (1987): Evaluation of protein nutritional status. J Pediatr Gastroenterol Nutr 6:7–9.

Rassin DK, Gaull GE (1977): Protein requirements and the development of amino acid metabolism in the neonate. In Green HL, Holliday MA, Munro HN (eds): "Clinical Nutrition Update: Amino Acids." Chicago: American Medical Association, pp 84–95.

Rassin DK, Gaull GE, Heinonen K, Raiha NCR (1977a): Milk protein quantity and quality in low-birth-weight infants. II. Effects on selected essential and non-essential amino acids in plasma and urine. Pediatrics 59:407–422.

Rassin DK, Gaull GE, Jarvenpaa A-L, Raiha NCR (1983): Feeding the low-birth-weight infant II. Effects of taurine and cholesterol supplementation on amino acids and cholesterol. Pediatrics 71:179–186.

Rassin DK, Gaull GE, Raiha NCR, Heinonen K (1977b): Milk protein quantity and quality in low-birth-weight infants. IV. Effects on tyrosine and phenylalanine in plasma and urine. J Pediatr 90:356–360.

Report of the Task Force on the Assessment of the Scientific Evidence Relating to Infant Feeding Practices and Infant Health (1984): Pediatrics 74:576–762.

Rodgers B (1978): Feeding in infancy and later ability and attainment: A longitudinal study. Med Child Neurol 20:421–426.

Rubin RA, Ordonez IA, Wurtman RJ (1974): Physiological dependence of brain methionine and S-adenosylmethionine concentrations on serum amino acid pattern. J Neurochem 23:227–231.

Snyder SH, Young AB, Bennet JP, Mulder AH (1973): Synaptic biochemistry of amino acids. Fed Proc 32:2039–2047.

Snyderman SE (1971): The protein and amino acid requirements of the premature infant. In Jonxis JHP, Visser HKA, Troelstra JA (eds): "Metabolic Processes in the Foetus and Newborn Infant." Leiden: Stenfert Kroese, pp 128–141.

Snyderman SE, Boyer A, Kogut MD, Holt LE (1969): The protein requirements of the premature infant I. The effect of protein intake on the retention of nitrogen. J Pediatr 74:872–880.

Snyderman SE, Boyer A, Roitman E, Holt LE Jr (1963): The histidine requirement of the infant. Pediatrics 31:786–801.

Steginik LD (1983): Amino acids in pediatric parenteral nutrition. Am J Dis Child 137:1008–1016.

Steginik LD, Im HA, Meyer PD (1982): N-acetyl-L-tyrosine as a tyrosine source during total parenteral nutrition on adult rats. Fed Proc 41:273.

Stein TP, Settle RG, Albina JA (1986): Metabilism of nonessential ^{15}N-labeled aminoacids and the measurement of human whole-body protein synthesis rates. J Nutr 116:1651–1659.

Sturman JA, Moretz RC, French JH, Wisniewski HM (1985): Postnatal taurine deficiency in the kitten results in a persistance of the cerebellar external granule cell layer: Correction by taurine feeding. J Neurosci Res 13:521–528.

Sturman JA, Wen GY, Wisniewski HM, Neuringer MD (1984): Retinal degeneration in primates raised on a synthetic human infant formula. Int J Dev Neurosci 2:121–130.

Werman R (1966): A review—Criteria for identification of a central nervous system transmitter. Comp Biochem Physiol 18:745–766.

Winters RW (1975): Summary of conference. In Winters RW, Hasselmeyer EG (eds): "Intravenous Nutrition in the High Risk Infant." New York: John Wiley & Sons, pp 467–475.

Winters RW, Heird WC, Dell RB, Nicholson JF (1977): Plasma amino acids in infants receiving parenteral nutrition. In Green HL, Holliday MA, Munro HM (eds): "Clinical Nutrition Update: Amino Acids." Chicago: American Medical Association, pp 147–154.

Wurtman RJ, Fernstrom JD (1976): Control of brain neurotransmitter synthesis by precursor availability and nutritional state. Biochem Pharmacol 25:1691–1696.

Zlotkin SH, Anderson GH (1982): The development of cystathionase activity during the first year of life. Pediatr Res 16:65–68.

Zlotkin SH, Bryan MH, Anderson GH (1981): Cysteine supplementation to cysteine-free intravenous feeding regimens in newborn infants. Am J Clin Nutr 34:914–923, 1981.

SECTION II: MODELS OF BRAIN DEVELOPMENT

Current Topics in Nutrition and Disease, Volume 16
Basic and Clinical Aspects of Nutrition and Brain Development,
pages 43–56
© *1987 Alan R. Liss, Inc.*

Changes in Brain Protein Metabolism With Developmental and Nutritional State

Abel Lajtha, Miriam Banay-Schwartz, and Anna Maria Giuffrida Stella

N.S. Kline Institute for Psychiatric Research, New York, New York 10035
(A.L., M.B.-S.) and Instituto di Chimica Biologica, Dell'Universita di
Catania, 95125 Catania, Italy (A.M.G.S.)

INTRODUCTION

The greater sensitivity of the nervous system to external influences during development has been shown in numerous studies. It is not as well known how general this higher sensitivity is, and the underlying reason for it. Are metabolic controls similar but not as strong or are different mechanisms operative; that is, are the differences only quantitative, and the same processes are affected but to a different degree, or are developmental sensitivity differences qualitative, in that there are differences in sensitive mechanisms affected by external influences.

Studies of nutritional influences clearly show that strong defense mechanisms are already present in the immature brain; malnutrition, for example, even in the immature organism, results in smaller changes in brain than in most other organs.

Since all processes—structures, enzymes, metabolites—do not change at the same rate, or even in the same direction, during development, heterogeneity in response to stimuli can be expected during development. Different metabolic steps are affected to different degrees, some being stimulated, others inhibited, and the pattern may depend on the stage of development.

This heterogeneity of developmental changes of metabolism and developmental changes in response to various factors can also be seen in studies of brain proteins. Not only does the composition of proteins change during development, but the properties of the individual components such as enzymes or membrane proteins probably change as well. Changes in development may involve interactions wtih other lipid components, posttranslational modifications (phosphorylation, glycosylation), or changes in molecular size. The consequence of such structural changes may be alteration in function (enzyme activity, receptor affinity) and alteration in metabolism, such as greater resistance to degradative processes. Many such developmental changes may influence brain protein metabolism and composition; most of them have not been explored in detail.

TURNOVER RATES

It is well established that the rate of protein synthesis as measured by the incorporation of labeled amino acids is greater in the developing brain than in adult tissue. In vivo, the rate of incorporation has been found to be about 0.6–0.8% per hour, with different amino acids, methods of administration, or incorporation times (Dunlop et al., 1977a; Fern and Garlick, 1974; Austin et al., 1972; Seta et al., 1973; Oja, 1967). Although this is a valid figure for the actual rate, it is an average of several rates; that is, it does not mean that incorporation into all proteins proceeds at this rate. Our approximation of pools and rates in adult tissue revealed two pools, a large (95% of total), more slowly metabolized pool, and a smaller pool with faster metabolism. The ratio of metabolic rate (9 d half-life for the large pool, 10 h half-life for the small) of 20:1 is about the same as the ratio of pool size (95%:5%) (Lajtha et al., 1976). Thus, initially, equal amounts of label will be incorporated into each pool, since the 20 times slower pool is also 20 times larger, and only in longer term experiments (with the rapid pool in isotopic equilibrium) will there be a greater amount of label in the large pool.

Incorporation in developing brain occurs at a rate that is more than twice as high as that in adult (Lajtha et al., 1979), but in first approximation it occurs in a single pool in the young, which therefore has a higher rate than the large slow pool, but a lower rate than the small active pool of the adult. Since the higher average rate in the young is not due to a small portion of very active proteins, most proteins in the immature brain must be synthesized at a rate that is higher than in the adult. This then suggests that the rate of synthesis of a protein is not constant, but changes during development.

The factors that determine developmental changes in protein synthesis rates have been examined in some detail (Brown and Cosgrove, 1983) in isolated systems, where the individual steps and factors can be analyzed more easily. It seems that several steps in synthesis are involved. It is of interest that in in vitro systems the developmental change appears to be greater than in vivo. We examined this finding in some detail in a recent set of papers (Shabazian et al., 1986a–c). Earlier, we had found that slices from the young brain incorporate amino acids at a rate close to that of the immature brain in vivo, but that slices from adult brain incorporate at only about 10% of the adult in vivo rate (Dunlop et al., 1977b). We examined whether such developmental and in vitro changes occur in only a few fractions or in most proteins. Fractionation according to cellular or subcellular elements, regions, solubility, or molecular weight (Shahbazian et al., 1986a,b,c) indicated that the metabolic rate, although heterogeneous, undergoes similar developmental change in most protein fractions. These findings indicate that the metabolism of most proteins undergoes similar developmental change. In the adult brain, the majority, 95% or more, have a lower rate of metabolism, but a small pool has higher metabolism than proteins in the immature brain. This pool could represent proteins that are not present in the young, or this fraction, unlike the bulk, could have higher metabolic rates in the adult. Since the components of the small active pool have not been identified, we do not know what distinguishes this pool with an increasing metabolic rate during development from the other pool with a decreasing metabolic rate. Several possibilities, such as posttranslational modifications or changes in molecular weight, distribution, association with lipids, or physical properties, or some combination of them, need to be examined.

Since the rate of synthesis of most brain proteins changes during development and, therefore, is not a constant characteristic for each protein species, and since these changes occur in a heterogeneous pattern, it is likely that not only developmental but also other factors influence cerebral protein synthesis, and that such influences will show a heterogeneous pattern. A particular factor could alter the metabolism of only a small fraction of proteins, and the fraction that is altered could vary in different brain regions or at different stages of development.

CHANGES IN PROTEIN BREAKDOWN

Much of the work examining changes in protein metabolism has been focused on measuring protein synthesis. The reasons for this may be largely technical—measurement of amino acid incorporation is more sensitive and easier to interpret than measurements of breakdown.

It is clear that protein composition and its alterations are determined both by synthesis and by breakdown. The two processes are likely to be controlled and influenced independently. Complex changes in proteolysis under different conditions have been observed. In fibroblasts, the rate of breakdown of slowly metabolized proteins decreases and that of rapidly metabolized pool increases during aging (Okada and Dice, 1984). In muscle degeneration, protein loss is due to a greater increase in catabolism, although synthesis is also increased (Li, 1980; Goldspink et al., 1983). The most often studied change in brain proteolysis has been the increase in breakdown in experimental allergic encephalomyelitis (Cammer et al., 1978; Smith et al., 1981). The increase of some proteolytic enzymes under these conditions is probably responsible for the loss of myelin proteins, as shown by the fact that inhibition of protease activity prevents the pathological changes (Brosnan et al., 1980; Smith and Amaducci, 1982). Increased protease content was also observed in multiple sclerosis plaques (Hirsch et al., 1981). Increased activity of a neutral protease (activated by Ca) is responsible for the axonolysis followed by demyelination in experimental spinal cord trauma (Banik et al., 1982).

In measuring the changes in protease content of the brain in various conditions, it is important to know that enzyme content and in vivo activity are not identical, since a number of enzymes are in excess but the major portion in vivo may be inactive. For similar reasons changes in enzyme content may not be a good measure of changes in in vivo activity. Comparing brain cathepsin D content with the activity needed for the observed rate of brain protein turnover in vivo, we have estimated that the content of this enzyme is about 250-fold in excess (Banay-Schwartz et al., 1987). Deducing changes of cerebral protein breakdown in vivo from changes of cerebral protease content as assayed in vitro is made difficult by the difference in their developmental patterns. During a developmental phase in which cerebral cathepsin D content increases (Banay-Schwartz et al., 1983), the rate of in vivo protein breakdown decreases (Dunlop et al., 1978).

Of interest in this respect is the difference in protein synthesis and breakdown as measured in vivo and in isolated systems. We compared the rate of amino acid incorporation in vivo to that in incubated slices of brain. In immature tissue, the two values were fairly close, in that incorporation in slices was about 70–90% of that in vivo. In adult tissue the difference was very large, and incorporation in slices was only 7–15% of that in vivo (Dunlop et al., 1977b). When the protein degradation rate was compared in vivo to that in slices, the rates in vivo were 80–130% of those in vivo, depending on age (Dunlop et al., 1981). Thus slices may be a suitable system for studying changes in protein breakdown under various conditions.

Changes During Development

Long-term incorporation studies in which most brain proteins were labeled at first, and subsequently most lost their label with time, indicated that most brain proteins are in a dynamic state in the brain, undergoing continuous synthesis and breakdown (Lajtha and Toth, 1966).

Not only was the rate of protein synthesis higher in young than in adult brain, but the protein breakdown rate in vivo was also higher in young brain, decreasing during development. In the cerebrum, breakdown decreased from 1.3% per hour to 0.8% per hour (Dunlop et al., 1982). In the young brain, the difference between synthesis (2.0%/h) and breakdown (1.3%/h), is the rate of protein deposition (0.7%/h). There was regional heterogeneity in turnover: in young cerebellum, both synthesis and breakdown were higher than in cerebrum, and rates in pineal and pituitary were higher than in young brain and remained higher in adults (Dunlop et al., 1977b, 1982).

It is of interest that in the period of development in which turnover decreases, protease content increases (Banay-Schwartz et al., 1983), indicating that more of the enzymes are occluded, with an increasing latent capacity to activate proteolysis upon tissue insult in the adult tissue. Since proteases are in great excess even in young brain, the lower content in young tissue is not likely to serve as protection against increase upon insult.

Since the ratio of RNA concentrations to protein synthesis rates remains constant during development (Dunlop et al., 1984a), RNA levels may control synethetic rate.

Alterations of Metabolism

The changes in metabolic rates during development indicate that a number of factors can influence protein metabolism, and the effects can be heterogeneous, in that not all proteins are affected to the same degree. Some of the influences on turnover have been reviewed (Lajtha and Dunlop, 1981). Perhaps the largest change in protein synthesis was caused by lowered temperature—each decrement of 1°C resulted in a 7% decrease in amino acid incorporation (Lajtha and Sershen, 1975). This dependence on temperature is important. A number of reports noted effects on brain protein metabolism by drugs that also influence body temperature, and the effects were most likley due not to the drug directly but to its effect on body temperature. Body temperature in young animals is less well maintained, and it has to be considered or controlled in experiments with them. An interesting finding is the small but significant inhibition of incorporation by cerebral puncture as used for intracerebral administration of drugs or labeled precursors (Dunn, 1975; Dunlop et al., 1984c).

Not all the factors that alter some aspect of function or metabolism alter protein metabolism as well. We found no effect that induced hepatic encephalopathy after portacaval shunt (Dunlop et al., 1984b) or after elevating neurotransmitter amino acids (Toth and Lajtha, 1984a). Some drugs have an influence on brain protein synthesis, such as nicotine (Sershen and Lajtha, 1979) or alcohol, which has effects on various steps of protein synthesis (Tewari and Sytinsky, 1985), and affects both breakdown and synthesis (Toth and Lajtha, 1981, 1984b).

Among endocrine influences, the effects of thyroid hormones (Nunez, 1985) and pituitary peptides (Reith et al., 1977) have been studied. The effect of ACTH is of interest since a number of experimental conditions and stressful situations may influence brain protein metabolism through changes in ACTH, ACTH fragments, or corticosteroids. It is likely that hormones also influence protein breakdown in brain since in other tissues, endocrine influences on protein breakdown have been observed. In muscle, glucocorticoids cause stimulation of protein breakdown, which can be prevented by insulin (Ballard and Francis, 1983). Glucocorticoids inhibit synthesis and breakdown of muscle proteins (McGrath and Goldspink, 1982; Odedra and Millward, 1982). Alloxan diabetes increases Ca-activated protease in muscle and decreases protein deposition (Brooks et al., 1983). Insulin at physiological concentrations has been shown to inhibit protein degradation (Sugden and Smith, 1982).

It is important to study breakdown effects as well, since changes in breakdown are often in a different direction from changes in synthesis. Muscle growth upon refeeding after starvation is due to a reduced rate of degradation to below normal and an increased rate of synthesis to above normal (Li and Warner, 1984). In liver, rapid recovery after malnutrition is caused by decreased breakdown (Conde and Scornik, 1976), and in kidney as well (Bur and Conde, 1982). At elevated temperatures (42°C), muscle protein degradation increases, whereas protein synthesis decreases (Baracos et al., 1984). Glucocorticoid effects on synthesis and breakdown are different (Odedra et al., 1983). In the rabbit Alzheimer model, aluminum adminis-tration alters brain protease content (Benuck et al., 1985).

Heterogeneity of Metabolism

The kinetic analysis of amino acid incorporation or release of label from prelabeled amino acid indicates that the bulk of proteins are metabolized at fairly close to average rates and that the fractions with very high or very low rates of metabolism are very small. In spite of this, the measurements of turnover of a few purified proteins and of the recovery of irreversibly inhibited enzymes show a fairly wide spectrum of turnover rates. An illustration of this is the metabolism of myelin proteins (Lajtha et al., 1977; Benjamins and Morell, 1978), where some differences were found in metabolism of individual proteins and some heterogeneity in the metabolism of a single protein, such as proteolipid protein (as if this protein would have fractions of faster and slower metabolism possibly dependent on its local-ization within the myelin sheath). A portion of myelin proteins was found to be very stable (Shapira et al., 1981). These and other studies seem to indicate that metabolic rates are heterogeneous—not only that some proteins are metabolized faster and others more slowly, but also that the metabolism of each protein may depend on its localization (neuronal or glial, outer or inner membrane surface, particulate or soluble, etc). Separation of brain proteins into various fractions based on solubility, molecular weight, cell type, particulate, etc., did show fairly similar average metabolic rates in each fraction (Shahbazian et al., 1986a,b,c) each possibly containing rapidly and slowly metabolized proteins. This metabolic heterogeneity—differences between proteins and differences in individual proteins depending on location and developmental stage—indicates that influences on metabolism have heterogeneity of effect; that is, a condition may alter the metabolism of only a few proteins, and the affected proteins may not be altered throughout the brain.

Studies of proteinase activity also indicate heterogeneity in protein catabolism in the brain. Some enzymes show high substrate specificity, e.g., some Ca-activated neutral proteases show high activity with vimentin or desmin but no activity with actin or tubulin (Nelson and Traub, 1982), and the 145,000-dalton subunits of neurofilaments are selectively converted only to the 143,000- and 140,000-dalton subunits (Nixon et al., 1983). Proteolysis may selectively activate an enzyme, such as calmodulin-dependent protein phosphatase (Tallant and Cheung, 1984), and may represent an important step in calcium-dependent neurotransmitter excoytosis (Baxter et al., 1983).

We examined the breakdown of several purified brain proteins by purified brain proteases. We found that some properties of the enzyme depend on the substrate: the pH optimum of brain cathepsin D is 3.2 with myelin basic protein as substrate; 4.0 with actin, calmodulin, S-100, and GFA; and over 5.0 with tubulin (Bracco et al., 1982a; Banay-Schwartz et al., 1985). The pH dependence curve is also somewhat variable, with S-100 breakdown relatively higher at an acidic pH range. The pattern of breakdown products formed depends on pH. The relative activities of cathepsin D preparations from various sources (rat brain, bovine brain, spleen) depends on the substrate. With cathepsin D, the breakdown of cytoplasmic tubulin is heterogeneous, with a faster and a slower component (Bracco et al., 1982a); membrane-bound tubulin in brain is resistant to cerebral cathepsin D, but susceptible to other proteases such as thrombin (Bracco et al., 1982b). We separated the individual neurofilament proteins (Hui et al., 1986) and measured their breakdown by cathepsin D. A difference in the rate of breakdown and in fragments produced was found, with a pH dependence of the breakdown pattern (Banay-Schwartz et al., 1987). The breakdown of lower molecular weight proteins was higher than that of the larger proteins. We found peptide hydrolase activity associated with opiate receptors (Hui et al., 1985) and we found that proteases such as cathepsin D are capable of neuropeptide breakdown (Azaryan et al., 1985).

Protein breakdown shows similar heterogeneity in other tissues and is also altered in a heterogeneous fashion. Illustrations of specific effects on substrates are the possibly receptor-linked protease initiation of phosphatidylinositol catabolism (Hirasawa et al., 1982), the activation of only one of three lysosomal "converting" proteases by starvation (Melloni et al., 1981), and the inhibition by colchicine of mainly particulate rather than cytosolic protein degradation (Crie et al., 1983). Of importance but as yet little-known is the role of neutral proteases in brain (Malik et al., 1983; Banik et al., 1983). These enzymes are likely to show heterogeneous action and response to factors similar to that found for cathepsins.

EFFECTS OF MALNUTRITION

The effects of protein deprivation and starvation on tissue protein synthesis have been investigated in some detail (Garlick et al., 1975). Like developmental changes, malnutrition can alter synthesis and/or breakdown (Conde and Scornik, 1977), and the change can be an increase or decrease. In brain, malnutrition results in regional inhibition of growth (Fish and Winick, 1969) and a decrease in cell number (Zamenhof et al., 1971), cell formation (Patel et al., 1973), nucleic acid content (Griffin et al., 1977), and myelination (Krigman and Hogan, 1976). The free amino acid pool levels are also altered (Mourek et al., 1970), as is amino acid compartmentation (Patel et al., 1975) and amino acid utilization (Miller et al., 1977). The effects of proteins are heterogeneous, but this aspect has not been studied in detail. Some transmitter enzyme levels are decreased (Patel et al., 1978; Eckhert et al., 1976), and S-100 protein is selectively decreased in specific areas (Moore et al., 1977). We found that in adult brain, the changes are small even after drastic starvation. The changes in young brain are significant, and if malnutrition persists for a major portion of growth, changes are permanent. The significant difference between brain and other organs is that in brain, malnutrition inhibits protein breakdown as well, thus decreasing the loss of proteins (Banay-Schwartz et al., 1979).

The effects may be different in brain from those in muscle, and not all proteins are similarly affected. Starvation initially decreases, and in later stages increases, muscle proteolysis, affecting the cathepsin D (protein) level and the level of endogenous inhibitors (Goodman et al., 1981; Samarel et al., 1981). The effect is somewhat dependent on pre-existing nutritional status (adiposity) and age. We could find only inhibition of protein breakdown in developing brain during malnutrition (Banay-Schwartz et al., 1979). The relative stability of brain protein metabolism as compared to that of other tissues has often been observed (Goodman et al., 1984). Malnutrition during lactation affects synaptic protein content quantitatively and qualitatively (Smith and Druse, 1982). The changes in myelin protein metabolism during malnutrition are much more extensive than in other proteins (Wiggins et al., 1974). That protein changes are different in various tissues is also shown by the lack of changes in liver protein turnover during aging (Goldspink and Kelly, 1984) but the decrease of turnover in muscle (Lewis et al., 1984) and in brain (Fando et al., 1980; Lajtha and Dunlop, 1981).

CONCLUSIONS

Protein metabolism in the brain is active, and most proteins are metabolized with a replacement rate of many times per year. The metabolic rates are heterogeneous, with high and low rates, although the fractions with very fast or very slow metabolism constitute only a small percentage of the total. The heterogeneity of metabolism is also regional; a membrane-bound fraction of a protein may be metabolized differently from its cytoplasmic fraction, or its neuronal fraction may differ from its glial fraction.

Although protein metabolism seems to be more stable in brain than in other organs, metabolism in brain also undergoes changes and is influenced by a number of factors. The major physiological changes occur during development, when the average rate of both synthesis and breakdown decreases, although some fractions show increases in their metabolic rates. The developmental changes thus are also heterogeneous, not affecting all proteins in all structures to the same degree.

Many factors affect cerebral protein turnover. Since synthesis and breakdown are separately controlled mechanisms, influences on these two processes are also different and can affect protein components such as myelin proteins, neurotransmitter enzymes, or structural components in a specific manner, thereby changing the protein composition of the organ. Body temperature is a mjaor determinant of metabolism, but several other influences have been observed, e.g., endocrine effects and effects of drugs such as alcohol and nicotine.

Adult brain proteins are fairly resistant to the effects of malnutrition, but if severe deficiency occurs early in development and over a long time, the changes are significant and long-lasting. Part of the stability of brain results from the decreases in breakdown that accompany decreases in rates of synthesis.

In its reactions to external influences, brain differs in degree and specificity from other organs. Effects such as those altering energy metabolism or membrane lipids will subsequently translate to effects on brain protein.

Factors affecting protein metabolism, metabolic rates and controls, steps involved in protein synthesis, properties of enzymes involved in breakdown, and the specificity of alterations have been studied at some detail. Studies on the functional significance of the observed changes have yet to be done.

REFERENCES

Austin L, Lowry OH, Brown JG, Carter JG (1972): The turnover of protein in discrete areas of rat brain. Biochem J 126:351–359.

Azaryan A, Barkhudaryan N, Galoyan A, Lajtha A (1985): Action of brain cathepsin B, cathepsin D, and high-molecular-weight aspartic proteinase on angiotensins I and II. Neurochem Res 10:1525–1532.

Ballard FJ, Francis GL (1983): Effects of anabolic agents on protein breakdown in L6 myoblasts. Biochem J 210:243–249.

Banay-Schwartz M, Bracco F, Dahl D, DeGuzman T, Turk V, Lajtha A (1985): The pH dependence of breakdown of various purified brain proteins by cathepsin D preparations. Neurochem Int 7:607–614.

Banay-Schwartz M, Bracco F, DeGuzman T, Lajtha A (1983): Developmental changes in the breakdown of tubulin by cerebral cathepsin D. Neurochem Res 8:51–61.

Banay-Schwartz M, Dahl D, Hui K-S, Lajtha A (1987): The breakdown of the individual neurofilament proteins by cathepsin D. Neurochem Res 12:361–367.

Banay-Schwartz M, Giuffrida AM, DeGuzman T, Sershen H, Lajtha A (1979): Effect of undernutrition on cerebral protein metabolism. Exp Neurol 65:157–168.

Banik NL, Hogan EL, Jenkins MG, McDonald JK, McAlhaney WW, Sostek MB (1983): Purification of a calcium-activated neutral proteinase from bovine brain. Neurochem Res 8:1389–1405.

Banik NL, Hogan EL, Powers JM, Whetstine LJ (1982): Degradation of cytoskeletal proteins in experimental spinal cord injury. Neurochem Res 7:1465–1475.

Baracos VE, Wilson EJ, Goldberg AL (1984): Effects of temperature on protein turnover in isolated rat skeletal muscle. Am J Physiol 246:C125–C130.

Baxter DA, Johnston D, Strittmatter WJ (1983): Protease inhibitors implicate metalloendoprotease in synaptic transmission at the mammalian neuromusclar junction. Proc Natl Acad Sci USA 80:4174–4178.

Benjamins J, Morell P (1978): Proteins of myelin and their metabolism. Neurochem Res 3:137–174.

Benuck M, Iqbal K, Wisniewski HM, Lajtha A (1985): Proteolytic activity in brains of rabbits treated with aluminum. Neurochem Res 10:729–736.

Bracco F, Banay-Schwartz M, DeGuzman T, Lajtha A (1982a): Brain tubulin breakdown by cerebral cathepsin D. Neurochem Int 4:541–549.

Bracco F, Banay-Schwartz M, De Guzman T, Lajtha A (1982b): Membrane-bound tubulin: Resistance to cathepsin D and susceptibility to thrombin. Neurochem Int 4:501–511.

Brooks BA, Goll DE, Peng Y-S, Greweling JA, Hennecke G (1983): Effects of alloxan diabetes on Ca$^+$-activated proteinase in rat skeletal muscle. Am J Physiol 244:C175–C181.

Brosnan CF, Cammer W, Norton WT, Bloom BR (1980): Proteinase inhibitors suppress the development of experimental allergic encephalomyelitis. Nature 285:235–237.

Brown IR, Cosgrove JW (1983): Analysis of protein synthesis in the brain using cell-free techniques. In Lajtha A (ed): "Handbook of Neurochemistry." New York: Plenum Press, pp 1–24.

Bur JA, Conde RD (1982): Decreased rate of protein breakdown during nutritional recovery of mouse kidney. Am J Physiol 243:E360–E364.

Cammer W, Bloom BR, Norton WT, Gordon S (1978): Degradation of basic protein in myelin by neutral proteases secreted by stimulated macrophages. A possible mechanism of inflammatory demyelination. Proc Natl Acad Sci USA 75:1554–1558.

Conde RD, Scornik OA (1976): Role of protein degradation in the growth of livers after a nutritional shift. Biochem J 158:385–390.

Conde RD, Scornik OA (1977): Faster synthesis and slower degradation of liver protein during developmental growth. Biochem J 166:115–121.

Crie JS, Ord JM, Wakeland JR, Wildenthal K (1983): Inhibition of cardiac proteolysis by colchicine. Biochem J 210:63–71.

Dunlop DS, Bodony R, Lajtha A (1984a): RNA concentration and protein synthesis in rat brain during development. Brain Res 294:148–151.

Dunlop DS, Kaufman H, Zanchin G, Lajtha A (1984b): Protein synthesis rates in rats with portacaval shunts. J Neurochem 43:1487–1489.

Dunlop DS, Lajtha A, Toth J (1977a): Measuring brain protein metabolism in young and adult rats. In Roberts S, Lajtha A, Gispen WH I (eds): "Mechanisms, Regulation and Special Functions of Protein Synthesis in the Brain." Amsterdam: Elsevier, pp 79–96.

Dunlop DS, McHale DM, Lajtha A (1982): The rate of protein degradation in developing brain. Biochem J 208:659–666.

Dunlop DS, McHale D, Lajtha A (1984c): Effect of cerebral puncture on brain protein synthesis in adult and young rodents. J Neurochem 42:897–899.

Dunlop DS, van Elden W, Lajtha A (1977b): Developmental effects on protein synthesis rates in regions of the CNS in vivo and in vitro. J Neurochem 29:939–945.

Dunlop DS, van Elden W, Lajtha A (1978): Protein degradation rates in regions of the central nervous system in vivo during development. Biochem J 170:637–642.

Dunlop DS, van Elden W, Plucinska I, Lajtha A (1981): Brain slice protein degradation and development. J Neurochem 36:258–265.

Dunn A (1975): Intracerebral injections inhibit amino acid incorporation into brain protein. Brain Res 99:405–409.

Eckhert C, Barnes RH, Levitsky DA (1976): The effect of protein-energy undernutrition induced during the period of suckling on cholinergic enzyme activity in the rat brain stem. Brain Res 101:372–377.

Frando JL, Salinas M, Wasterlain CG (1980): Age-dependent changes in brain protein synthesis in the rat. Neurochem Res 5:373–383.

Fern EB, Garlick PJ (1974): The specific radioactivity of the tissue free amino acid as a basis for measuring the rate of protein synthesis in the rat in vivo. Biochem J 142:413–419.

Fish I, Winick M (1969): Effect of malnutrition on regional growth of the developing rat brain. Exp Neurol 25:534–540.

Garlick PJ, Millward DJ, James WPT, Waterlow JC (1975): The effect of protein deprivation and starvation on the rate of protein synthesis in tissues of the rat. Biochim Biophys Acta 414:71–84.

Goldspink DF, Kelly FJ (1984): Protein turnover and growth in the whole body, liver, and kidney of the rat from the foetus to senility. Biochem J 217:507–516.

Goldspink DF, Garlick PJ, McNurlan MA (1983): Protein turnover measured in vivo in muscles undergoing compensatory growth and subsequent denervation. Biochem J 210:89–98.

Goodman MN, Lowell B, Belur E, Ruderman NB (1984): Sites of protein conservation and loss during starvation: Influence of adiposity. Am J Physiol 246:E383–E390.

Goodman MN, McElaney MA, Ruderman NB (1981): Adaptation to prolonged starvation in the rat: Curtailment of skeletal muscle proteolysis. Am J Physiol 241:E321–E327.

Griffin WST, Woodward DJ, Chandra R (1977): Malnutrition and brain development: Cerebral weight DNA, RNA, protein and histological correlations. J Neurochem 28:1269–1279.

Hirasawa K, Irving RF, Dawson RMC (1982): Proteolytic activation can produce a phosphatidylinositol phosphodiesterase highly sensitive to Ca^{2+}. Biochem J 206:675–678.

Hirsch HE, Blanco CE, Parks ME (1981): Fibrinolytic activity of plaques and white matter in multiple sclerosis. J Neuropathol Exp Neurol 40:271–280.

Hui K-S, Gioannini T, Hui M, Simon EJ, Lajtha A (1985): An opiate receptor-associated aminopeptidase that degrades enkephalins. Neurochem Res 10:1047–1058.

Hui K-S, Hui M, Chiu F-C, Banay-Schwartz M, DeGuzman T, Sacchi RS, Lajtha A (1986): Separation and purification of individual neurofilament proteins by reverse-phase high-performance liquid chromatography. Anal Biochem 153:230–234.

Krigman MR, Hogan EL (1976): Undernutrition in the developing rat: Effect upon myelination. Brain Res 107:239–255.

Lajtha A, Dunlop DS (1981): Turnover of protein in the nervous system. Life Sci 29:755–767.

Lajtha A, Dunlop DS, Patlak C, Toth J (1979): Compartments of protein metabolism in the developing brain. Biochim Biophys Acta 561:491–501.

Lajtha A, Latzkovits L, Toth J (1976): Comparison of turnover rates of proteins of the brain, liver and kidney in mouse in vivo following long-term labeling. Biochim Biophys Acta 425:511–520.

Lajtha A, Sershen H (1975): Changes in the rates of protein synthesis in the brain of goldfish at various temperatures. Life Sci 17:1861–1868.

Lajtha A, Toth J (1966): Instability of cerebral proteins. Biochem Biophys Res Commun 23:294–298.

Lajtha A, Toth J, Fujimoto K, Agrawal HC (1977): Turnover of myelin proteins in mouse brain in vivo. Biochem J 164:323–329.

Lewis SEM, Kelly FJ, Goldspink DF (1984): Pre- and post-natal growth and protein turnover in smooth muscle, heart and slow- and fast-twitch skeletal muscles of the rat. Biochem J 217:517–526.

Li JB (1980): Protein synthesis and degradation in skeletal muscle of normal and dystrophic hamsters. Am J Physiol 239:E401–E406.

Li JB, Wassner SJ (1984): Effects of food deprivation and refeeding on total protein and actomyosin degradation. Am J Physiol 246:E32–E37.

Malik MN, Fenko MD, Iqbal K, Wisniewski HM (1983): Purification and characterization of two forms of Ca^{2+}-activated neutral protease from calf brain. J Biol Chem 258:8955–8962.

McGrath JA, Goldspink DF (1982): Glucocorticoid action on protein synthesis and protein breakdown in isolated skeletal muscles. Biochem J 206:641–645.

Melloni E, Pontremoli S, Salamino F, Sparatore B, Michetti M, Horecker BL (1981): Changes during fasting in the activity of a specific lysosomal proteinase, fructose-1,6-bisphosphatase convering enzyme. Proc Natl Acad Sci USA 78:1499–1502.

Miller M, Leahy JP, McConville F, Morgane PJ, Resnick O (1977): Phenylalanine utilization in brain and peripheral tissues during development in normal and protein malnourished rats. Brain Res Bull 2:189–195.

Moore BW, Menke R, Prensky AL, Fishman MA, Agrawal HC (1977): Selective decreases of S-100 in discrete anatomical areas of undernourished rat brain. Neurochem Res 2:549–553.

Mourek J, Agrawal HC, Davis JM, Himwich WA (1970): The effects of short-term starvation on amino acid content in rat brain during ontogeny. Brain Res 19:229–237.

Nelson WJ, Traub P (1982): Purification and further characterization of the Ca^{2+}-activated proteinase specific for the intermediate filament proteins vimentin and desmin. J Biol Chem 257:5544–5553.

Nixon RA, Brown BA, Marotta CA (1983): Limited proteolytic modification of a neurofilament protein involves a proteinase activated by endogenous levels of calcium. Brain Res 275:384–388.

Nunez J (1985): Thyroid hormones. In Lajtha A (ed): "Handbook of Neurochemistry." vol. 8, 2nd ed. New York: Plenum Press, pp 1–28.

Odedra BR, Bates PC, Millward DJ (1983): Time course of the effect of catabolic doses of corticosterone on protein turnover in rat skeletal muscle and liver. Biochem J 214:617–627.

Odedra B, Millward DJ (1982): Effect of corticosterone treatment on muscle protein turnover in adrenalectomized rats and diabetic rats maintained on insulin. Biochem J 204:663–672.

Oja SS (1967): Studies on protein metabolism in developing rat brain. Ann Acad Sci Fenn (Med) 131:7–81.

Okada AA, Dice JF (1984): Altered degradation of intracellular proteins in aging human fibroblasts. Mech Ageing Dev 26:341–356.

Patel AJ, Atkinson DJ, Balazs R (1975): Effect of undernutrition on metabolic compartmentation of glutamate and on the incorporation of [^{14}C]leucine into protein in the developing rat brain. Dev Psychobiol 8:453–464.

Patel AJ, Balazs R, Johnson AL (1973): Effect of undernutrition on cell formation in the rat brain. J Neurochem 20:1151–1165.

Patel AJ, Del Vecchio M, Atkinson DJ (1978): Effect of undernutrition on the regional development of transmitter enzymes: Glutamate decarboxylase and choline acetyltransferase. Dev Neurosci 1:41–53.

Reith MEA, Schotman P, Gispen WH (1977): Pituitary peptides and brain protein synthesis. In Roberts S, Lajtha A, Gispen WH (eds): "Mechanisms, Regulation and Special Functions of Protein Synthesis in the Brain." Amsterdam: Elsevier, pp 383–398.

Samarel AM, Ogunro EA, Ferguson AG, Allenby P, Lesch M (1981): Rabbit cardiac immunoreactive cathepsin D content during starvation-induced atrophy. Am J Physiol 240:H222–H228.

Sershen H, Lajtha A (1979): The effect of nicotine on the metabolism of brain proteins. Neuropharmacology 18:763–766.

Seta K, Sansur M, Lajtha A (1973): The rate of incorporation of amino acids into brain proteins during infusion in the rat. Biochim Biophys Acta 294:472–480.

Shahbazian FM, Jacobs M, Lajtha A (1986a): Amino acid incorporation in relation to molecular weight of proteins in young and adult brain. Neurochem Res 11:647–660.

Shahbazian FM, Jacobs M, Lajtha A (1986b): Rates of amino acid incorporation into particulate proteins in vivo and in slices of young and adult brain. J Neurosci Res 15:359–366.

Shahbazian FM, Jacobs M, Lajtha A (1986c): Regional and cellular differences in rat brain protein synthesis in vivo and in slices during development. Int J Dev Neurosci 4:209–215.

Shapira R, Wilhelmi MR, Kibler RF (1981): Turnover of myelin proteins of rat brain, determined in fractions separated by sedimentation in a continuous sucrose gradient. J Neurochem 36:1427–1432.

Smith DM, Druse MJ (1982): Effects of maternal protein deficiency on synaptic plasma membranes in offspring. Dev Neurosci 5:403–411.

Smith ME, Chow SH, Rolph RH (1981): Partial purification and characterization of neutral proteases in lymph nodes of rats with experimental allergic encephalomyelitis. Neurochem Res 6:901–912.

Smith ME, Amaducci LA (1982): Observations on the effects of protease inhibitors on the suppression of experimental allergic encephalomyelitis. Neurochem Res 7:541–548.

Sugden PH, Smith DM (1982): The effect of glucose, acetate, lactate, and insulin on protein degradation in the perfused rat heart. Biochem J 206:467–472.

Tallant EA, Cheung WY (1984): Activation of bovine brain calmodulin-dependent protein phosphatase by limited trypsinization. Biochemistry 23:973–979.

Tewari S, Sytinsky S (1985): Alcohol. In Lajtha A (ed): "Handbook of Neurochemistry." New York: Plenum Press, pp 219–261.

Toth E, Lajtha A (1981): Alcohol effects on cerebral protein turnover in mice. Subst Alcohol Actions/Misuse 2:321–329.

Toth E, Lajtha A (1984a): Brain protein synthesis rates are not sensitive to elevated GABA taurine, or glycine. Neurochem Res 9:173–179.

Toth E, Lajtha A (1984b): Effect of chronic ethanol administration on brain protein breakdown in mice in vivo. Subst Alcohol Actions/Misue 5:175–183.

Wiggins RC, Benjamins JA, Krigman MR, Morell P (1974): Synthesis of myelin proteins during starvation. Brain Res 80:345–349.

Zamenhof S, van Marthens E, Grauel L (1971): DNA (cell number) and protein in neonatal rat brain: Alteration by timing of maternal dietary protein restrictions. J Ntr 101:1265–1270.

Current Topics in Nutrition and Disease, Volume 16
Basic and Clinical Aspects of Nutrition and Brain Development,
pages 57–73
© 1987 Alan R. Liss, Inc.

Animal Models of Malnutrition Applied to Brain Research

Janina R. Galler and Karla B. Kanis

Center for Behavioral Development and Mental Retardation, Boston
University School of Medicine, Boston, Massachusetts 02118

INTRODUCTION

Animal models have a rich and productive history in the biomedical sciences. They have been used to elucidate the etiology, consequences, and treatment of human disease states and to characterize the processes of normal development. However, experimental models are at best compromised symbols of the human condition that attempt to represent a complex and often less readily available system. Thus, ''animal comes to represent the patient, the tissue slice the intact living brain and the isolated nerve ending the intact synapse'' (Baldessarini and Fischer, 1975). The intent of this chapter is to provide a comprehensive overview of the advantages and limitation of animal models of human malnutrition. The rat has been used most often for this purpose and less frequently other species including mice and primates.

The uses of animal models for studying the effects of malnutrition on brain and mental function have been published previously (Smart, 1984; Crnic, 1976; Levine and Weiner, 1975; Turkewitz and Fleisher, 1984; Beynen and West, 1986). One major advantage of using animal models to study malnutrition has been the ability to conduct experiments which could not ethically be undertaken in human populations. Studies of the consequences of malnutrition in human populations have required investigators to take advantage of natural disasters, such as famines (Stein et al., 1975). With the exception of planned intervention programs, human populations exposed to malnutrition are not subject to experimental study, making it difficult if not impossible to conclude whether adverse outcomes are the result of malnutrition or the result of associated factors such as poverty and infection (Richardson, 1980; Galler, 1987). An advantage of animal models is, therefore, the ability to control for many extranutritional factors which affect human populations at risk for developing malnutrition. A related advantage of animal models is the ability to undertake studies of brain function both in vivo and in vitro. In humans, this has been possible predominantly by indirect measures, including head circumference or electrophysiologic function (Barnet et al., 1978; Stoch et al., 1982; Bartel et al., 1979) and, in limited circumstances, by the direct measurement of brain weight and components of organs derived from postmortem examination of the most severe cases (Rosso et al., 1970). Finally, the shorter life span of animals and lower cost compared to human studies have made experimental research attractive to the investigator.

The rationale for making use of animal models is relatively well founded when biological functions in homologous structures are being studied, although the timing of events differs across species (Dobbing, 1971). Thus, despite certain differences between species, underlying brain mechanisms may be expected to be similar across species. However, this is not necessarily the case for higher mental functions which are not so easily extrapolated from rat to man. Despite apparent similarities in certain behaviors of animals and humans, such analogous behaviors in the different species are most likely associated with different underlying mechanisms (Maier and Schnierla, 1933). For example, learning in rats may not be directly comparable to learning in humans even though it is by far the most frequently studied outcome in animal studies of malnutrition (Crnic, 1976; Levitsky, 1979). It has, therefore, been suggested that behaviors to be studied in the animal model should closely parallel those in the human condition and follow a similar developmental course, such as in the case of mother-infant interaction (Denenberg and Thoman, 1976). This approach increases the accuracy of extrapolating findings from the animal model and was used by these investigators to develop an appropriate animal model of the high-risk infant. Clearly, a related disadvantage of animal models is the inability to study certain effects of malnutrition which are known to have a major impact on the development of human children, such as delays in language development (Cravioto and DeLicardie, 1972). Certain behaviors, including social behaviors, which have been described as being impaired in response to malnutrition, cannot be easily studied in rodents and have been most suitably studied using primates (Chappel et al., in press).

Another disadvantage of animal models concerns the possiblity that animal models may be "too pure" (Smart, 1984) because of excessive control of laboratory conditions. For example, infection is a common phenomenon among chronically malnourished children and the two conditions have a synergistic effect on growth (Scrimshaw et al., 1959). Although infection has not generally been described in animals exposed to brief periods of malnutrition, we have reported an increased incidence of infectious dermatitis in rats suffering from chronic malnutrition over many generations (Galler et al., 1979). Alternatively, the animal model has been criticized for not being pure enough (Plaut, 1970; Crnic, 1976) because of the inability to eliminate impaired social and environmental conditions in the early rearing environment of the malnourished rat pup. These factors, including impaired mother-pup interactions which are known to accompany most forms of malnutrition early in life, may have effects on brain and behavioral development independent of the effects of malnutrition. The latter point will be discussed in detail in the section on extranutritional variables.

In summary, the use of animal models to elucidate the effects of malnutrition on brain and mental function has provided valuable insights into the mechanisms and consequences of undernutrition and associated and interacting factors. Interpretation of the results of animal experimentation requires that the investigator carefully characterize the processes being studied in the human. Ideally, multiple models using different means of inducing malnutrition should be utilized in order to provide a more comprehensive view of consistencies and discrepancies between the various methodologies (Fleisher and Turkewitz, 1984). This will allow the investigator to determine which effects are attributable to malnutrition and which are derived from other influences associated with the specific treatment used to induce malnutrition. Multiple tests should be administered at different stages of development to confirm the possiblity of developmental lags (Castro and Rudy, in press). In addition to the type of malnutrition, the investigator must pay particular attention to the timing of the insult relative to the critical period of brain growth spurt, its severity, and duration (Dobbing, 1971). In this way, findings observed in subhuman species can be extrapolated to the human by carefully matching for nutritional status and comparable periods of brain growth.

METHODS USED TO INDUCE MALNUTRITION IN ANIMALS

A variety of methods have been applied to induce malnutrition in the fetal or suckling animal. The methods used most frequently have included 1) feeding the mother a diet low in protein or 2) adequate in composition but reduced in quantity, 3) reducing the number of nipples available for the suckling pups, 4) increasing the litter size, 5) rotating the pups between lactating and non-lactating dams or between lactating dams and an incubator, and 6) artificially feeding the pups in a controlled environment. The effects of each of these procedures is dependent on the timing of the nutritional deficit. Thus, the most severe effects are known to occur when malnutrition is present during the critical period of rapid brain growth and development. In the rat, this corresponds to gestation and the first 3 postnatal weeks. In addition, the duration and degree of nutritional deficiency also determine the nature of the insult to the developing offspring (Dobbing, 1971). It is important to note that weight deficits per se may not correspond directly to effects on brain function, which may occur even without significant weight reduction in response to malnutrition. This dissociation has been described using several techniques.

One of the most common methods of inducing malnutrition during the prenatal period is feeding the pregnant female a low-protein diet (Kanis et al., 1987, Massaro et al., 1977, Miller and Resnick, 1980, Zamenhof et al., 1973). During pregnancy and periods of rapid growth and development, rats require in excess of 12% protein, so that a diet containing between 6 and 8% protein will significantly retard normal rates of growth. Protein levels lower than 6% result in increased numbers of resorptions and stillbirths, whereas protein levels of 10% showed no lasting effects on the offspring (Altman et al., 1970; Nowak and Munro, 1977). A 6% casein diet provided during gestation produced pups significantly lighter at birth than adquately nourished control pups. Thus, the malnourished pups resembled "small-for-gestational age" infants seen in the human condition (Resnick and Morgane, 1983). Dietary protein levels during gestation of 7% (Massaro et al., 1977) or 7.5% (Galler, 1979) also resulted in birth weights that were significantly lower than controls.

There is some controversy about the effects of an 8% protein diet during gestation. Zamenhof and Guthrie (1977) found that when mothers were fed an 8% protein diet 1 month prior to mating and throughout gestation, 70% of the newborn rat pups weighed less than 2 standard deviations below the mean weight control pups; a weight deficit of 1.5 g (25%) was reported. In contrast, other investigators (Resnick et al., 1982; Resnick and Morgane, 1983; Kanis et al., 1987) fed the 8% diet to females 5 weeks prior to mating and during gestation but did not find any significant reduction in birth weight as compared with matched control pups. Nevertheless, deficits in neurochemical parameters, including elevated neurotransmitter levels, characterized the malnourished pups despite the normal birth weights (Resnick and Morgane, 1983). These deficits were present at birth and persisted into adulthood although an adequate diet was supplied from birth onward. This confirms the permanent response of the brain to malnutrition during the prenatal period despite normal birth weight.

Postnatal malnutrition can be induced in pups by providing dams with a 6–8% protein diet during the suckling period (Frankova, 1973; Crnic, 1980; Vendite et al., 1985). A low protein diet at this time resulted in less milk output and in changes in the composition of maternal milk, including a reduction in protein available to the pups (Mueller and Cox, 1946; Crnic and Chase, 1978; Sturman et al., 1986). Weight deficits of pups in response to a low protein diet appeared by postnatal day 5 and persisted throughout the lactation period. At weaning, between days 21 and 28, pups reared by low protein females showed a range of weight deficits from 25 to 45% (Crnic,

1980; Frankova, 1973; Massaro et al., 1974; Vendite et al., 1985). Some studies have examined the effects of a low protein diet during both gestation and lactation (Resnick and Morgane, 1984b; Finger et al., 1986; Goodlett et al., 1986; Wiener et al., 1983). Animals born to and reared by mothers on a 6% casein diet had up to an 80% weight deficit, while animals born to and reared by 8% dams showed a 50% deficit at weaning. Sykes and Cheyne (1976) reported that the combined impact of malnutrition during both prenatal and postnatal periods was much greater than nutritional deficiency restricted to either period alone. However, using an 8% casein diet, Miller and Resnick (1980) found that weight deficits at weaning were attributable primarily to lactational malnutrition. Thus, impaired growth rates after birth appear to be predominantly associated with postnatal nutrition or the combination of prenatal and postnatal malnutrition, whereas deficits in brain composition and function may occur in response to prenatal malnutrition even in the absence of impaired physical growth (Resnick et al., 1982, Miller and Resnick, 1980).

A model believed to more closely simulate the human condition of malnutrition is the restriction of dietary intake of lactating females (Smart and Dobbing, 1971; Smart et al., 1973; Hseuh et al., 1973, 1974; Chow, 1974; Whatson and Smart, 1978; Crnic, 1980; Menendez-Patterson et al., 1982; Rathbun and Druse, 1985; Rogers et al., 1986). The total food intake of these females is usually restricted to half the ad libitum intake of control females, thereby depriving the dam of both protein and calories. The restricted diet has been induced at the time of conception (Hseuh et al., 1974) or at the end of the first week of gestation (Smart and Dobbing, 1971; Smart et al., 1973) and maintained throughout pregnancy. Neither study found significant differences in the number of live pups born, dead pups, and resorptions between females provided with the 50% restricted diet and those on the control diet. However, birth weights showed significant deficits of 12 to 19% (Smart et al., 1973; Menendez-Patterson et al., 1982).

The restricted diet provided to the lactating female during the postnatal period reduces the amount of milk available to the suckling pups, but does not alter the composition of the diet ingested by the pups (Crnic and Chase, 1978). Postnatal restriction to 50% of normal dietary intake resulted in weight deficits of 25 to 45% at weaning, closely approximating weight deficits reported in response to low protein diets (Hseuh et al., 1973; Rathbun and Druse, 1985; Rogers et al., 1986; Smart and Dobbing, 1971; Smart et al., 1973; Whatson and Smart, 1978). Smart et al. (1973) reported an additive effect of gestational and postnatal dietary restriction on physical growth, learning, and forebrain size, although cerebellum was effected only by the postnatal treatment.

The effects of malnutrition have also been studied for more than one generation, since malnutrition in human populations is most often a chronic, intergenerational process. The intergenerational malnutrition using low protein or restricted diets resulted in weight deficits at birth and throughout the suckling period (Cowley and Griesel, 1963; Stewart, 1973; Zamenhof and van Marthens, 1978; Galler, 1979; Resnick and Morgane, 1984a). Since birth weights and body size remained similarly reduced after one or more generations, there was no cumulative effect of malnutrition on growth, present over several generations, although there was evidence that behavioral and neurochemical deficits may have increased from one generation to the next. Refeeding with a control diet produced normal birth weights in the successive generation of offspring regardless of the number of generations of malnutrition (Stewart et al., 1980; Galler and Seelig, 1981). However, offspring in the subsequent generations (F2, F3) showed continued impairment in brain and behavioral function even after dietary rehabilitation.

Other methods have been developed to induce malnutrition in the offspring without malnourishing the mother. Rearing pups in abnormally large litters reduces the amount of milk available to each pup in the litter. Neonatal mortality has been reported as being increased in large litters of 16 pups compared with small litters of 8 pups (Fleischer and Turkewitz, 1979b). Weights of pups from large litters were significantly lower than those from control litters by the end of the first postnatal week (Kennedy, 1957; Widdowson and McCance, 1960; Wurtman and Miller, 1976). Weaning weights of pups from large litters of 16 to 22 pups were approximately 60% of values reported for pups from small litters of 4 to 8 pups (Widdowson and McCance, 1960; Wurtman and Miller, 1976; Fleischer and Turkewitz, 1979b; Crnic, 1980; Galler et al., 1980). Wurtman and Miller (1976) found no weight differences between subjects reared in groups of 2, 4, 8, or 12 pups per litter, whereas pups reared in litters of 16 weighed significantly less than pups from the smaller litters. There was also significantly higher variability in daily weights of pups from large litters since treatment effects were not uniform across all pups in the litter (Galler and Turkewitz, 1975). This has important implications for brain research since the selection of excessively light or heavy subjects may bias findings.

Partial mammectomy of the lactating female also reduces the ratio of teats to pups, as in the case of large litter rearing (Codo and Carlini, 1979; Crnic, 1980; Galler and Turkewitz, 1977). Since litter size is restricted to six to eight pups, the effects of crowding are not present. When three alternate pairs of mammae (Galler and Turkewitz, 1977) or the six posterior nipples (Codo and Carlini, 1979) were removed, pup weights during the lactational period were reduced by 10 to 20% relative to controls. When more mammae were removed, the mortality rate of the pups was significantly increased in one study without additional weight loss in the surviving litter members

(Galler and Turkewitz, 1977). Therefore, this technique can be used only to produce relatively mild degrees of undernutrition.

Another technique to produce early malnutrition is the rotation of pups between lactating and non-lactating females, known as "aunts" (Slob et al., 1973; Lynch, 1976; Fleischer and Turkewitz, 1979a; Crnic, 1980; Galler et al., 1980; Castro et al., in press) or between lactating mothers and an incubator (Crnic, 1980), thereby limiting the amount of time each day that pups spend with a lactating female. This technique, particularly the reassignment to non-lactating aunts, has the advantage of restricting pup intake while continuing to provide maternal attention and stimulation to the offspring. At weaning, animals rotated to lactating females for 8 or 12 hours daily showed a 40–50% reduction in weight compared with pups who suckled with lactating females for 24 hours daily (Castro et al., in press; Crnic, 1980; Fleischer and Turkewitz, 1979a; Galler et al., 1980; Slob et al., 1973).

Miller and Dymsza (1963) fed pups artificially while keeping them with a non-lactating foster mother. This technique allowed the pups to receive the requisite maternal care while the composition and quantity of the diet was varied. From postnatal day 2 to day 7, pups fed rat's milk by this method grew as well as the pups fed by lactating dams. In more recent studies using artificial feeding methods, pups were removed from the mother and raised in a temperature-controlled housing arrangement with an intragastric cannula to supply the nutrition (Hall, 1975; Smart et al., 1983, 1984). Hall (1975) developed an artificial rearing technique in order to measure feeding behavior in pups without prior suckling experience. Feeding behavior was not impaired, although at day 18, artificially reared pups weighed significantly less than did control pups nurtured by lactating females. Smart et al. (1983, 1984) provided artificially reared pups with an adequate amount of milk substitute to support normal body-weight gain or a restricted amount of the same diet in order to produce malnutrition while controlling for maternal care. The artificially reared pups given the restricted diet weighed significantly less than pups given an adequate diet or mother-reared control pups. By day 25, these animals weighed 41% of the weights of mother-reared or artificially reared pups raised on the adequate diet. However, the patterns of growth and metabolism differed between the mother-reared and adequate-diet pups, leading these investigators to conclude that the technique had limited usefulness as an animal model, probably because of the nutritional content of the milk substitute product.

In summary, a variety of techniques have been used to produce malnutrition in the developing rat. The most frequently used methods are low protein diets fed to the pregnant or lactating female or a reduction in the total food intake of the female. These methods can be applied to produce prenatal and postnatal malnutrition, but have the disadvantage of malnourishing the mother which may in turn alter her maternal behavior during suckling. A number of methods that do not directly affect the mother's nutritional status have been used to produce postnatal malnutrition. These methods include rearing to large litters, reducing the number of teats available to the suckling animals, rotating between lactating and non-lactating females, and artificially feeding. The effect of each of these techniques on the mother-pup interaction is discussed in the next section.

EXTRANUTRITIONAL VARIABLES

In human children, brain and behavioral deficits resulting from early malnutrition may be the direct outcome of nutritional deficiency or may occur as a result of other factors such as changes in mothering which occur in association with the episode of malnutrition (Galler et al., 1984). We will describe normal patterns of maternal behavior in rats, emphasizing a developmental pattern parallel to the human condition and the changes in maternal behavior present under conditions of malnutrition during the suckling period. We conclude that the role of maternal care and malnutrition cannot be separated even in rat models, and we suggest an intrinsic compensatory response by the mother to correct for the effects of nutritional deficits in her offspring. This conclusion underlines the importance of documenting conditions in the early rearing environment when undertaking animal studies of malnutrition. Thus, changes in maternal behavior may have effects on long-term outcome which interact with or increase the direct effects of the episode of malnutrition.

Normal Patterns of Maternal Behavior

Patterns of mother-infant interaction (often referred to as maternal behavior in animal studies) have been recognized in a wide variety of animals in both field studies and experimental laboratories. In general, these studies have demonstrated that behavioral patterns in the lactating female serve the needs of the newborn young and are synchronized with the physical and behavioral development of the young. Most of the research on mother-infant interaction in animals has been conducted with rats and, to a lesser extent, with monkeys. Maternal behavior in the rat has been explored throughout the reproductive cycle, from conception through weaning of the young. In the rat, this period covers nearly 2 months; during the first 22 days (suckling period), she takes care of her young. Three phases of mother-infant interaction have been identified, which are affected by endocrine as well as environmental influences: the initiation of maternal behavior about 24 hours prior to birth, its maintenance during the following 2 to 3 weeks following parturition, and its decline as weaning approaches (Rosenblatt, 1969, 1975).

These phases of maternal behavior are synchronized with stages in the physical and behavioral development of the young and represent a dyadic mother-pup relationship. Each phase requires analysis in terms appropriate to the events of that phase, and the separate phases need to be related to one another in a development sequence.

The initiation phase of maternal behavior extends from 24 hours before birth to the 3rd day postpartum. This phase has been established as the "critical period" for the mother-infant relationship during which secure bonding is established. Interference between the suckling mother and her young at this time results in an immediate decline in maternal behavior and death of the offspring. Under normal conditions, extensive nursing, retrieving (carrying the young back to the nest when they have strayed), licking the pups to stimulate bowel function, and nest-building are present during this developmental phase. The onset of these maternal behaviors occurs immediately after birth and is regulated primarily by hormonal factors including the rise in estrogen in the mother. Male and virgin female rats will also develop "maternal" behaviors when exposed to pups, but only when placed in constant contact with the foster young for 5 or 6 days (Rosenblatt, 1967). Although maternal responses are dominant in this phase, maternal behavior is also influenced by characteristics of the pups. Thus, it has been reported that the newborn and the placenta possess attractive stimuli that evoke maternal behavior from the female (Denenberg and Whimbey, 1963). However, some features of the newborn (such as movement) inhibit the mother from eating her young after she has eaten the placenta. It has often been observed that newly parturient rodents under stress will consume their live pups possibly because of interference with the normal inhibitory response. In mice and rats, dead pups present in the home cage have been shown to diminish maternal responsiveness to the remaining live pups (Noirot, 1964). Other characteristics of the pup which may influence maternal behavior during the initiation phase are size and level of maturity. An example of this is the observation that newborn pups are capable of increasing maternal behaviors which are normally declining during the 3rd week postpartum (Nicoll and Meites, 1959; Wiesner and Sheard, 1933).

During the maintenance phase (from the 4th to about the 14th day postpartum), maternal behavior is largely dependent on the physical characteristics and behavior of the young for maintenance of her responses. The pup actively suckles and seeks out the mother during this phase. Tests of cage orientation conducted on pups during this period confirm an increasing ability to find their way back to the nest when displaced from it over days 5 to 12 of life (Turkewitz, 1966; Galler and Seelig, 1981).

The decline phase of maternal behavior begins around the 15th or 16th day postpartum and extends until the 21st to 28th days. During this period, the young undergo changes in feeding paterns corresponding to weaning at about day 16. This is a period of rapid growth for the pup, and they show improvement in locomotion, progressing from walking to running and climbing. These changes also coincide with the opening of the eyelids and the beginning of hearing. Social interactions between pups within a litter and between mother and the litter also become more varied, involving grooming and play activity. This increased independence on the part of the pups is associated with a diminished response by the mother. Thus, nest-building declines, followed by a reduction in pup retrieval several days later and, finally, by a reduction in nursing.

In summary, the development of postpartum maternal behavior in the rat follows a predictable sequence during the 3 to 4 weeks following birth. During initiation, maternal behaviors are predominantly dependent on maternal factors, especially hormone levels, which heighten the mother's sensitivity to her pups after birth. During the maintenance and decline phases, pup characteristics are the major contributors to ensuring the continuation of maternal behaviors. As the pups become more independent, the frequencies of maternal behaviors decline. All of these factors have an impact on the nutritional status of the young. Because of the greater plasticity of behavioral development in humans, patterns of maternal responsiveness cannot be predicted with the same degree of certainty as in animals. However, maternal behavior in the human is also influenced by the degree of development of the infant and by its nutritional status (Galler et al., 1984).

Changes in Maternal Behavior Accompanying Malnutrition

In early studies of the long-term effects of malnutrition during the gestation and suckling of rat pups, factors other than nutrition which were associated with the early rearing environment of the pup received little or no attention. It has since been recognized that all procedures applied to induce malnutrition also affect the relationship between the mother and her pups. Changes in the maternal behavior of lactating females are described in association with a variety of methods applied to induce malnutrition during the suckling period.

Low protein and restricted maternal diets malnourish the mother which per se may effect her responsiveness to her young. A number of investigators have directly examined maternal behavior under these conditions and have confirmed that maternal malnutrition during the suckling period is associated with changes in the mother-pup relationship, including increased nursing and physical contact. When maternal diet is low in protein during lactation, high levels of nursing and physical contact have been reported which persisted until the end of the suckling period at 21 days. When the diet was adequate in protein content, nursing declined after the first week postpartum (Massaro et al., 1974; Wiener et al., 1977; Hall et al., 1979; Crnic, 1980). Nursing time and physical contact between mothers and pups were also increased when a low protein diet was provided over many generations (Galler and Propert, 1981a). Similar results, including increased time spent in the nest by malnourished mothers, were reported in response to maternal calorie restriction (Smart and Preece, 1973). Thus, techniques which result in malnutrition of the lactating female result in similar changes in maternal behavior, characterized by an increased percentage of time actively nursing throughout the suckling period.

Large litter rearing was first reported as being associated with a decrease in maternal attentiveness to the pups (Grota and Ader, 1969). Thus, lactating females rearing large litters were reported as spending less time with their litters and as being less likely to retrieve their young and to build adequate nests. However, Crnic (1980) recently studied maternal behavior using large litters to produce malnutrition of the young, and she found increased nursing through day 20 of the litter period. She also found no differences in retrieval or in nest quality between large and small litters. The discrepancy between the two studies may be attributed to differences in testing conditions, including the use of an escape area in the first study, whereas the second study was restricted to observations in the maternal cage. In the case of large litter rearing, crowding and competition for a limited number of nipples, among other factors, also modified the early experience of the suckling rat pups.

Because of these documented changes in the mother-pup relationship, a number of newer techniques were developed to produce malnutrition in rat pups with the aim of eliminating alterations in maternal behavior. To date, none of these methods has achieved this objective. Galler and Turkewitz (1977) subjected female rats to partial mammectomy before pregnancy and compared their interaction with their pups to that of non-mammectomized and sham-operated controls. These investigators found that following mammectomy, nursing was increased through the end of the litter period in contrast to values obtained for both groups of controls. Since the lactating female was not malnourished, these findings demonstrated that the changes in maternal behavior were a response to malnutrition of the pups. Similar observations were reported by Crnic (1980) in her study comparing several techniques, including partial mammectomy. These data contrast with those of Codo and Carlini (1979) who found no differences in maternal behavior between mothers with four or six functional mammae who reared six pups per litter and control animals with the full set of mammae. However, these observations were limited to the first 12 postpartum days, although most studies have shown that differences in maternal behavior in response to malnutrition were present in the second half of the litter period.

A similar conclusion of increased maternal suckling may be reached by reviewing the evidence related to the technique of rotating rat pups between lactating and non-lactating "aunts" (Slob et al., 1974). When Lynch (1976), Fleischer and Turkewitz (1979b), and Crnic (1980) examined maternal behavior using this approach to producing malnutrition, they found that both mothers and aunts spent more time in the nest with malnourished pups than with control pups in the second half of the litter period. In these studies, the lactating females spent more time nursing malnourished pups than control pups. Thus, changes in maternal behavior in these studies may represent a response to concurrent malnutrition of the young.

Increased nursing and physical contact have also been reported among females rearing pups malnourished during the gestational period or chronically, but fed an adequate diet postnatally. Thus, neither mother nor pups were concurrently malnourished. Massaro et al. (1977) reported increased nursing and contact in litters whose mothers were fed a low protein diet during gestation only. Similarly, litters with histories of many generations of low protein malnutrition which were cross-fostered to control females at birth showed increased maternal nursing, physical contact, and time spent in the nest (Galler and Propert, 1981a). Galler and Propert (1981b) also showed that the altered pattern of mother-pup interaction was a result of the nutritional history of the mother, rather than the pups. Thus, in a 2 × 2 crossover design, rehabilitated mothers suckled rehabilitated or well-nourished control pups and control mothers similarly suckled rehabilitated or control pups. Increased nursing and physical contact were observed only in rehabilitated mothers, and not control mothers. The persistence of increased nursing in malnourished rats that have been rehabilitated after many generations of malnutrition may represent genetic selection of individuals best able to compensate for malnutrition.

The changes in maternal behavior reported in these studies can be seen as compensation for the reduced food intake of the young by increasing opportunities for suckling. Alternatively, the response may be compensation for other effects of malnutrition, such as reduced body size, body temperature of the pups, or the impaired or delayed onset of ultrasonic vocalizations of the pups (Hunt et al., 1976; Hennessy et al., 1978). The interpretation of a compensatory response is supported by the work of Galler and Propert (1982), who reported that among malnourished litters, more weight gain and better survival during the first 28 days of life were associated with high amounts of physical contact between the mother and pups in the first 12 hours after birth. Conversely, mothers that did not have adequate contact with their young as early as the first 3 hours of life had a significantly higher death rate among their offspring.

In summary, alterations in the mother-pup relationship appear to be an integral aspect of malnutrition of the pups during the litter period. For the most part, these changes appear to compensate for the effects of malnutrition and include increased nursing of pups and physical contact between mothers and pups throughout the litter period. Similar changes are also present in rats with gestational or intergenerational malnutrition that were then rehabilitated at birth with an adequate diet. It is instructive to note the similarity betwen results of animals studies and certain observations reported in studies of human populations. Increased time spent nursing and increased physical contact have been found in both species when the infant is malnourished (Galler et al., 1984). Clearly, the situation in humans is more complex than in rats, especially since pre-existing inadequacies in the mother-infant relationship may contribute to the episode of malnutrition and its outcome. This difference emphasizes the need to analyze animal models comprehensively, including documentation of extranutritional factors which may independently affect brain function. Despite this, the animal model, when used properly, provides a useful analysis of human malnutrition and its impact on brain development.

REFERENCES

Altman J, Das GD, Sudarshan K (1970): The influence of nutrition on neural and behavioral development. I. Critical review of some data on the growth of the body and the brain following dietary deprivation during gestation and lactation. Dev Psychobiol 3:281–301.

Baldessarini RJ, Fischer J (1975): Biological models in the study of false neurotransmitters. In Ingle D, Shein H (eds): "Model Systems in Biological Psychiatry." Cambridge, Mass.: MIT Press, pp 51–79.

Barnet AB, Weiss IP, Sotillo MV, Ohrlich ES, Sakurovich ZM, Cravioto J (1978): Abnormal auditory evoked potentials in early infancy malnutrition. Science 201:450–452.

Bartel PR, Griesel RD, Freiman I, Rosen EU, Geefhuysen J (1979): Long-term effects of kwashiorkor on the electroencephalogram. Am J Clin Nutr 32:753–757.

Beynen C, West CE (1986): The suitability of animal models for research in human nutrition: A workshop report. In Taylor TG, Jenkins NK (ed): "Proceedings of the XIII International Congress of Nutrition, 1985." London: John Libbey and Company.

Castro CA, Rudy JW (1987): Early-life malnutrition selectively retards the development of distal- but not proximal-cue navigation. Dev Psychobiol, in press.

Chow BF (1974): Effect of maternal dietary protein on anthropometric and behavioral development of the offspring. Adv Exp Med Biol 49:183–219.

Codo W, Carlini EA (1979): Postnatal undernutrition in rats: Attempts to develop alternative methods to food deprived pups without maternal behavior alteration. Dev Psychobiol 12:475–484.

Cowley JJ, Griesel RD (1963): The development of second generation low-protein rats. J Genet Psychol 103:233–242.

Cravioto J, DeLicardi ER (1972): Environmental correlates of severe clinical malnutrition and language development in survivors from kwashiorkor and marasmus. In: "Nutrition, the Nervous System and Behavior." PAHO Publication no. 251. pp 73–94.

Crnic LS (1976): Effects of infantile undernutrition on adult learning in rats: Methodological and design problems. Psychol Bull 83:715–728.

Crnic LS (1980): Models of infantile malnutrition in rats: Effects on maternal behavior. Dev Psychobiol 13:615–628.

Crnic LS, Chase HP (1978): Models of infantile undernutrition in rats: Effects on milk. J Nutr 108:1755–1760.

Denenberg VH, Thoman EB (1976): From animal to infant research. In Pjossen TD (ed): "Intervention Strategies for High Risk Infants and Young Children." Baltimore: University Press, pp 85–106.

Denenberg VH, Whimbey AE (1963): Behavior of adult rats is modified by experiences their mothers had as infants. Science 142:1192–1193.

Dobbing J (1971): Undernutrition and the developing brain: The use of animal models to elucidate the human problem. Psychiatr Neurol Neurochir 74:433–442.

Finger S, Almli CR, Green L, Wolf C, Morgane PJ (1986): Severe early malnutrition and DRL performance in the rat. Physiol behav 38:731–734.

Fleischer SF, Turkewitz G (1979a): Behavioral effects of rotation between lactating and nonlactating females. Dev Psychobiol 12:245–254.

Fleischer SF, Turkewitz G (1979b): Effect of neonatal stunting on development of rats: Large litter rearing. Dev Psychobiol 12:137–149.

Fleischer SF, Turkewitz G (1984): The use of animals for understanding the effects of malnutrition on human behavior: Models vs a comparative approach. In Galler JR (ed): "Human Nutrition, A Comprehensive Treatise." New York: Plenum Press, pp 37–61.

Frankova S (1973): Effect of protein-calorie malnutrition on the development of social behavior in rats. Dev Psychobiol 6:33–43.

Galler JR (1979): Behavioral development following intergenerational and postnatal malnutrition. In Brozek J (ed): "Behavioral Effects of Energy and Protein Deficits." NIH Publication no. 79–1906. pp. 22–38.

Galler JR (1987): The interaction of nutrition and environment in behavioral development. In Dobbing J (ed): "Early Nutrition and Later Achievement. New York: Academic Press.

Galler JR, Fleischer SF, Turkewitz G, Manes M (1980): Varying deficits in visual discrimination performance associated with different forms of malnutrition in rats. J Nutr 110:231–240.

Galler JR, Fox JG, Murphy JC, Melanson DE (1979): Ulcerative dermatitis in rats with over fifteen generations of protein malnutrition. Br J Nutr 41:611–618.

Galler JR, Propert KJ (1981a): Maternal behavior following rehabilitation of rats with intergenerational malnutrition. 1. Persistant changes in lactation-related behaviors. J Nutr 111:1330–1336.

Galler JR, Propert KJ (1981b): Maternal behavior following rehabilitation of rats with intergenerational malnutrition. 2. Contributions of mothers and pups to deficits in lactation related behavior J Nutr 111:1337–1342.

Galler JR, Propert KJ (1982): Early maternal behavior predictive of the survival of suckling rats with intergenerational malnutrition. J Nutr 112:332–337.

Galler JR, Ricciuti HN, Crawford MA, Kucharski LT (1984): The role of the mother-infant interaction in nutritional disorders. In Galler JR (ed): "Nutrition and Behavior." New York: Plenum Press, pp 269–304.

Galler JR, Seelig C (1981): Home-orienting behavior in rat pups: The effect of two and three generations of rehabilitation following intergenerational malnutrition. Dev Psychobiol 14:541–548.

Galler JR, Turkewitz G (1977): Use of partial mammectomy to produce malnutrition in the rat. Biol Neonate 31:260–265.

Galler JR, Turkewitz G (1975): Variability of the effects of rearing in a large litter on the development of the rat. Dev Psychobiol 8:325–331.

Goodlett CR, Valentino ML, Morgane PJ, Resnick O (1986): Spatial cue utilization in chronically malnourished rats: Task-specific learning deficits. Dev Psychobiol 19:1–15.

Grota LJ, Ader R (1969): Continuous recording of maternal behavior patterns in the Rattus norvegicus. Anim Behav 17:722–729.

Hall RD, Leahy JP, Robertson WM (1979): The effects of protein malnutrition on the behavior of rats during the suckling period. Dev Psychobiol 12:455–466.

Hall WG (1975): Weaning and growth of artificially reared rats. Science 190:1313–1315.

Hennessy MB, Smotherman WP, Kolp L, Hunt L, Levine S (1978): Stimuli from pups of adrenalectomized and malnourished female rats. Physiol Behav 20:509–513.

Hseuh AM, Simonson M, Chow BF, Hanson HM (1974): The importance of the period of dietary restriction of the dam on behavior and growth in the rat. J Nutr 104:37–46.

Hseuh A, Simonson M, Kellum M, Chow B (1973): Perinatal undernutrition and the metabolic and behavioral development of the offspring. Nutr Rep Int 7:437–445.

Hunt LE, Smotherman WP, Wiener SG, Levine S (1976): Nutritional variables and their effect on the development of ultrasonic vocalizations in rat pups. Physiol Behav 17:1037–1039.

Kanis KB, Galler JR, Teicher MH, Baldessarini R (1987): Mother-pup interaction altered following prenatal malnutrition and dopamine-depletion, despite normal pup growth rates. Fed Proc 46:574.

Kennedy GC (1957): The development with age of hypothalamic restraint upon the appetite of the rat. J Endocrinol 16:9–17.

Levine S, Wiener S (1975): A critical analysis of data on malnutrition and behavioral deficits. Adv Pediatr 22:113–136.

Levitsky DA (1979): Malnutrition and the hunger to learn. In Levitsky DA (ed): "Malnutrition, Environment, and Behavior, New Perspectives." Ithaca: Cornell University Press, pp 161–179.

Lynch A (1976): Postnatal undernutrition: An alternative method. Dev Psychobiol 9:39–48.

Maier NRF, Schnierla TC (1933): "Principles of Animal Psychology." New York: McGraw-Hill.

Massaro TF, Levitsky DA, Barnes RH (1974): Protein malnutrition in the rat: Its effects on maternal behavior and pup development. Dev Psychobiol 7:551–561.

Massaro TF, Levitsky DA, Barnes RH (1977): Protein malnutrition induced during gestation: Its effect on pup development and maternal behavior. Dev Psychobiol 10:339–345.

Menendez-Patterson A, Fernandez S, Florez-Lozano J, Marin B (1982): Effect of early, pre- and postnatal acquired malnutrition on development and sexual behavior in the rat. Pharmacol Biochem Behav 17:659–664.

Miller M, Resnick O (1980): Tryptophan availability: The importance of prepartum and postpartum dietary protein on brain indolamine metabolism in rats. Exp Neurol 67:298–314.

Miller SA, Dymsza HA (1963): Artificial feeding of neonatal rats. Science 141:517–518.

Mueller AJ, Cox WM (1946): The effect of changes in diet on the volume and composition of rat milk. J Nutr 31:249–259.

Nicoll C, Meites J (1959): Prolongation of lactation in the rat by litter replacement. Proc Soc Exp Biol Med 101:81–82.

Noirot E (1964): Changes in responsiveness to young in the adult mouse: The effect of external stimuli. J Comp Physiol Psychol 57:97–99.

Nowak TS, Munro HN (1977): Effects of protein-calorie malnutrition on biochemical aspects of brain development. In Wurtman RJ, Wurtman JJ (eds): "Nutrition and the Brain." New York: Raven Press 2:193–260.

Plaut SM (1970): Studies of undernutrition in the young rat: Methodological considerations. Dev Psychobiol 3:157–167.

Rathbun WE, Druse MJ (1985): Maternal undernutrition during lactation: Effect on amino acids in brain regions of offspring. J Neurochem 45:1802–1808.

Resnick O, Morgane PJ (1983): Animal models for small-for-gestational-age (SGA) neonates and infants-at-risk (IAR). Dev Brain Res 10:221–225.

Resnick O, Morgane PJ (1984a): Generational effects of protein malnutrition in rat. Dev Brain Res 15:219–227.

Resnick O, Morgane PJ (1984b): Ontogeny of the levels of serotonin in various parts of the brain in severely protein malnourished rats. Brain Res 303:163–170.

Resnick O, Morgane PJ, Hasson R, Miller M (1982): Overt and hidden forms of chronic malnutrition in the rat and their relevance to man. Nueorsci Biobehav Rev 6:55–75.

Richardson SA (1980): The long range consequences of malnutrition in infancy: A study of children in Jamaican West Indies. In Wharton B (ed): ''Topics in Pediatrics.'' Vol. 2, ''Nutrition in Childhood.'' London: Pitman, pp 163–176.

Rogers PJ, Tonkiss J, Smart JL (1986): Incidental learning is impaired during early-life undernutrition. Dev Psychobiol 19:113–124.

Rosenblatt JS (1967): The nonhormonal basis of maternal behavior in the rat. Science 156:1512–1514.

Rosenblatt JS (1969): The development of maternal responsiveness in the rat. Am J Orthopsychiatry 39:36–56.

Rosenblatt JS (1975): Prepartum and postpartum regulation of maternal behavior in the rat. Parent-Infant Interaction. 33:17–37.

Rosso P, Hormazabal J, Winick M (1970): Changes in brain weight, cholesterol, phospholipid, and DNA content in marasmic children. Am J Clin Nutr 23:1275–1279.

Scrimshaw NS, Gordon JE, Taylor CE (1959): Interactions of nutrition and infection. Am J Med Sci 237:367.

Slob AK, Snow C, Natris-Mathot E (1973): Absence of behavioral deficits following neonatal undernutrition in the rat. Dev Psychobiol 6:177–186.

Smart JL (1984): Animal models of early malnutrition: Advantages and limitations. In Brozek J, Schurch B (eds): ''Malnutrition and Behavior: Critical Assessment of Key Issues.'' Switzerland: Nestle Foundation, pp 444–464.

Smart JL, Dobbing J (1971): Vulnerability of developing brain. II. Effects of early nutritional deprivation on reflex ontogeny and development of behaviour in the rat. Brain Res 28:85–95.

Smart JL, Dobbing J, Adlard BP, Lynch A, Sands J (1973): Vulnerability of developing brain: Relative effects of growth restriction during the fetal and suckling periods on behavior and brain composition of adult rats. J Nutr 103:1327–1338.

Smart JL, Preece J (1973): Maternal behavior of undernutrition mother rats. Anim Behav 21:613–619.

Smart JL, Stephens DN, Katz HB (1983): Growth and development of rats artificially reared on a high or a low plane of nutrition. Br J Nutr 49:497–506.

Smart JL, Stephens DN, Tonkiss J, Auestad NS, Edmond J (1984): Growth and development of rats artificially reared on different milk-substitutes. Br J Nutr 52:227–237.

Stein Z, Susser M, Saenger G, Marolla F (1975): ''Famine and Human Development: The Dutch Hunger Winter of 1944–1945.'' New York: Oxford University Press.

Stewart RJC (1973): A marginally malnourished rat colony. Nutr Rep Int 7:487–493.

Stewart RJC, Sheppard H, Preece R, Waterlow JC (1980): The effect of rehabilitation at different stages of development of rats marginally malnourished for ten to twleve generations. Br J Nutr 43:403–412.

Stoch MB, Smythe TM, Moodie AD, Bradshaw D (1982): Psychosocial outcome and CT findings after growth undernutrition during infancy: A twenty year developmental study. Dev Med Child Neurol 24:419–436.

Sturman JA, Devine E, Resnick O, Morgane PJ (1986): Maternal protein malnutrition in the rat: Effect on protein and two enzymes in the milk. Nutr Res 6:437–442.

Sykes SE, Cheyne JA (1976): The effects of prenatal and postnatal protein malnutrition on physical and motor development of the rat. Dev Psychobiol 9:285–295.

Turkewitz G (1966): The development of spatial orientation in relation to the effective environment in rats. Ph.D. diss., New York University.

Vendite D, Wotchuk S, Souza DO (1985): Effects of undernutrition during suckling on footshock escape behavior and on related neurochemical parameters in rats. J Nutr 115:1418–1424.

Whatson TS, Smart JL (1978): Social behavior of rats following pre- and early postnatal undernutrition. Physiol Behav 20:749–753.

Widdowson EM, McCance RA (1960): Some effects of accelerating growth. 1. General somatic development. Proc R Soc Lond [Biol] 162:188–206.

Wiener SG, Fitzpatrick KM, Levin R, Smotherman WP, Levine S (1977): Alterations in the maternal behavior of rats rearing malnourished offspring. Dev Psychobiol 10:243–254.

Wiener SG, Robinson L, Levine S (1983): Influence of perinatal malnutrition on adult physiological and behavioral reactivity in rats. Physiol Behav 30:41–50.

Wiesner B, Sheard N (1933): "Maternal Behavior in the Rat." London: Oliver and Boyd.

Wurtman JJ, Miller SA (1976): Effect of litter size on weight gain in rats. J Nutr 106:697–701.

Zamenhof S, Guthrie D (1977): DIfferential responses to prenatal malnutrition among neonatal rats. Biol Neonate 32:205–210.

Zamenhof S, van Marthens E (1978): The effects of chronic undernutrition over generations on rat development. J Nutr 108:1719–1723.

Zamenhof S, van Marthens E, Grauel L (1973): Prenatal nutritional factors affecting brain development. Nutr Rep Int 7:371–382.

Current Topics in Nutrition and Disease, Volume 16
Basic and Clinical Aspects of Nutrition and Brain Development,
pages 75–98
© 1987 Alan R. Liss, Inc.

Nutrients and Humoral Substances in the Microenvironment Influence the Development and Aging of Glial Cells in Culture

Antonia Vernadakis, Nikos Sakellaridis, and Dimitra Mangoura

Departments of Psychiatry and Pharmacology, University of Colorado
School of Medicine, Denver, Colorado 80262

INTRODUCTION

The brain is a complex organ composed of neuronal "wiring" cells and the more supportive glial and connective tissue cells. Brain function is highly dependent upon the interrelationships between the cell types and their interaction with the microenvironment. A schematic representation of the various intercellular interactions is shown in Figure 1 (Vernadakis and Sakellaridis, 1985). It has been shown that neurons, neuroglia, and connective tissue cells secrete factors into the microenvironment which in turn influence the function of the other cells, i.e., neurotransmitter and neurohumoral substances, hypothalamic releasing factors, nucleotide messengers, etc. Age-related changes in any component of this cellular unit will shift the balance, interrupt intercellular relationships, and ultimately affect neuronal function.

In this chapter, we will focus on changes in glial cells, one component of the neuronal-glial-connective-tissue unit. Recent advances in culture methodology have allowed meaningful investigations of glial cells. Research to be reported here shows that glial cells in culture undergo development and aging and are responsive to nutrients and humoral substances present in the in vitro microenvironment.

DEVELOPMENTAL CHANGES IN GLIAL CELLS IN CULTURE

We have used the chick embryo as an experimental animal to study neural growth and differentiation in vivo and in culture. We have examined changes in the activites of two glial cell enzymes, glutamine synthetase (GS) and $2',3'$-cyclic nucleotide $3'$-phosphohydrolase (CNP) in chick embryonic brain

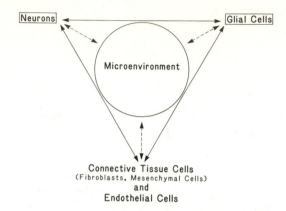

Fig. 1. Schematic representation of cell–cell interactions in the central nervous system tissue (from Vernadakis and Sakellaridis, 1985).

and in cultures derived from chick embryonic brain. Glutamine synthetase has been used as a marker for astrocytes (Riepe and Norenberg, 1977; Norenberg and Martinez-Hernandez, 1979), and CNP has been used as a marker for oligodendrocytes (Poduslo and Norton, 1972; Poduslo, 1975). Since the oligodendrocytic plasma membrane gives rise to brain myelin (Bunge, 1968) and since the regional distribution of CNP appears to be paralleled by the distribution of the myelinated fibers (Kurihara and Tsukada, 1967), it is reasonable to conclude that CNP is localized in the myelin sheath and on the oligodendrocyte plasma membrane. Therefore, CNP can be used as a marker for myelination as well (Kurihara and Tsukada, 1968). In addition, we examined whether the developmental profiles of the two enzymes differ in cultures consisting of both neurons and glial cells and in glia-enriched cultures in an attempt to evaluate the influence of neurons on the developmental profile of these glial cell enzymes in culture.

The developmental profiles of the two glial cell enzymes assayed in the chick embryo brain follow a similar pattern, increasing with age. This increase in activity was very pronounced after the 15th day of incubation in both enzymes. The pattern for GS activity was almost identical for the cerebrum and cerebellum, whereas the CNP activity in the cerebellum showed a 40-fold increase compared to a relatively moderate 3-fold increase for the cerebrum (Figs. 2, 3). Developmental changes in CNP activity in the chick brain and spinal cord have been reported by Kurihara and Tsukada (1968). They found that the greatest increase in activity occurred between 18 days of incubation and 3 days after hatching in the whole brain and between 18 and 21 days of incubation in the spinal cord. As mentioned previously, CNP has been associated with myelin membranes (Kurihara and Tsukada,

1968) and also has been detected in oligodendroglial membranes (Poduslo and Norton, 1972; Poduslo, 1975). The rise of CNP activity between days 15 and 20 of embryonic age can be associated with the myelination occurring during this embryonic period.

The developmental profile of CNP in culture is of considerable interest in that CNP activity appears to decrease in cultures derived from either 7-day-old chick embryo whole brain or 15-day-old chick embryo cerebral hemispheres (Figs. 4, 5). This finding is in contrast to recent reports on cultures derived from rat brain. Bansal and Pfeiffer (1985) have reported the developmental expression of CNP in cultures derived from 19- to 21-day-old fetal rat brains and also reported the CNP activity in developing whole rat brain from birth to 120 days after birth. The developmental profile of CNP enzymatic activity and amount of CNP protein in culture paralleled that observed in rat brain in which the period of most active development was 7–25 days after birth. However, as we also have observed in our chick embryo model, CNP activity was lower in culture as compared to in vivo rat brain preparation.

Wernicke and Volpe (1986) have also reported growth of oligodendrocytes in cultures derived from neonatal rat cerebral hemispheres using CNP and glycerol 3-phosphate dehydrogenase (GPDH) as glia markers. As also reported by Breen and de Vellis (1974) and Breen et al. (1978), GPDH activity was stable and low during the first 3 weeks in culture. However, over the next 12 days, a marked increase in activity was observed in the study by Wernicke and Volpe (1986); a 15-fold rise occurring between 20 to 32 days in culture. In contrast to the slow rise of GDPH, CNP activity progressively increased in culture.

Thus, the growth of oligodendrocytes in culture appears to follow different developmental profiles in the rat and chick, at least as related to CNP activity. Whether the oligodendrocytes from chick brain are more sensitive to the lack of neuronal input than those from rat is a possible consideration, and we will discuss it below. On the other hand, the possibility that fetal calf serum contains some substance which inhibits oligodendrocyte proliferation cannot be excluded.

Bologa and associates have studied the development of oligodendrocytes in culture (see review Bologa, 1985) using galactocerebroside (GC) and myelin basic protein (MBP) as markers for oligodendrocytes (Raff et al., 1978; Sternberger et al., 1978). In cultures derived from embryonic mouse brain, oligodendrocytes differentiate very early into GC^+MBP^+ cells (Bologa et al., 1982b); while in cultures of neonatal mouse brain, oligodendrocytes differentiate very early into GC^+MBP^+ cells later and in a small percentage (Bologa et al., 1981). The difference in the differentiation of oligodendrocytes in these two types of cultures could not be accounted for by

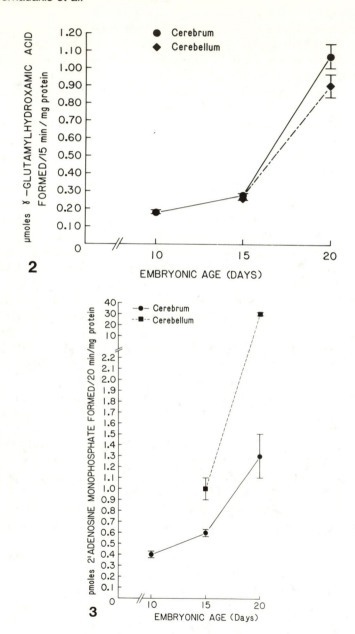

2

3

the presence of other cells, such as astrocytes and neurons. The appearance, quantity, and developmental pattern of astrocytes using glial fibrillary acidic protein (GFAP) as marker (Bignami and Dahl, 1977) were similar in both culture systems (Bologa et al., 1982a). However, the appearance, number, and development of neurons using neuron-specific γ-enolase (NSE) are different (Marangos et al., 1975) in embryonic and neonatal mouse brain cell cultures (Bologa et al., 1982a, 1983). While neonatal mouse brain cell cultures are very poor in neurons, in embryonic cultures, many NSE$^+$ neurons are present. Bologa and associates suggest that neurons are involved in the enhancement of the ability of oligodendrocytes to differentiate and to express myelin-related components in culture.

In contrast to the lack of growth of oligodendrocytes in cultures derived from the chick brain, astrocyte growth in culture parallels the in vivo growth, as shown by the progressive increase in GS activity (Figs. 6, 7). Wernicke and Volpe (1986), also using GS activity as an astrocytic marker, have reported a progressive increase in astrocyte growth in culture. It appears that astrocyte growth may not be dependent on neuronal input but rather on information that astrocytes carry in their own nuclei. Moreover, astrocyte growth in culture is similar at least in the two experimental animal species studied.

RESPONSIVENESS OF GLIAL CELLS TO MICROENVIRONMENT IN CULTURE

Tissue culture systems have considerable advantages in examining cell interrelationships, since cells in culture are devoid of some of their *in vivo* complexities. Cell-cell relationships and also microenvironment-cell relationships can be assesssed by systematically focusing on specific factors that may regulate developmental processes. Considerable research interest in these phenomena is reflected by various methodologies as reported in the literature: different culture media (see review by Bottenstein, 1985), including conditioned media (Monard et al., 1973), and different forms of coating the culture dishes, i.e., gelatin (Yaffe, 1973), poly-L-lysine (Booher and

---

Fig. 2. (Facing page) Changes in glutamine synthetase activity in cerebrum and cerebellum dissected from chick embryos with embryonic age. Activity is expressed in μmol of γ-glutamylhydroxamic acid formed in 15 min/mg protein and plotted vs. embryonic age expressed in days. Points represent mean ± S.E. of four to six samples (from Sakellaridis et al., 1983).

Fig. 3. Changes in 2′,3′-cyclic nucleotide 3′-phosphohydrolase activity in cerebrum and cerebellum dissected from chick embryos with embryonic age. Activity is expressed in pmoles of 2′-adenosine monophosphate formed in 20 min/mg protein and plotted vs. embryonic age expressed in days. Points represent mean ± S.E. of four to six samples (from Sakellaridis et al., 1983).

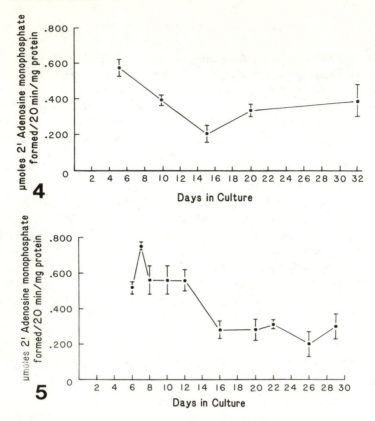

Fig. 4.   Changes with days in culture in 2',3'-cyclic nucleotide 3'-phosphohydrolase activity in neuronal-glial cultures dissociated from cerebral hemispheres of 7-day-old chick embryos. Activity is expressed in μmol of 2'-adenosine monophosphate formed in 20 min/mg protein and plotted vs. days in culture. Points represent mean ± S.E. of three to four separate culture dishes (from Sakellaridis et al., 1983).

Fig. 5.   Changes with days in culture in 2',3'-cyclic nucleotide 3'-phosphohydrolase activity in glia-enriched cultures dissociated from cerebral hemispheres of 15-day-old chick embryos. Activity is expressed in μmol of 2'-adenosine monophosphate formed in 20 min/mg protein and plotted vs. days in culture. Points represent mean ± S.E. of three to four separate culture dishes (from Sakellaridis et al., 1983).

Sensenbrenner, 1972), polyornithine (Adler and Varon, 1981; Varon et al., 1983), matrix (Igarashi and Yaoi, 1975), killed cell substrata (Hawrot, 1980), and simultaneous plating of two autologous cell populations (McCarthy and Partlow, 1976a,b).

We have examined the influence of various components of the micro-environment on glial cell growth: humoral factors present in fibroblast and neuron-conditioned media and cell contact provided by fibroblast or

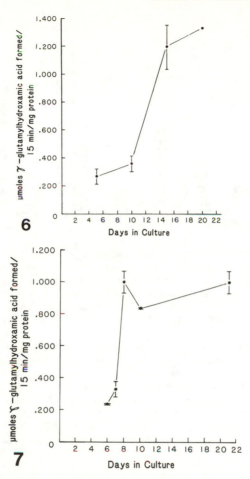

Fig. 6.   Changes with days in culture in glutamine synthetase activity in neuronal-glial cultures dissociated from cerebral hemispheres of 7-day-old chick embryos. Activity is expressed in μmol of γ-glutamylhydroxamic acid formed in 15 min/mg protein and plotted vs. days in culture. Points represent mean ± S.E. of three to four separate culture dishes (from Sakellaridis et al., 1983).

Fig. 7.   Changes with days in culture in glutamine synthetase activity in glia-enriched cultures dissociated from cerebral hemispheres of 15-day-old chick embryos. Activity is expressed in μmol of γ-glutamylhydroxamic acid formed in 15 min/mg protein and plotted vs. day in culture. Points represent mean ± S.E. of three to four separate culture dishes (from Sakellaridis et al., 1983).

neuronal substrata. We have found that replacement of D-valine with L-valine in the medium in order to eliminate the growth of fibroblasts greatly retards astrocytic growth in cultures derived from newborn mouse cerebral

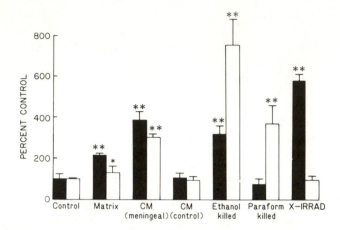

Fig. 8. Specific glutamine synthetase activity and incorporation of ³H-thymidine in glial cells dissociated from newborn mice and cultured in D-valine medium under conditions with various components derived from brain fibroblast cultures. D-valine-cultured glial cells were plated on: plastic (control); on matrix derived from confluent brain fibroblast cultures (matrix); on plastic with 50% media conditioned by confluent brain fibroblast cultures (CM meningeal); on plastic with 50% media conditioned by confluent D-valine-cultured glial cells (CM control); on a layer of confluent brain fibroblast cultures killed with ethanol (ethanol killed); on a layer of confluent brain fibroblast cultures killed with 0.2% paraformaldehyde (paraform killed); on a layer of confluent brain fibroblast cultures (X-irrad). At 2 weeks after plating, cultures were treated with 2 μCi per dish ³H-thymidine for 24 hr. Cultures were washed three times and grown for 4 days longer, then harvested for glutamine synthetase assay, tritium counting, and DNA assay. Substrata alone were assayed for subtracting background biochemical values. Solid bars are glutamine synthetase activity per DNA. Open bars are ³H-thymidine incorporation per DNA. Values are the mean ± S.E. of five dishes. *P < 0.05, **P < 0.0005, relative controls. Controls were 19.7 μmol product/hr/μg DNA and 1.4 × 10³ DPM/μg DNA (from Estin and Vernadakis, 1986).

hemispheres (Estin and Vernadakis, 1986). On the other hand, when medium conditioned by brain fibroblast cell cultures was added to the glial cultures, glial growth was enhanced as assessed by GS activity as a marker for astrocytes. Furthermore, matrix derived from brain fibroblast cell cultures enhanced the growth of glial cells (Fig. 8). The role of extracellular matrix in various cell growth phenomena has been extensively investigated in recent years (Gospodarowicz et al., 1981; Overton, 1978; Rojkind et al., 1980; Weiss et al. 1975; Wicha et al., 1982; Yaoi and Kanaseki, 1972).

In the same study (Estin and Vernadakis, 1986), we found that glial growth was enhanced when the cells were plated on an ethanol or paraformaldehyde-killed cell layer of fibroblasts (Fig. 8). On the other hand, in another study (Sakellaridis et al., 1984), we found that growth of glial cells derived from 15-day-old chick embryo cerebral hemispheres and plated on an established neuron-enriched alive culture derived from 6-day-old chick embryonic brain was markedly inhibited as shown by a decrease in GS and CNP activities. In contrast, when a cell population derived from dissociated 6-day-old chick embryonic brain was plated on a glia-enriched culture, the growth of glial cells was enhanced (Figs. 9–12) (Sakellaridis et al., 1984). To investigate further this neuronal influence on glial cell growth, we exposed established glial cell cultures from 15-day-old chick embryo cerebral hemispheres to different concentrations of medium conditioned by a neuron-enriched cell population derived from 6-day-old chick embryo brain (Sakellaridis et al., 1986). We found that in cultures exposed to neuron-conditioned medium, GS activity was decreased and CNP activity was increased (Figs. 13, 14). In the same study we observed that with increasing concentration of fetal calf serum (5% up to 20%) CNP activity decreased, whereas GS activity markedly increased. These findings taken together further emphasize the differential responsiveness of astrocytes and oligodendrocytes to microenvironmental influences such as neuronal input or nutrients present in the culture medium.

The direct involvement of neurons has been shown in the proliferation and differentiation of Schwann cells (Aguayo et al., 1976; Weinberg and Spencer, 1976; Wood and Bunge, 1975). Privat et al. (1981) have reported that after injury, the presence of axons is required for the development of a normal oligodendrocyte population. Roussel et al. (1983) have shown that brain extract elicits stimulation of the proliferation of oligodendrocytes, whereas Pruss et al. (1981) obtained a similar effect with fibroblast growth factor or with a growth factor from the bovine pituitary.

In a recent study, Bologa et al. (1986) found that myelin basic protein production by oligodendrocytes in culture was greatly enhanced by treatment with either pure neurons from 16-day-old rat embryo cortical cultures, rat neuron-conditioned medium, or chick neuron-conditioned medium but not hormonally supllemented medium or medium conditioned by astrocytes and fibroblasts. These authors also conclude, as we also found in our CNP study, that MBP by oligodendrocytes is regulated by a non-specific soluble neuronal factor. Sensenbrenner and associates (Pettman et al., 1980) have reported that extracts prepared from 12-day-old chick embryo enhanced the maturation of astroglial cells in cultures prepared from newborn rat brain cerebral hemispheres. Also, they found that brain extract enhances the development of oligodendrocyte-like cells (Pettman et al., 1980; Sensenbrenner et al., 1982). The dependence of oligodendrocyte growth in cultures on neuronal input is further emphasized in myelination studies in culture (Wood et al., 1980; Wood and Williams, 1984).

Of importance are studies showing interactionof astroglia-oligodendroglia in culture. Evidence has been reported on the stimulation of optic nerve

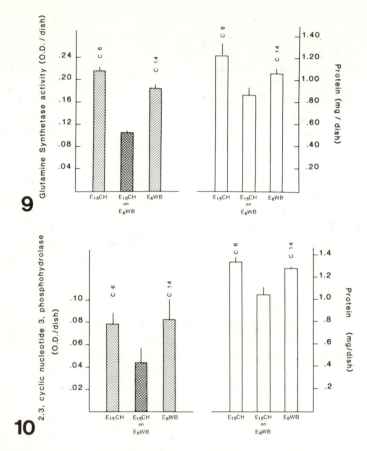

Fig. 9. Glutamine synthetase (GS) activity (left) and protein content (right) in cultures. $E_{15}CH$: Cultures derived from 15-day-old chick embryo cerebral hemispheres, plated on plastic (6 days in culture). E_6WB: Cultures derived from 6-day-old chick embryo whole brain, plated on plastic (14 days in culture). $E_{15}CH$ on E_6WB: Cells dissociated from $E_{15}CH$ plated on a neuron-enriched living cell substratum from E_6WB. GS activity is expressed as optical density recorded per culture dish/15 min. Protein content is expressed as mg/dish. Data are the mean ± S.E. of four to six samples (from Sakellaridis et al., 1984).

Fig. 10. $2',3'$-Cyclic nucleotide $3'$-phosphohydrolase (CNP) activity (left) and protein content (right) in cultures. $E_{15}CH$: Cultures derived from 15-day-old chick embryo cerebral hemispheres, plated on plastic (6 days in culture). E_6WB: Cultures derived from 6-day-old chick embryo whole brain, plated on plastic (14 days in culture). $E_{15}CH$: Cells dissociated from $E_{15}CH$ and plated on a neuron-enriched living cell substratum derived from E_6WB. CNP activity is expressed as optical density recorded per culture dish/20 min. Protein content is expressed as mg/dish. Bars represent the mean ± S.E. of four to six samples. No statistically significant changes exist between any groups of cultures (from Sakellaridis et al., 1984).

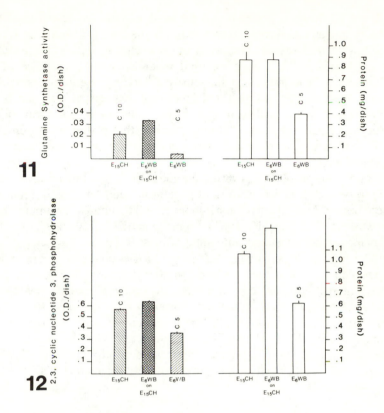

Fig. 11. Glutamine synthetase (GS) activity (left) and protein content (right) in cultures. $E_{15}CH$: Cultures derived from 15-day-old chick embryo cerebral hemispheres, plated on plastic (10 days in culture): E_6WB: Cultures derived from 6-day-old chick embryo whole brain, plated on plastic (5 days in culture); E_6WB on $E_{15}CH$: Cells dissociated from E_6WB plated on a glia-enriched living cell substratum from $E_{15}CH$. GS activity is expressed as optical density recorded per culture dish/15 min. Protein content is expressed as mg/dish. Data are the mean ± S.E. of four to six samples (from Sakellaridis et al., 1984).

Fig. 12. 2′,3′-Cyclic nucleotide 3′-phosphohydrolase (CNP) activity (left) and protein content (right) in cultures. $E_{15}CH$: Cultures derived from 15-day-old chick embryo cerebral hemispheres, plated on platic (10 days in culture). E_6WB: Cultures derived from 6-day-old chick embryo whole brain, plated on plastic (5 days in culture). E_6WB on $E_{15}CH$: Cells dissociated from E_6WB plated on a glia-enriched living cell substratum from $E_{15}CH$. CNP activity is expressed as optical density recorded per culture dish/20 min. Protein content is expressed as mg/dish. Bars represent the mean ± of four to six samples (from Sakellaridis et al., 1984).

oligodendroglia progenitor cell proliferation by a soluble factor produced by optic nerve astrocytes (Noble and Murray, 1984) and, conversely, the inhibitory effect on oligodendrocyte differentiation of a factor found in fetal calf serum (Raff et al., 1983). As reported earlier, we also found that increasing concentrations of fetal calf serum in the culture medium decreased CNP activity but increased GS activity in culture (Sakellaridis et al., 1986). Bhat and Pfeiffer (1985) have reported evidence for the presence of an non-dialysable, heat-labile, trypsin-sensitive factor present in extracts of astrocyte-enriched cultures that enhances the expression parameters of myelinogenesis when added to rat brain cultures enriched in oligo-dendrocytes. Bhat and Pfeiffer (1985) propose that pathological perturba-tions in factors produced by astrocytes could result in dysmyelination or demyelination.

Lim and associates (1973, 1980) have identified a glial maturation factor (GMF) to be a high-molecular-weight protein in adult rat and pig brain and found to be biologically active on newborn rat glial cultures. From pig brain, other workers (Kato et al., 1981) report purified active factors in two molecular-morphological and mitogenic effects.

Cellular interactions involving cell surface have been implicated in various morphogenetic and inductive events during development. The cellular basis of these interactions may take the form of syncytial events (passage of electrical currents or small molecules through gap junctions) (Revel and Brown, 1975; Lawrence et al., 1978), the release of short-acting soluble factors (Grobstein, 1968), or may involve interactions of extracellular-facing elements associated with the plasma membranes of adjacent cells (Fishman and Brady, 1976) and "cell surface-mediated cellular interactions" (Ciment and de Vellis, 1982).

CHANGES IN GLIAL CELLS WITH AGING IN CULTURE

For many years the consensus has been that memory and cognitive decline of the aged was simply the result of attrition of nerve cells which are estimated to be lost at the rate of 50–100,000 cells per day. However, although neuronal loss must play a role in the memory and cognitive decline in aging, it is now clear that this is not the complete explanation. As discussed earlier, the neuron is only one component of the complex circuitry of the brain. Other significant cellular components are the neuroglial cells and the conective tissue cells such as endothelial cells, fibroblasts, and mesenchymal cells. All of these cells, neurons, neuroglia, and connective tissue cells intercommunicate through their microenvironment and function as a unit. Age-related changes in any component of this cellular unit will shift the balance, interrupt intercellular relationships, and ultimately affect neuronal function.

Several studies using cell culture as a model have been exploring cell changes with aging. More specifically, using somatic cells as a model, changes with cell passage in culture have been interpreted to reflect changes with aging (Strehler, 1977).

Using the concepts derived from the fibroblast in vitro model of aging, in early studies, we used the glioma cell line (C-6, 2B clone) at early passage (20–25) and late passage (50–90) as a model to study changes in glial cells with aging in culture (Parker et al., 1980; Vernadakis et al., 1982). We have found differences in doubling time (12–16 hr for late passage vs. more than 24 hr for young passage), cell size and protein content (late passage greater than young), and responsiveness to hormones. Moreover, we observed that cells at early passages (20–30) were predominantly oligodendrocytic, using CNP as a marker, whereas cells at later passages (80–90) were predominantly astrocytic, using GS as a marker. We have proposed that this shifting in cell types with cell passage may reflect an in vitro aging phenomenon, i.e., astrogliosis in vitro. We have continued to subculture these cells, and in cell passage 117, GS activity continues to be high.

More recently, we have been studying aging in glial cells using dissociated cultures from newborn and aged (18 month) mice (Vernadakis et al., 1984, 1986). In these preliminary studies, we compared changes in glial cells derived from young and aged mouse brain with days in culture and with cell passage. Again we used GS and CNP as glial markers and also used the astrocytic marker, glial fibrillary acidic protein (GFA) and GPDH (de Vellis, 1973; McGinnis and de Vellis, 1974). After 3–4 weeks in culture, when cells were at confluency, cultures were trypsinized, and the dispersed cells were replated at a density of 1 million per ml. At present, cell passages 0–11 have been studied. Differences have been observed in the rate of dispersed cells adhering to the culture dish in that in the cultures derived from aged mouse brain, the dispersed cells did not adhere to the dish for at least 9–10 days and suggest possible differences in cell membrane properties between young and old cells. Small patches or "islands" of large flat cells began to appear sporadically on the dish (Fig. 15). By 2–3 weeks in culture, an almost confluent monolayer of flat cells was formed, on top of which a smaller number of round, dark, process-bearing cells, presumptively oligo-dendrocytes, were seen (Fig. 15). GFA-positive and GPDH-rhodamine-positive cells were present in both types of cell cultures, newborn and aged mouse, up to passage 4 (Fig. 16). However, with progressive cell passage, the number of GFA-positive cells declined significantly as did the intensity and pattern of immunoreactivity. Attempts to stain these cultures with GFA antiserum failed to yield GFA-positive cells.

Phase microscopy has revealed different patterns of growth in cells cultured under various substratum conditions: plastic stratum, glass coverslips, or sandwiched between plastic and glass. The cell population on glass coverslips consisted of carpets of flat epithelioid cells with fusiform,

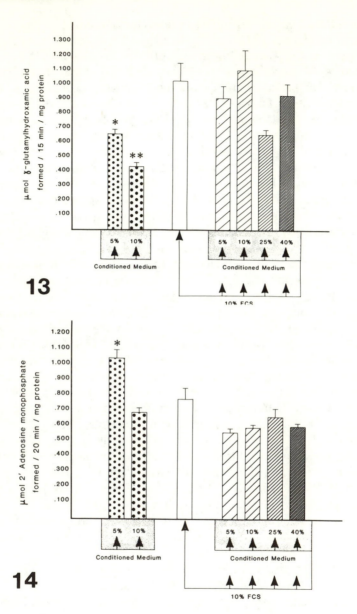

bipolar cells lying on top. In the special microenvironment provided in the space between the glass coverslip and the plastic petri floor, cells of three types were found: at early passages (P5 to P7), large veil-like epithelioid cells; at late passages (P10 or P11) large epithelioid, phase dark cells with processes resembling mature astrocytes, and cells with small somata similar to oligodendrocytes. The cell populations grown on plastic consisted predominantly of spindle-shaped cells and a smaller number of polyhedral cells. An increasing number of the polyhedral cells were multinucleated at the late passages, especially in the cultures derived from the aged mouse (Fig. 17). Somatic polyploidy occurs widely in both plants and animals, but its function is unclear. Extensive evidence from studies of fibroblasts during in vitro aging supports the view that polyploidy increases during in vitro aging (Kaji and Matsuo, 1981; Matsuo et al., 1982).

The decline in GFA-positive cells with cell passage is of interest and warrants further exploration. The question to be considered is whether there is a decline in GFA astrocytes or whether there is a cellular change in the GFA molecule so that the antibody no longer recognizes it and thus the decline in GFA-positive immunoreactivity. Lindsay et al. (1982) character-ized astrocyte cultures derived from corpus callosum of adult rat after surgical lesion and a period of postoperative "priming" in vivo. They

---

Fig. 13. (Facing page) GS activity in glia-enriched cultures from 15-day-old chick embryo cerebral hemispheres exposed to different combinations of culture media. From left to right: DMEM with 5% NCM; DMEM with 10% NCM; DMEM with 10% FCS; DMEM with 10% FCS and 5% NCM; DMEM with 10% FCS and 10% NCM; DMEM with 10% FCS and 25% NCM; DMEM with 10% FCS and 10% NCM; DMEM with 10% FCS and 25% NCM; DMEM with 10% FCS and 40% NCM. Cultures were harvested at day 9, and GS activity is expressed as μmol of γ-glutamylhydroxamic acid formed/15 min/mg protein. Data are the mean $\pm$ S.E. of four to six samples. GS activity was significantly lower in cultures with 5 or 10% NCM only, as compared to cultures with 5 or 10% NCM + 10% FCS, or 10% FCS alone (*P < 0.01 and **P < 0.001). Total protein content (mg/dish): 5% NCM, 0.411 $\pm$ 0.03; 10% NCM, 0.504 $\pm$ 0.06; 10% FCS, 0.808 $\pm$ 0.05; 5% NCM + 10% FCS, 0.729 $\pm$ 0.04; 10% NCM + 10% FCS, 0.698 $\pm$ 0.05; 25% NCM + 10% FCS, 0.666 $\pm$ 0.02; 40% NCM + 10% FCS, 0.791 $\pm$ 0.04 (from Sakellaridis et al., 1986).

Fig. 14. CNP activity in glia-enriched cultures from 15-day-old chick embryo cerebral hemispheres exposed to different combinations of culture media. From left to right: DMEM with 5% NCM; DMEM with 10% NCM; DMEM with 10% FCS; DMEM with 10% FCS and 5% NCM; DMEM with 10% FCS and 10% NCM; DMEM with 10% FCS and 25% NCM; DMEM with 10% FCS and 40% NCM. CNP activity is expressed as μmol of 2'-adenosine monophosphate formed/20 min/mg protein. Data are the mean $\pm$ S.E. of four to six samples. CNP activity was significantly higher in cultures with 5% NCM alone as compared to cultures with 5% NCM and 10% FCS or 10% FCS alone (P < 0.01). Total protein content (mg/dish): 5% NCM, 0.480 $\pm$ 0.01; 10% NCM, 0.560 $\pm$ 0.02; 10% FCS, 0.671 $\pm$ 0.04; 5% NCM + 10% FCS, 0.793 $\pm$ 0.02; 10% NCM + 10% FCS, 0.634 $\pm$ 0.03; 25% NCM + 10% FCS, 0.699 $\pm$ 0.05; 40% NCM + 10% FCS, 0.716 $\pm$ 0.02 (from Sakellaridis et al., 1986).

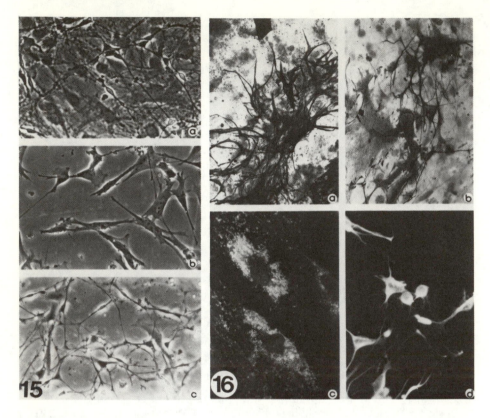

Fig. 15. a) Glial cell cultures derived from dissociated newborn mouse cerebral hemisphere: A 15-day primary culture (P_0) under phase contrast. Dark process-bearing cells (oligo-dendrocytes) are seen on top of the flat background cells (astrocytes and connective tissue cells). ×470. b) "Flat" cell cultures derived from 18-mo-old mouse cerebral hemispheres: 9-day culture under phase contrast. ×470. c) Glial cell cultures derived from 18-mo-old mouse cerebral hemispheres: 14-day primary culture (P_0) under phase contrast. Primarily process-bearing cells and flat background cells are seen. ×470 (from Vernadakis et al., 1984).

Fig. 16. a) GFA-positive cells from dissociated newborn mouse cerebral hemispheres, passage 3, 22 days in culture. ×1,860. b) GFA-positive cells from dissociated aged mouse (18 mo) cerebral hemispheres, passage 2, 11 days in culture. ×1,900. c) GPDH-rhodamine-positive cells from dissociated newborn mouse cerebral hemispheres, passage 4, 8 days in culture. ×2,700. d) GPDH-rhodamine-positive cells from dissociated aged (18 mo) mouse cerebral hemispheres, passage 5, 25 days in culture. ×1,900 (from Vernadakis et al., 1984).

describe two distinct morphologies in early cultures: process-bearing cells with small rounded perikarya and very large flattened cells with a readily discernible nuclei. By 3 weeks in culture, 90% of the GFA-stained cells adopted a flattened morphology, and after 4 or more weeks in culture,

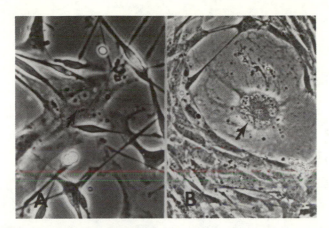

Fig. 17.   Phase contrast photomicrographs of cultures prepared from mouse cerebral hemi-spheres. Cells were from late passage (P10 or P11) and were grown on the floor of plastic culture petri dish. A) Cultures from newborn mouse, cell passage 10, 24 days in culture. B) Cultures from aged mouse (18 mo), cell passage 11, 24 days in culture. Arrow indicates multinucleated cell. × 500 (from Vernadakis et al., 1986).

process-bearing cells were virtually absent. In our cultures, flat epithelioid cells, as described by Lindsay et al. (1982), were observed on the plastic floor of the culture dish. Meller and Waelsch (1984) have recently reported cyclic morphological changes of glial cells in long-term cultures of rat brain. After four subcultures and 8–10 weeks of cultivation, the following cell types could be distinguished: 1) flat epithelioid cells proposed to be precursors of 2) astroglial GFA-positive cells, and 3) oligodendroglia. After 6 weeks, the most prominent cells were the flat epithelioid cells. Our findings also show that with cell passage, the appearance of flat epithelioid cells increases.

The biochemical characterization of the cultures revealed some interesting differences between cells derived from newborn and aged mouse brain (Figs. 18–21). In cultures derived from newborn mouse cerebral hemispheres, CNP activity increased and remained rather constant with cell passage (Figs. 18, 19). In contrast, in cultures derived from aged mouse cerebral hemispheres, CNP increased at P2, decreased at P4, and remained at that level at all subsequent cell passages. Thus, the responsiveness of CNP-containing glia, presumptively oligodendrocytes, to cell passage remained more or less constant. In contrast, the changes in GS activity with cell passage were dramatic (Figs 20, 21). This marked GS activity coincided temporarily with the appearance of large polyhedral multinucleated cells (Fig. 17). Lapham (1962) has reported that in reactive protoplasmic astrocytosis, there is an

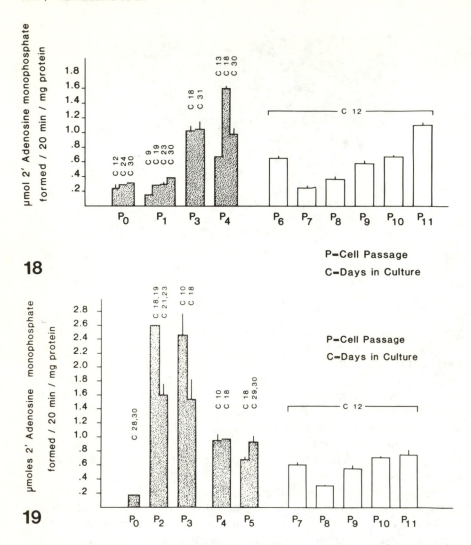

Fig. 18. Cyclic nucleotide phosphohydrolase activity in glial cell cultures. Cells were dissociated from newborn mouse cerebral hemispheres and used either as primary cultures passage 0 (P_0) or passaged cultures (passages 1 to 11). Data for passaged P_0 to P_{4-5} were from Vernadakis et al., 1984 and are presented here for comparison to P_{6-11}. Points with lines represent the mean ± S.E. for three to five cultures.

Fig. 19. As in Figure 18 except that cells were dissociated from aged mouse (18 mo) cerebral hemispheres.

increased number of nuclei without increased proliferation and proposes that nuclear division in reactive protoplasmic astrocytes may have a special adaptive significance with greater functional capacity.

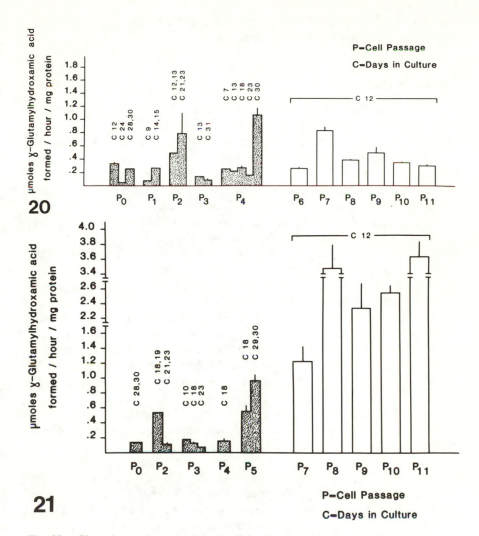

Fig. 20.   Glutamine synthetase activity in glial cell culture. Details as in Figure 18.
Fig. 21.   As in Figure 20 except that cells were dissociated from aged mouse (18 mo) cerebral hemispheres.

In our study, multinucleated cells may be GS-containing glial cells and in culture there may be a shift in the astrocyte population with a decline in GFA-positive cells and an increase in GS-containing cells; this possibility remains to be explored. Based on our glioma studies (Parker et al., 1980) and also studies by Raff et al. (1983) and Hallermayer and Hamprecht (1984) showing shifting of glial types in culture, it is conceivable that in our study the decline in GFA-positive glial cells and the increase in GS activity represent a shift toward GS-containing glial and other cells (to be identified), reflecting a phenomenon of cellular aging.

CONCLUSIONS

The research findings reported here show that using specific glial markers, one can study the influence of the microenvironment on the development and aging of glial cells in culture. Glial cells in culture undergo developmental changes similar to those observed in vivo. Moreover, both astrocytes and oligodendrocytes show differential responsiveness to the microenvironmental inputs such as nutrients, humoral substances secreted by neuronal and non-neuronal cells, and cell surface-mediated interactions.

It appears that oligodendrocytes are dependent at least in part on neuronal input, as shown by enhanced oligodendrocyte growth and differentiation by neuron-conditioned medium or the presence of neurons in culture. Conversely, oligodendrocyte growth is markedly low in cultures lacking neurons, and this is evident both in cultures derived from embryonic or newborn nervous tissue and from adult tissue.

In contrast to oligodendrocytes, astrocytes do not appear to be dependent on neuronal input, and, in fact, substrata of neuron-enriched alive culture or neuron-conditioned medium inhibit astrocyte growth. However astrocyte growth is greatly enhanced by nutrients in fetal calf serum as shown by increased GS activity with progressively increasing concentration of fetal calf serum in the culture medium.

A cell-cell relationship is also apparent in the influence of astrocytes to enhance oligodendrocyte growth and differentiation and may be mediated through an astrocyte-secreted factor.

Glial cell aging appears to occur in culture. There is a decline in oligodendrocytic growth and a shift in the types of astrocytes, thus assimilating glial cell changes reported with aging in vivo. More specifically, the marked increase in GS-containing astrocytes can be interpreted to reflect "gliosis" in vitro and to assimilate the phenomenon of "gliosis" in vivo. We suggest that gliosis may be a glial aging phenomenon reflecting a compensatory response of glial cells to neuronal loss in vivo and absence of neurons in culture.

ACKNOWLEDGMENTS

This chapter is dedicated to the Developmental Psychobiology Research Group of the Department of Psychiatry, University of Colorado School of Medicine that has generously supported our experimental work on glial cells.

REFERENCES

Adler R, Varon S (1981): Neurite guidance of polyornithine-attached materials of ganglionic origin. Dev Biol 81:1–11.

Aguayo A, Charron L, Brag G (1976): Potential of Schwann cells from unmyelinated nerved to produce myelin: A quantitative ultrastructural and radiographic study. J Neurocytol 5:565–573.

Bansal K, Pfeiffer SE (1985): Developmental expression of 2′,3′-cyclic nucliotide 3′-phosphohydrolase in dissociated fetal rat brain cultures and rat brain. J Neurosci Res 14:21–34.

Bhat S, Pfeiffer SE (1985): Stimulation of oligodendrocytes by extracts from astrocyte-enriched cultures. J Neurosci Res 15:19–27.

Bignami A, Dahl D (1977): Specificity of the glial fibrillary acidic protein for astroglia. J Histochem Cytochem 25:466–469.

Bologa L (1985): Oligodendrocytes, key cells in myelination and target in demyelinating diseases. J Neurosci Res 14:1–20.

Bologa L, Aizenman Y, Chiappelli F, de Vellis J (1986): Regulation of myelin basic protein in oligodendrocytes by a soluble neuronal factor. J Neurosci Res 15:521–528.

Bologa L, Bisconte JC, Joubert R, Marangos PJ, Derbin C, Rioux F, Herschkowitz N (1982a): Accelerated differentiation of oligodendrocytes in neuronal rich embryonic mouse brain cell cultures. Brain Res 252:129–136.

Bologa L, Joubert R, Bisconte JC, Margules S, Deugnier MA, Derbin C, Herschkowitz N (1983): Development of immunonologically identified brain cells in cultures: Quantitative aspects. Exp Brain Res 53:163–167.

Bologa L, Siegrist HP, Z'graggen A, Hofmann K, Wiesmann U, Dahl D, Herschkowitz N (1981): Expression of antigenic markers during the development of oligodendrocytes in mouse brain cell cultures. Brain Res 210:217–229.

Bologa L, Z'graggen A, Rossi E, Herschkowitz N (1982b): Differentiation and proliferation: Two possible mechanisms for the regeneration of oligodendrocytes in cultures. J Neurol Sci 57:419–434.

Booher G, Sensenbrenner M (1972): Growth and cultivation of dissociated neurons and glial cells from embryonic chick, rat and human in flask cultures. Neurobiology 2:97–105.

Bottenstein JE (1985): Growth and differentiation of neural cells in defined media. In Bottenstein JE, Sato G (eds): "Cell Culture in the Neurosciences." New York: Plenum, pp 3–43.

Breen GAM, de Vellis J (1974): Regulation of glycerol phosphate dehydrogenase by hydrocortisone in dissociated rat cerebral cell cultures. Dev Biol 41:255–266.

Breen GAM, McGinnis JF, de Vellis J (1978): Modulation of the hydrocortisone induction of glycerol phosphate dehydrogenase by N^6,O^2-dibutyryl cyclic AMP, norepinephrine, and isobutylmethylxanthine in rat brain cell cultures. J Biol Chem 253:2554–2562.

Bunge RP (1968): Glial cells and the central myelin sheath. Physiol Rev 48:197–251.

Ciment G, de Vellis J (1982): Cell surface-mediated cellular interactions: Effects of B1O4 neuroblastoma surface determinants on C6 glioma cellular properties. J Neurosci Res 7:371–386.

de Vellis J (1973): Mechanisms of enzymatic differentiation in the brain and in cultured cells. In Rockstein M, Sussman ML (eds): "Development and Aging of the Nervous System." New York: Academic Press, pp 171–198.

Estin C, Vernadakis A (1986): Primary glial cells and brain fibroblasts: Interactions in culture. Brain Res Bull 16:723–731.

Fishman PH, Brady RO (1976): Biosynthesis and function of gangliosides: Gangliosides appear to participate in the transmission of membrane-mediated information. Science 194:906–915, 1976.

Gospodarowicz D, Vlodasky I, Savion N (1981): The role of fibroblast growth factor and the extracellular matrix in the control of proliferation and differentiation of corneal endothelial cells. Vision Res 21:87–103.

Grobstein C (1968): Developmental significance of interface materials in epithelio-mesenchymal interaction. In Fleischmajer R and Billingham RE (eds): "Epithelial-Mesenchymal Interactions." Baltimore: Williams & Wilkins, pp 173–176.

Hallermayer K, Hamprecht B (1984): Cellular heterogenicity in primary cultures of brain cells revealed by immunocytochemical localization of glutamine synthetase. Brain Res 295:1–11.

Hawrot E (1980): Cultured sympathetic neurons: Effects of cell-derived and sympathetic substrata on survival and development. Dev Biol 65:136–151.

Igarashi Y, Yaoi Y (1975): Growth-enhancing protein obtained from cell surface of culture fibroblasts. Nature 254:248–250.

Kaji K, Matsuo K (1981): Aging of chick embryo fibroblasts in vitro. V. Time course studies on polyploid nucleus accumulation. Exp Cell Res 131:410–412.

Kato T, Fukui Y, Turriff DE, Nakagawa S, Lim R, Arnason BCW, Tanaka R (1981): Glia maturation factor in bovine brain: Partial purification and physiochemical characterization. Brain Res 212:393–402.

Kurihara T, Tsukada Y (1967): The regional and subcellular distribution of 2',3'-cyclic nucleotide 3'-phosphohydrolase in the central nervous system. J Neurochem 14:1167–1174.

Kurihara T, Tsukada Y (1968): 2',3'-Cyclic nucleotide 3'-phosphohydrolase in the developing chick brain and spinal cord. J Neurochem 15:827–832.

Lapham LW (1962): Cytological and cytochemical studies of neuroglia in a study of the problem of amitosis in reactive protoplasmic astrocytes. Am J Pathol 41:1–21.

Lawrence TS, Beers WM, Gilula NB (1978): Transmission of hormonal stimulation by cell-to-cell communication. Nature 272:501–506.

Lim R (1980): Glia maturation factor. Curr Top Dev Biol 16:305–322.

Lim R, Mitsunobu K, Li WKP (1973): Maturation-stimulated effect of brain extract and dibutyryl cyclic AMP on dissociated embryonic brain cells in culture. Exp Cell Res 79:243–246.

Lindsay RM, Barber PC, Sherwood MRC, Zimmer J, Raisman G (1982): Astrocyte cultures from adult rat brain: Derivation, characterization and neurotrophic properties of pure astroglial cells from corpus callosum. Brain Res 243:329–343.

Marangos PJ, Zomzely-Neurath C, Luk DCM, York C (1975): Isolation and characterization of the nervous system specific protein 14-3-2 from rat brain. J Biol Chem 250:1884–1891.

Matsuo M, Kaji K, Utakoji T, Hosoda D (1982): Ploidy of human embryonic fibroblasts during in vitro aging. J Gerontol 37:33–37.

McCarthy KD, Partlow LM (1976a): Neuronal stimulation of ^{3}H-thymidine incorporation by primary cultures of highly purified non-neuronal cells. Brain Res 114:415–426.

McCarthy KD, Partlow L (1976b): Preparation of pure neuronal and non-neuronal cultures form embryonic chick eympathetic ganglia: A new method based on both differential cell adhesiveness and the formation of homotypic neuronal aggregates. Brain Res 114:391–414.

McGinnis JF, de Vellis J (1974): Purification and characterization of rat brain glycerol phosphate dehydrogenase. Biochem Biophys Acta 364:17–27.

Meller K, Waelsch M (1984): Cyclic morphological changes of glial cells in long-term cultures of rat brain. J Neurocytol 13:29–47.

Monard D, Solomon F, Rentsch M, Gysin R (1973): Glial-induced morphological differentiation in neuroblastoma cells. Proc Natl Acad Sci USA 70:1894–1897.

Noble M, Murray K (1984): Purified astrocytes promote the in vitro division of a bipotential glial progenitor cell. EMBO J 3:2243–2247.

Norenberg MD, Martinez-Hernandez A (1979): Fine structural localization of glutamine synthetase in astrocytes of rat brain. Brain Res 161:303–310.

Overton J (1978): Differential response of embryonic cells to culture on tissue matrices. Tissue Cell 11:89–98.

Parker KP, Norenberg MD, Vernadakis A (1980): Transdifferentiation of C6 glial cells in culture. Science 208:179–181.

Pettman B, Delaunoy JP, Courageot J, Devilliers G, Sensenbrenner M (1980): Rat brain glial cells in culture: Effects of brain extracts on the development of oligodendroglial-like cells. Dev Biol 75:278–287.

Poduslo SE (1975): The isolation and characterization of a plasma membrane and myelin fraction derived from oligodendroglia of calf brain. J Neurochem 24:647–664.

Poduslo SE, Norton WT (1972): Isolation and some chemical properties of oligodendroglia from calf brain. J Neurochem 19:727–736.

Pruss KM, Barlett PF, Gavrilovai J, Lisak RP, Rattray S (1981): Mitogens for glial cells: A comparison of the response of cultured astrocytes, oligodendrocytes and Schwann cells. Dev Brain Res 2:19–35.

Privat A, Valat J, Fulcrand J (1981): Proliferation of neuroglial cell lines in the degenerating optic nerve of young rats: Radioautographic study. J Neuropathol Exp Neurol 40:46–60.

Raff MC, Miller RH, Nobel M (1983): A glial progenitor cell that develops in vitro into an astrocyte or an oligodendrocyte depending on culture media. Nature 303:390–399.

Raff MC, Mirsky R, Fields KL, Lisak RP, Dorfman SH, Silbergerg DH, Gregson NA, Leibowitz S, Kennedy MC (1978): Galactocerebroside is a specific cell-surface antigenic marker for oligodendrocytes in culture. Nature 274:813–816.

Revel JP, Brown SS (1975): Cell junction in development, with particular reference to the neural tube. Cold Spring Harbor Symposia Quant Biol 40:443–455.

Riepe RE, Norenberg MD (1977): Muller cell localization of glutamine synthetase in rat retina: An immunohistochemical study. Nature 268:654–655.

Rojkind M, Gatmetan Z, Mackensen S, Giambrone H, Ponce P, Reid LM (1980): Connective tissue biomatrix: Its isolation and utilization for long-term cultures of normal rat hepatocytes. J Cell Biol 87:255–263.

Roussel G, Sensenbrenner M, Labourdette G, Wittendorp-Rechenmann E, Pettman B, Nussbaum JL (1983): An immunohistochemical study of two myelin-specific proteins in enriched oligodendroglial cells combined with an autoradiographic investigation using ^{3}H-thymidine. Dev Brain Res 8:193–204.

Sakellaridis N, Bau D, Mangoura D, Vernadakis A (1983): Developmental profiles of glial enzymes in the chick embryo: In vivo and in culture. Neurochem Intern 5:685–690.

Sakellaridis N, Mangoura D, Vernadakis A (1986): Effects of neuron-conditioned medium and fetal calf serum content on glial growth in dissociated cultures. Dev Brain Res 27:31–41.

Sakellaridis N, Mangoura D, Vernadakis A (1984): Glial cell growth in culture: Influence of living substrata. Neurochem Res 9:1477–1491.

Sensenbrenner M, Barakat I, Delaunoy JP, Labourdette G, Pettman B (1982): Influence of brain extracts on nerve cell development. In Pfeiffer SE (ed): "Neuroscience Approached Through Cell Culture," Vol. 1. Boca Raton, Fla.: CRC Press, pp 87–105.

Sternberger NH, Itoyana Y, Kies MW, de F Webster H (1978): Myelinic basic protein demonstrated immunocytochemically in oligodendroglia prior to myelin sheath formation. Proc Natl Acad Sci USA 75:2521–2524.

Strehler RL (1977): "Time Cells and Aging." New York: Academic Press.

Varon S, Adler R, Manthorpe M, Skaper S (1983): Culture strategies for trophic and other factors directed to nerve cells. In Pfeiffer SE (ed): "Neuroscience Approached Through Cell Culture." West Palm Beach, Fla.: CRC Press, pp 53–77.

Vernadakis A, Davies D, Sakellaridis N, Mangoura D (1986): Growth patterns of glial cells dissociated from newborn and aged mouse brain with cell passage. J Neurosci Res 15:79–85.

Vernadakis A, Mangoura D, Sakellaridis N, Linderholm S (1984): Glial cells dissociated from newborn and aged mouse brain. J Neurosci Res 11:253–262.

Vernadakis A, Parker K, Arnold EB, Norenberg MD (1982): Role of glial cells in CNS aging. In Giacobini E, Giacobini G, Filogamo G, Vernadakis A (eds): "The Aging Brain: Cellular and Molecular Mechanisms of Aging in the Nervous System." New York: Raven Press, pp 57–68.

Vernadakis A, Sakellaridis N (1985): Role of glial cells in neurotransmission mechanisms. In Parvez H, Parvez S, Gupta D (eds): "Progress in Neuroendocrinology." Vol. 1. VNU Science Press, The Netherlands, pp 17–44.

Weinberg H, Spencer P (1976): Studies on the control of myelinogenesis. II. Evidence for neuronal regulation of myelin production. Brain Res 113:363–378.

Weiss L, Poste G, Mackearmin A, Willet K (1975): Growth of mammalian cells on substrates coated with cellular microexudate. J Cell Biol 64:135–145.

Wernicke JF, Volpe JJ (1986): Glial differentiation in dissociated cell cultures on neonatal rat brain: Noncoordinate and density-dependent regulation of oligodendroglial enzymes. J Neurosci Res 15:39–47.

Wood P, Bunge R (1975): Evidence that sensory axons are mitogenic for Schwann cells. Nature 256:662–664.

Wood P, Okada E, Bunge R (1980): The use of networks of dissociated rat dorsal root ganglion neurons to induce myelination by oligodendrocytes in culture. Brain Res 196:247–252.

Wood DM, Williams AD (1984): Oligodendrocyte proliferation and CNS myelination in cultures containing dissociated embryonic neuroglia and dorsal root ganglia neurons. Dev Brain Res 12:225–241.

Yaffe D (1973): Rat skeletal muscle cells. In Kruse PF, Patterson MM (eds): "Tissue Culture: Methods and Applications." New York: Academic Press, pp 106–114.

Yaoi Y, Kanaseki T (1972): Role of microexudate carpet in cell division. Nature 237:283–285.

Current Topics in Nutrition and Disease, Volume 16
Basic and Clinical Aspects of Nutrition and Brain Development,
pages 99–130
© *1987 Alan R. Liss, Inc.*

Cerebellar Development and Nutrition

Francesco Vitiello and Giorgio Gombos

Istituto di Fisiologia Umana, Facoltà di Medicina e Chirurgia, Bari, Italy
(F.V.) and Centre de Neurochimie du CNRS, 5 Rue Blaise Pascal, 67000
Strasbourg, France (G.G.)

INTRODUCTION

There is no longer any doubt that a quantitative deficit or a qualitative
unbalance of food intake produces alterations in the nervous system ontogeny
and function. Often the nutritional unbalance is associated with other factors
which also have negative effects on central nervous system (CNS) development; thus, the distinction between lesions produced by malnutrition and
lesions produced by these concurrent factors sometimes proves to be
difficult. A further element, to consider when we compare published data,
concerns differences in experimental designs in studies on experimentally
induced malnutrition or undernutrition. Taking all this into account, we can,
however, still establish some general principles:

1) The type and extent of the nutritionally produced lesion and the cellular
elements involved depend upon the qualitative and quantitative departure
from optimal nutrition, its duration, the stage in the life span when it is
applied, and the region of CNS considered (Vitiello et al., 1980; Balàzs et
al., 1986). Though we now know a good deal about these CNS alterations,
we do not yet have a precise picture of the specificity of CNS alterations in
relation to the chronology of the nutritional deficit.

2) At present, functional deficits can be correlated with morphological
alterations only in some cases, since relationships between structure and
function in brain are not always well defined and a single morphological
structure cannot always be identified as the "structure" essential for a certain
function. In this context the crucial questions are the following: Will we be
able to correlate all the functional alterations with the morphological and
biochemical modifications, vis-à-vis elementary physiology and complex
behavior? Are all the morphological alterations detectable? The
neuropathological findings in the CNS of nutritionally deprived animals very
rarely show focal lesions. Thus, it is possible that undernutrition produces
diffuse, often imperceptible, anatomical changes and deficits throughout the
entire brain, the functional consequences of which are not easy to predict.

3) Some morphological and/or biochemical alterations can be at least partially prevented and sometimes corrected; others cannot. Similarly, some functional deficits, but not all, appear to be reversible.

Can all the alterations be made reversible and how? For practical therapeutic reasons, it would be interesting to know exactly when and how we should intervene to repair or prevent the lesions produced by the malnutrition, i.e., if we knew precisely when (vulnerable period) and how the major brain damage is provoked by malnutrition we could hopefully protect the brain by short-term therapeutic intervention.

In almost all the experimental studies, nutritional deprivation is imposed during early life (prenatally or postnatally), thus leaving unanswered the question whether non-lethal starvation can alter structure, composition, and function of an already normally developed brain. While we cannot rule out the possibility that other less evident alterations of the CNS can be provoked by severe malnutrition in adult brain, in general a nutritional deficit appears to be particularly harmful when it occurs during phases of maximal rate of CNS development. Evidently at this stage the vulnerable situations are either very frequent or a single developmental phase is particularly vulnerable, possibly because the number of damaged cells is very high.

Malnutrition could affect different CNS developmental processes: either cell multiplication or cell migration or cell differentiation and maturation. Interference with any of these phenomena could have long-lasting effects by altering synaptogenesis and, hence, the formation of neuronal circuits. Plasticity phenomena or compensatory mechanisms, however, could also produce functional restoration. In addition, CNS development is an asynchronous, non-linear phenomenon, and the different developmental processes occur at different times and at different rates in different regions. This is why the specific effects of malnutrition on each CNS developmental phase are better studied in a relatively simple, and "homogeneous," experimental model (i.e. a region of the brain where the effects on different phases of cell formation, multiplication, migration, differentiation and maturation, and histogenesis can be easily distinguished).

Alterations of the whole CNS following nutritional deficits have been extensively and recently reviewed (Vitiello et al., 1980; Balàzs et al., 1986). This chapter will focus on a single CNS region with a comprehensive view of its normal development and of that altered by malnutrition.

We have chosen rodent cerebellum because studies on structural alterations during ontogeny are greatly facilitated by its "simple" cytoarchitecture and because its morphology in the adult and during development is well known. In addition, cerebellar ontogeny in rodents mostly occurs after birth (see below); this is a considerable technical advantage when external noxae are applied to alter a developmental pattern permitting comparison of different methods for producing the nutritional imbalance and affording the possibility of precisely selecting the periods of undernutrition and of rehabilitation. From the biochemical point of view, chemical events can be more easily correlated with morphological processes in cerebellum than in other CNS regions because cerebellum is much more homogeneous in cellular composition than the rest of the brain.

NORMAL RAT CEREBELLUM
The Adult Cerebellum

The adult cerebellar cortex (folium) consists of three layers, the molecular layer, the Purkinje cell (Pc) layer, and the granular layer, and contains six neuronal types (Ramon y Cajal, 1911; Palay and Chan-Palay, 1974). Pc is the principal neuronal type. Four other cell types are interneurons of the folium: Golgi neurons (Gn) and granule cells which are located in the granular layer, basket and stellate cells which are located in the molecular layer. The sixth neuronal cell type, the Lugaro cell, is rare.

Cells were counted around fissure E in the vermis (the fissure between lobes V and VI separating the anterior part of vermis from the posterior) in 35-day-old "normal" cerebella (Clos et al., 1977), i.e., when the adult cellular composition of the folium appears established. Of the cells, 80% are neurons and, of these, granule cells account for 85%, while inhibitory interneurons (stellate cells and basket cells) and macroneurons (Pc and Gn) represent about 5%; deep cerebellar nuclei neurons (DCNN) account for no more than 1% of the neuronal population. Thus, the granule cell is the most abundant cell type in adult cerebellum. In the rat, for each Pc there are, on the average, around 300 granule cells (but only 0.3 Gn and 0.6–1 stellate and basket cells) (Clos et al., 1977). The granule cell axons, the so-called parallel fibers, form synapses with the dendritic spines of all the other interneurons and with those of a row of Pc (whose dendritic tree is arranged in a single plane perpendicular to the axis of the folium). Stellate cells form synapses with the Pc dendritic shaft, while basket cells form synapse with the Pc soma and axonal hillock. Each Gn forms a local circuit which does not directly include Pc, since it receives input from parallel fibers and sends its axon to the granule cell dendrites within the glomeruli. (Glomeruli are junctional complexes which include granule cell dendrites, Gn axons, and mossy fiber terminals; see below.)

Input into the folium follows two major fiber systems: the so-called climbing fibers, which originate in the inferior olive and establish synapses with Pc dendrites (one climbing fiber per Pc), and the so-called mossy fibers, which mostly consist of terminals (rosettes) of spinocerebellar and pontocerebellar projections and which terminate in the glomeruli. Additional input is given by monoamine-containing axons which originate from neurons in the locus ceruleus, raphe nuclei, and substantia nigra, (Hökfelt and Fuxe, 1969; Bloom et al., 1971; Hoffer et al., 1973).

Pc axons are responsible for the whole output of the cerebellar cortex; they have collateral recurrent branches which reach Pc somata and neurons in the granular layer, while the main axons make synapses with DCNN except in the vestibulocerebellum where they terminate directly on neurons of the vestibular nucleus in the brain stem. Thus, the cerebellar output from vestibulocerebellum is via Pc axons and that from the rest of cerebellum is via DCNN axons.

The cerebellar glial population consists of oligodendrocytes (which are abundant in white matter and are also present in granular and Pc layers) and of protoplasmic and fibrillar astrocytes. Protoplasmic astrocytes with characteristic morphology are the "velate astrocytes" in the granular layer and the so-called Golgi epithelial cells, satellites cells of Pc. The so-called Bergmann fibers, which cross the molecular layer and terminate under the pia mater (Palay and Chan-Palay, 1974), are long processes of Golgi epithelial cells. Glial cells account for 10% of the folium cell population, the Golgi epithelial cells and the astrocytes of the granular layer account for about one-half of these, the remaining cells being the so-called satellite oligodendrocytes (Clos et al., 1977). In the white matter, only two cellular types are found (besides endothelial elements): oligodendrocytes and astrocytes (mostly fibrous astrocytes). They are present in a proportion of six cells (four oligodendrocytes and two astrocytes) for each Pc (Clos et al., 1977). The cellular composition of white matter does not vary from the 35th to the 160th postnatal day.

Cerebellar Development

In different vertebrates the development of cerebellum proceeds with a similar sequence of events but at different rates. The developmental stage of the organ at birth in different species can be correlated with the capacity for locomotion and motor coordination of the newborn of the species. In precocial animals (such as chick and guinea pig), the cerebellum is well developed at birth, whereas in atricial animals (such as rodents and man), which are helpless at birth, cerebellum is immature and its histogenesis and morphogenesis mainly occur during postnatal life. Birth by itself apparently does not trigger the postnatal events of cerebellar ontogeny, since in rats in which gestation is prolonged for 3 days beyond its normal duration, these events occur at the usual time counted from the day of fecundation (Zagon, 1975).

The times and sites of origin of cerebellar glial and nerve cells, their migration routes to specific positions in the cortex, their patterns of differentiation and growth, and their synaptogenesis have been described in a variety of species, ranging from frogs to primates. This review will be restricted to the development of rodent cerebellum, but it is reasonable to assume that the major steps in cerebellar neurogenesis are similar in most mammalians.

Prenatal cerebellar development. Cerebellum originates from a bilateral eminence in the metencephalon, the so-called cerebellar plate, which, in the rat, is clearly recognizable at the 13th embryonal day (ED) and by ED 15 becomes larger and more clearly separated from the underlying zone. In the ventricular germinal zone (the deepest region of the cerebellar plate), the differentiation of DCNN begins on ED 13 and ED 14. From ED 15 and ED 16, a second wave of differentiation involves cells which are situated beneath the DCNN zone and which, from ED 17 on, mature into Pc. Immediately before birth three major events occur (Altman, 1982): 1) cells migrate from the primitive neuroepithelium of the rhombic lip over the surface of the cerebellar plate to form the external germinal layer (EGL); 2) Pc precursors migrate across the DCNN zone towards the cerebellar plate surface; and 3) starting from ED 19, the neuroblasts which will differentiate into Gn are formed. The EGL arises on ED 17 and then spreads rostrally reaching the anterior pole of the cerebellum by ED 20–ED 21. At the same time, immature Pc perykaria position themselves beneath the EGL. At birth (which occurs after a 21-day gestation) only around 3% of the cells found in adult cerebellum are already present (Balàzs et al., 1971; Gombos et al., 1980), and the only postmitotic neurons present are the Pc, Gn, and DCNN (Altman, 1972a).

Postnatal cerebellar development. In newborn rat, the cerebellar cortex consists of the EGL, a thin band of fibers, and a multicellular layer composed of immature Pc and Gn. In addition, the Golgi epithelial cells which were formed perinatally (Del Cerro and Swarz, 1976; Clos et al., 1979) and a few other cells that can be identified as glial are present (Ghandour et al., 1980b, 1981).

During the first week of postnatal life, Pc move to form a single row, due to the fact, according to Altman (1982), that the first migrating granule cells (see below) "squeeze" (between their somata and their parallel fibers) the multicellular arrangement of Pc until these cells are aligned in a single layer. In fact, when the formation of the earliest granule cells is inhibited by either X-rays or viruses or anti-mitotics applied at the earliest postnatal ages, Pc remain positioned in multicellular arrangements (Altman, 1982). Pc axons are already present at the time of birth, while the axonal collaterals which spread transversally to the cell bodies of neighboring Purkinje cells develop shortly after birth. The formation of the apical growth cone starts on PD 4–5 and continues throughout the second week when primary dendrites begin to form in the molecular layer. During the first postnatal week, climbing fibers make "early synapses" with the perisomatic processes on PC soma. These "early synapses" disappear by PD 7–8, and the definitive synapses between climbing fibers and the "stubby spines" on Pc dendrites are formed. In the third postnatal week, the dendritic tree of the Pc continues to branch, secondary and tertiary dendrites develop, and the parallel fibers begin to make synapses with the dendritic spines (spiny branchlets) in the molecular layer.

The formation of synapses between climbing fibers and Pc dentrites is accompanied by a weeding out of redundant climbing fibers until only one fiber per Pc remains. Pc axon recurrent branches go through a similar reduction.

The other prenatally formed neurons of the folium derived from the ventricular germinal zone are the Gn, which, in rodent cerebellum, differentiate very slowly throughout the first 30 postnatal days (Miale and Sidman, 1961).

Granule, stellate, and basket cells develop from the stem cells of the EGL. The histogenesis of interneurons in the EGL has been described in chick (Mugnaini and Forströnen, 1967), mouse (Miale and Sidman, 1961), rat (Altman, 1972a,b,c), cat (Purpura et al., 1964), monkey (Kornguth et al., 1967, 1968), and human (Rakic and Sidman, 1970; Friede, 1973). In all vertebrates the proliferation of the external germinal cells increases the EGL thickness from a monocellular layer to a layer six to eight cells deep. The EGL persists for a period depending on the species. In rat and mouse, for example, it disappears 20–21 days after birth, i.e., at the time of weaning.

In rat, granule cells are formed throughout the period of cell proliferation (i.e., from day 0 to the 21st PD), but most of them are formed during the second postnatal week. Similarly, basket and stellate cells are mostly formed between PD 6–8 and 8–11, respectively. The newly formed interneurons migrate toward the depth of the folium. Basket and stellate cells remain in the molecular layer, while granule cells go deeper, probably using Bergmann glia processes as a guide (Rakic, 1971), cross the Purkinje cell layer, and reach the internal granular layer (IGL).

Granule cell migration is a special type of cell migration, which we may define as "growth-migration." It lasts about 2 days and during this period, the morphology of the cell undergoes striking changes (Altman, 1982). In the deepest part of the EGL granule, cells are bipolar, with two processes oriented parallel to the surface of the folia (this will be the arrangement of the mature parallel fibers), but then a third cytoplasmic process grows vertically from the cell down into the molecular layer, and the nucleus migrates into the process. Thus, the cell becomes T-shaped, and the parallel fibers, as they develop, are stacked in the molecular layer. When the granule cell reaches its position in the IGL, its dendrites establish synapses with the presynaptic partner, the mossy fiber, as described by Larramendi (1969) and Hàmori and Somogyi (1983). Almost simultaneously, the parallel fibers make synapses with the dendritic spines in the molecular layer. From the arrangement of the granule cells, it seems that the IGL is formed in an "inside-out" order: the deepest granule cells are generated first and, similarly, each parallel fiber is stacked above those already formed (Altman, 1972b).

The IGL develops (mostly during the first 3 postnatal weeks) with a phase of maximal growth rate during the second week as a result of 1) migration through the Pc layer of the granule cells formed in the EGL and growth and differentiation of their dendrites and 2) proliferation and maturation of glial cells. In the adult, around 60% of the IGL volume consists of cell processes (Paula-Barbosa and Sobrinho-Simoes, 1976).

The development of cerebellar glia is still a matter for discussion. One of the major debates is whether their site of production is in the EGL (Meller and Glees, 1969; Privat, 1975) or in the ventricular germinal zone (Ramon y Cajal, 1911; Swarz and Del Cerro, 1977). In recent years, however, immunocytochemical methods have been used to follow the formation and maturation of distinct astrocytic and oligodendrocytic populations from very early stages to adulthood (for a review see Ghandour et al., 1983). These (Ghandour et al., 1981) and autoradiographic (Swarz and Del Cerro, 1977) data suggest that cerebellar glial cells do not derive from the EGL, but are formed in the periventricular germinal layer. Thus, EGL is a monopotential germinal site where only neuroblasts are formed.

Another characteristic of cerebellum is that gliogenesis and neurogenesis appear to occur simultaneously (Ghandour et al., 1980b, 1981), while in other CNS regions, gliogenesis follows, briefly overlapping, neurogenesis (Ramon y Cajal, 1911; Brizzee et al., 1964). Moreover, both cerebellar astrocytes and oligodendrocytes develop and mature simultaneously. Their proliferation occurs during the first 2 postnatal weeks, with a maximum between PD 4 and 7, while their maturation mostly occurs from PD 7 to 21; the bulk of compact myelin accumulates during the fourth and the fifth postnatal weeks. During the first postnatal week those Golgi epithelial cells (Bergmann glia) which are formed postnatally grow typical perisomatic processes which rapidly increase in number (Del Cerro and Swarz, 1976; Clos et al., 1979). Some of them are reabsorbed; others grow across the molecular layer to reach the pia mater and form the radial "Bergmann fibers." These fibers rapidly differentiate, increase in number and thickness, and grow characteristic "leaf-like appendages" (Palay and Chan-Palay, 1974). Bergmann glia maturation has been schematically divided into six phases (see Clos et al., 1979). At the end of the first week, Bergmann glia form a continuous and "overcrowded" palisade, which is partially remodelled during the following 2 weeks to assume the adult appearance around day 21.

In man, Pc differentiation follows the same pattern as in other mammals, but growth is slower (Zacevic and Rakic, 1976). During the fourth fetal month, Pc are still distributed in multiple rows and become aligned between the 16th and the 28th week of gestation; at the same time they develop their dendritic tree. PC assume their adult form at the end of the first postnatal year. The EGL is still present during the second postnatal year (Dobbing and Sands, 1973).

CEREBELLAR ONTOGENY IN UNDERNOURISHED RATS
Experimental Models of Undernutrition

Since the report by Sugita (1918) (who devised some of the techniques still used to obtain a nutritional unbalance), several methods have been developed for producing food deficiency at different developmental stages (in utero, during the suckling period, after weaning). Rat is the most widely investigated species, probably because the "growth spurt period" (hence the vulnerable phase) of its CNS mainly occurs during postnatal life, facilitating the application of a "direct" (i.e., not mediated by the mother) undernutrition (Dobbing, 1974). Moreover, some regions of the rat CNS (the cerebellum, for example) are very immature at birth; hence it is easier to study the effects of the nutritional deficit on the very early ontogenetic events.

Fetal malnutrition can be produced by feeding pregnant females on diets either deficient in total calories or only in proteins. An early severe malnutrition started from gestational day 7–10 produces a reduction in the number of term pregnancies and an increase in the proportion of stillborn offspring (Zamenhof et al., 1971b), while less extreme restrictions of food intake during the same period are compatible with fetus survival but affect growth of body and brain.

Experimental undernutrition in lactating rats is produced by different methods (or combinations of them) which all aim to reduce the milk available to the pups (either by increasing the number of animals nursed by each mother, or by separating the pups from their mother for part of the day, or by feeding the dams protein- or calorie-restricted diets). More severe food deprivation can be obtained by combining two of these methods (Wiggins et al., 1974). It is generally believed that maternal undernutrition affects the quantity of milk without altering its composition (Mueller and Cox, 1946), but a different milk quality has been also reported (Crnic and Chase, 1978). In some experimental models pre- and postnatal undernutrition is obtained by underfeeding the mothers during pregnancy (starting from the sixth day of gestation) and lactation (Altman et al., 1971; Patel et al., 1973; Clos et al., 1977). Under these conditions the fetus seems relatively spared at the expense of the mother (Smart and Dobbing, 1971), even if there are limits to the protection offered (see below) (Zamenhof et al., 1971a,b).

All these methods probably do not produce a "pure" malnutrition, since in each of them food deficiency is accompanied by the alteration of other environmental factors (i.e., mother-pup interaction or handling of pups during the experiment) which are very important during development (Balàzs et al., 1986). Increasing the litter size, for example, results in decreased mother-pup contact and separating the pups from the mother for part of the day deprives them of social, thermal, and sensory stimulation as well as food. The question has been raised whether an undernourished mother is able to attend to the offspring as carefully as a "normal" mother. Thus, no single model appears to be an exclusively nutritional model and possibly only the comparison of the results obtained with different models may indicate which of the effects is mainly, or solely, attributable to the nutritional deficiency.

Undernutrition after weaning is usually obtained by reducing, to different levels, either the intake of proteins or of proteins and calories together. The first situation is analogous to human kwashiorkor, the second to marasmus.

In this review, we will only discuss malnutrition imposed in the early postnatal and preweaning period since we focused our studies on a part of the CNS which develops mostly during this period. In our hands, regardless of the technique by which malnutrition was imposed, the alterations observed were the same in all cases. This strongly indicates that the crucial factor is not the method for imposing malnutrition but the period at which malnutrition was imposed.

Cerebellar Growth

Malnutrition imposed on pregnant rats starting from gestation day 6 causes weight reduction (wet and dry) of the offspring cerebrum at birth, but does not significantly affect that of cerebellum (Zamenhof et al., 1971a,b). These effects are the same whether malnutrition is produced by a diet deficient in protein and/or an insufficient total calorie intake. If the nutritional deficit is maintained during lactation, the growth impairment also involves cerebellum. This impairment increases with age, and persists even after a 4-month postweaning rehabilitation period started from the fifth postnatal week. Similar effects on rat postnatal cerebellar growth are obtained by imposing the nutritional deficit exclusively after birth and during the suckling period, i.e., during the first 3 or 4 postnatal weeks. The alterations of cerebellar growth are the same whether malnutrition was produced by increasing the number of pups per dam, or by undernourishing the mother, or by removing pups from the mother for several hours each day. In all these cases, the weight gain of cerebellum is significantly impaired, and no recovery occurs on postweaning rehabilitation (Chase et al., 1969; Dobbing et al., 1971). A similar lack of recovery is obtained for hippocampus and cerebral cortex, while other cerebral regions partially or fully recover (Fuller and Wiggins, 1984).

Reduction of cerebellar and cerebral growth is proportionally smaller than the reduction of body growth whether the undernutrition is imposed pre- and postnatally or exclusively postnatally (Brown and Guthrie, 1968).

The growth deficit is roughly the same in all parts of the cerebellum, which, thus, appears uniformly smaller than in normal animals, with a normal foliation index, giving the fallacious impression of a small-for-age, but otherwise normal, organ. In contrast, other conditions which alter cerebellar ontogeny, such as dysthyroidisms, affect the different cerebellar lobules to a different extent.

Postweaning (in contrast to preweaning or prenatal) undernutrition has little or no effect on the weight of cerebellum and other cerebral regions (Winick and Noble, 1966).

Cerebellar Cell Proliferation and Final Cell Composition

Cell formation (or cell accumulation) in the cerebellum can be followed by measuring its DNA content (Balàzs et al., 1971; Gombos et al., 1980).

At birth the DNA content of rat cerebellum is around 3% of the adult value. In agreement with morphological data (Altman, 1972a), DNA in normal animals increases slowly until PD 7 and then rapidly during the second postnatal week; the adult value is attained between PD 16 and PD 21 (Balàzs et al., 1971; Gourdon et al., 1973; Vitiello et al., 1985a).

In cerebella from undernourished animals the pattern is similar but DNA content is lower throughout development (Gourdon et al., 1973; Patel et al., 1973; Vitiello et al., 1985c) and remains lower even after postweaning nutritional rehabilitation (Dobbing et al., 1971; Vitiello et al., 1985c). During the first 3 postnatal weeks DNA concentration per gram of wet tissue is lower than in controls, but it slowly comes back to normal values by day 21 (Gourdon et al., 1973), indicating that, in undernourished animals, the smaller size (weight) of the adult cerebellum is mostly due to reduction of its cell number (DNA).

The severe and permanent deficit in cerebellar cell number (about 25% as compared with controls) is the same whether the nutritional deficit is imposed during the prenatal life or only after birth (Vitiello et al., 1985c).

The rate of DNA synthesis (measured as incorporation of labeled thymidine) is even more reduced (maximal decrease -70 to -80%)

than the final cell number (-25%) (Patel et al., 1973). This could be explained by different mechanisms.

A reduction in the number of germinal cells in the EGL of undernourished rats, probably contributes to this phenomenon (Barnes and Altman, 1973a) but is not sufficient to completely explain it. Another possibility is that cell death, which usually accompanies cell formation during nervous tissue ontogeny (Cowan, 1973), is reduced much more than the reduced mitotic activity. However, this is apparently not the case, since during the whole period of cell proliferation the number of pyknotic figures in the EGL of undernourished rats are proportionally identical or at certain times (i.e., at PD 12), even higher than controls (Lewis, 1975). But a higher number of degenerative figures than in controls is still detected in the ventricular subependymal layer of adult undernourished animals (Lewis et al., 1977), suggesting that in these animals the rate of disappearance of degenerating cells is slowed down (Koppel et al., 1983). Again other possibilities could be that less thymidine is available to brain and/or that the synthesis of thymidine triphosphate is slowed down. This hypothesis can be ruled out since, in undernutrition, the availability of thymidine to brain tissue is normal, and the rate of thymidine nucleotide synthesis is slowed down only slightly and cannot account for the significant decrease in DNA synthesis (Balàzs et al., 1979). So far the most satisfactory explanation is that there is elongation of the S phase (i.e., the phase of DNA synthesis) of the cell cycle. In the proliferating cells of cerebellar EGL (Lewis et al., 1975), the dentate gyrus of the hippocampus, and the lateral ventricle subependymal layer in the forebrain (Lewis et al., 1979) of rats undernourished during lactation, the cell cycle appears to be altered in a particular way: the G_1 phase is curtailed sometimes severely, the G_2 phase, and the whole cell cycle time are normal or, after PD 12, moderately prolonged, while the S phase is lengthened so as to compensate for the shorter G_1 phase.

In the rat, cell multiplication continues in the adult in the subependymal layer of cerebral lateral ventricles. Acute food deprivation or chronic undernutrition in young adult rats (6 weeks old) produces different effects on these cells from those described above, but similar effects as those seen in other tissues. The duration of the whole cell cycle increases by 40–75%, the S phase increases proportionally more (70–85%), but the length of the G_1 phase is either normal (in acute food deprivation) or increased (in chronic undernutrition), but never reduced.

The most interesting aspect of the data summarized above is that they indicate that in rapidly multiplying neural cells, G_1 (i.e., the phase corresponding to the activation of protein synthesis in the newly formed cell) is the phase "vulnerable" to nutritional deficit. An irreversible reduction of protein synthesis in postmitotic neural cells might also explain the smaller-than-normal cells in the CNS of some undernourished animals.

The effect of food deficiency on cell proliferation in the CNS (cerebellum and forebrain) is smaller than in other organs, where both the whole cell cycle and the S phase appear to be markedly prolonged (Deo and Ramalingaswami, 1965).

The deficit in final cell number indicated by the lower DNA content of the undernourished cerebellum does not involve all cell types to the same degree. Cell counts were made around fissure E in the vermis at PD 35, after a pre- and postnatal undernutrition period, and at PD 160, following a 4-month rehabilitation period (Barnes and Altman, 1973b; Clos et al., 1977; Bedi et al., 1980a,b). The results were the following:

Undernutrition (even imposed prenatally) does not affect the total number of the macroneurons of the folium (Pc and Gn). This absence of effect on macroneurons is easily understandable when undernutrition is imposed postnatally (after that these cells are formed [Altman, 1982]), but it is difficult to explain when the food deficit is imposed prenatally, since prenatal food deficit affects forebrain cell multiplication which, for most neurons, occurs prenatally (Dobbing, 1974). Possibly, cell proliferation in prenatal cerebellum is partially spared from the nutritional insult because of mobilization and utilization of nutrients from the mother reserves which are sufficient for the needs of cerebellum (where few cells are formed prenatally) but remain inadequate for those of forebrain (where most of the nerve cells are formed prenatally).

The same conditions of undernutrition greatly altered the proportions of other neuronal types. A 12% decrease of granule cell, a severe reduction (−35%) of basket cell, and no change of stellate cell number have been reported. The most striking observation is the 35% decrease of basket cell number, in contrast to a proportionally smaller reduction of granule cells. Quantitatively, basket cells are not a major neuronal type, but they play a significant role in cortical circuitry, since their axons constitute the principal inhibitory inputs to Pc somata and axonal hillock (Palay and Chan-Palay, 1974). The loss of the equilibrium between excitatory (granule cells and climbing fibers) and inhibitory (basket cells) inputs to the sole efferent pathway from the folium, the Pc, could alter the functional maturation of cerebellum.

The number of all glial cell types in both cortex and white matter is irreversibly reduced by prenatal and postnatal undernutrition, and the deficit is more severe than that of neurons. Golgi epithelial cells and astrocytes in the internal granular layer are decreased by 20 and 25%, respectively, and satellite oligodendrocytes by 60%. In white matter, both the astrocyte and the oligodendrocyte number is lower (70% of controls). Because the glial damage is more severe than that of neurons, the glial/neuronal cell ratio becomes lower (-30%) than in controls at both PD 35 and PD 160.

To our knowledge no data exist on the effects of an exclusively postnatal undernutrition on glial cells, but it is tempting to suggest that in this case Golgi epithelial cells (Bergmann glia), which develop mostly in the perinatal period, would be spared.

Cell Growth and Maturation

Formation of the IGL.   In undernutrition, the chronology of growth is normal. The IGL surface area on cerebellar section, which is slightly reduced compared with controls up to PD 10, becomes normal between PD 10 and 21, but at PD 35 it is again significantly lower than controls. The IGL surface deficit is proportional to the severity of the nutritional insult and does not recover on rehabilitation (Barnes and Altman, 1973b).

The decreased surface area during the early postnatal period could be due to a delay in cell migration, as described in rat olfactory bulb following protein deprivation (Debassio and Kemper, 1985), and the lower IGL surface value at PD 35 could be due to the decreased number of cells (granule and glial cells) formed and to reduced growth of their processes.

Apparently, however, malnutrition and hyponutrition do not affect the direction and the distance or the timing of cell migration in cerebellum, since the presence of "ectopic" granule cells (which could have indicated that granule cells did not migrate correctly) has not been reported. According to the hypothesis of Rakic (1971), granule cells migrate along the Bergmann fibers. If we assume that Rakic's hypothesis is correct, these results indicate that in malnutrition, Golgi epithelial cells and Bergmann fibers, though less abundant and mature than in controls from the end of the first postnatal week, are present in a sufficient number to allow normal granule cell migration. Alternatively, we can hypothesize that the Bergmann glia guiding role is not essential for granule cell migration.

Cell growth and differentiation.   It is generally accepted that in brain, like in other organs, the phase of maximal cell growth rate follows that of cell proliferation. In rodent cerebellum, however, these two phases overlap, probably due to the brief "growth spurt period" of the region and because of the unusual "growth-migration" of the granule cells. In cerebellum, both cell proliferation and maximal cell growth occur from birth to the 21st postnatal day; during this period dramatic changes in cellular and biochemical composition occur. After the end of the proliferative phase, cells continue to mature (morphologically and biochemically), and the cerebellar circuitry is definitively set up by the fourth postnatal week.

The maturation of cerebellar cells has been studied not only by using morphological methods, but also by following the developmental curves of several biochemical parameters of growth and some markers specific for cell types.

Morphogenesis of Purkinje cells. Two excitatory inputs to Pc, the parallel fibers on the spiny branchlets and the climbing fibers on the stubby spines, and one inhibitory input, the stellate cell terminals on the dendritic shaft, converge on the Pc dendritic tree, while inhibitory basket cell terminals make axo-somatic synapses on Pc somata. It is thus conceivable that an alteration in the Pc dendritic branching and/or the establishment of synaptic connections with this part of the cell could be directly relevant to the information processing capacity of the cerebellum.

Several reports on the effects of undernutrition on Pc dendritic branching have appeared (for a review, see Shoemaker and Bloom, 1977), but in many cases the quantification of such effects has been hampered by the lack of suitable indices of the branching patterns of dendritic networks, thus allowing exclusively qualitative descriptions.

Using the "network analysis" technique, Berry et al. (1975) were able to quantify some aspects of the nutritional insult to the Pc dendritic tree. The experiments were carried out in 30-day-old rats starved from birth by limiting the suckling time (McConnell and Berry, 1978b) and in 80-day-old animals after 50 days of nutritional rehabilitation (McConnell and Berry, 1978a). At PD 30, in addition to a reduction in the cross-sectional area of the vermis and to an increased density of both granule cells (which in these experiments are reduced in number by 29%) and Pc, the authors found a significant increase in the density of the Pc dendritic field with a dramatic decrease in the overall network size, due to the reduction in the total number of dendritic segments and in the length of distal segments. The topological analysis revealed that in undernourished animals the dendritic tree developed by terminal branching, as in normal animals, but deviated from the usual, purely random, branching pattern. The authors suggest that at least two mechanisms might be responsible for these effects.

1) The loss of granule cells. A great deal of evidence, in fact, indicates that size and morphology of a dendritic field are influenced by the environment in which dendrites develop. Deafferentation studies carried out in a number of brain regions, including cerebellum (Altman and Anderson, 1971; Bradley and Berry, 1976), have shown that the extent of dendritic growth is related to the afferent input available. Since Pc receive a large proportion of their input from parallel fibers, the reduction in granule cell number should affect network size.

One hypothesis of dendritic growth (Vaughn et al., 1974) suggests that the formation of dendritic segments is a result of the interaction of dendritic growth cone filopodia and incoming axons. Thus, segment length will be inversely proportional and the order of branching at nodes directly proportional to the axonal density in the environment. This hypothesis has been tested in cerebellum in several situations of hypogranularity produced by X-irradiation (Berry and Bradley, 1976) or methylazoxymethanol administration (Bradley and Berry, 1978) and has been found correct. In contrast, in underfed animals, the reduction in segment length is not accompanied by an increase in the frequency of high-order branching nodes, indicating that in this case it is unlikely that the hypoplasia of Pc dendrites is produced by a reduced density of axons in the area surrounding the developing dendritic growth cone. A more reasonable explanation is that undernutrition directly affected Pc dendritic growth.

2) In 30-day-old undernourished animals, Pc bodies are significantly smaller than in controls, suggesting that food deficiency also has a direct influence on neuronal metabolism. This could account for the reduction in dendritic segment length observed in undernutrition.

A 28% decrease in overall size of the Pc dendritic network persists after rehabilitation, due primarily to a deficit in segment frequency which does not recover between day 30 and day 80. On the contrary, segment length shows some recovery, suggesting that dendritic remodeling has occurred during the rehabilitation period. This ability to partially recover is in good agreement with recent morphological data showing that in normal cerebellum the Pc dendritic tree significantly increases in size and is remodeled after weaning until PD 150 (Anderson and Flumerfelt, 1985). The failure to observe a total recovery of dendritic growth could be explained by the fact that although Pc metabolism is "normalized," the normalization occurs in an environment which, because of the irreversible deficit in granule cell, and hence parallel fiber number, is no longer suitable to correct development of dendrites.

All these observations suggest that for Pc dendritic growth, as for other events of cerebellar development, a "critical period" exists and that an alimentary deficit occurring during this period produce alterations which cannot, or can only partially, recover on future nutritional rehabilitation.

Morphogenesis of Golgi epithelial cells (Bergmann glia). Undernutrition (from the gestational day 6) produces, at birth and during the first postnatal week, an acceleration of Bergmann glia maturation, which is demonstrated by the presence of a higher than normal percentage of cells already displaying fiber polarization (Clos et al., 1979). The number of these "mature" cells is abnormally high until PD 10, but afterwards (PD 14 to PD 21) the number of relatively immature-for-age cells becomes higher than in controls, indicating a delayed maturation of Bergmann glia during the late phase of postnatal cerebellar development.

RNA and proteins. In "normal" rat cerebellum the chronology of RNA accumulation is very similar to that of DNA. At birth the cerebellum contains about 7% of the adult total RNA. The phase of maximal accumulation occurs during the second postnatal week, and by PD 16–18 the adult value is attained and remains constant thereafter (Gourdon et al., 1973; Gombos et al., 1980; Vitiello et al., 1985a). Since the amount of RNA accumulated during the first three postnatal weeks is smaller than that of the DNA formed in the same period, the RNA/DNA ratio continuously decreases from birth to PD 14, when it reaches a plateau. This pattern is due to the formation, during postnatal cerebellar growth, of a large number of cells, the granule cells, which contain very little cytoplasm and rough endoplasmic reticulum.

The rapid growth phase for protein occurs between PD 7–8 and 21; 80% of the adult value is attained at the end of the third week. Protein continues to accumulate after the end of cell multiplication, parallel with the dry weight increase.

Undernutrition does not alter the chronology of RNA accumulation, nor the normal developmental pattern of the RNA/DNA ratio (Vitiello et al., 1985b,c), but the cerebellar amount of RNA significantly and irreversibly decreases.

The same results are obtained for protein, only the total amount is decreased, without any reduction in the concentration per cell (per mg DNA) and per unit of dry weight (Vitiello et al., 1985b,c). Also the concentration of membrane protein is normal (Rabié and Legrand, 1973).

In conclusion, it appears that undernutrition does not affect protein concentration in cerebellum, in contrast with other situations, like dysthyroidism, which also alter the development of this region (Legrand, 1982–1983).

Na$^+$,K$^+$-ATPase and 5'-nucleotidase. Na$^+$,K$^+$-ATPase and 5'-nucleotidase are constituents of the plasma membrane of all cellular types, although 5'-nucleotidase, also present in endoplasmic reticulum, is apparently more abundant in glial cell membranes (Kreutzberg et al., 1978) and has been recently detected by immunocytochemical methods mainly in oligodendroglia and myelin (Cammer et al., 1985).

We have measured the effect of undernutrition on these two enzyme in the cerebellum of AF Wistar rats from our laboratories in the following way. All rats born on the same day were pooled then distributed to form nursing litters of eight (controls) or 18 pups (postnatal undernutrition during lactation) per each dam. Dams were fed ad libitum (Kennedy, 1957). After weaning (PD 25), the pups were also fed ad libitum (rehabilitation). The results obtained (Figs. 1, 2) did not significantly differ from data obtained with rats undernourished pre- and postnatally according to the method described by Patel et al. (1973), which consisted of reducing by 50% the normal balanced diet of the mother from the sixth day of gestation until the day when the pups were sacrificed (not shown).

In normal rat, the total and specific (per mg of protein) activities of

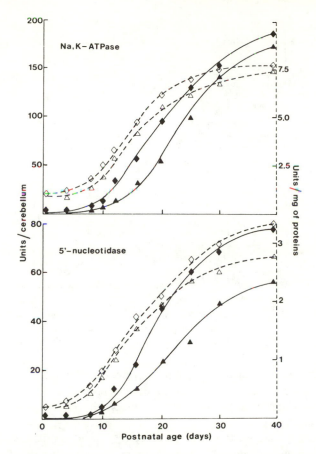

Fig. 1.   Accumulation of Na$^+$,K$^+$-dependent, ouabain-inhibited ATPase and 5'-nucleotidase activities in the cerebellum of undernourished ($\triangle$ $\blacktriangle$) and control ($\diamond$ $\blacklozenge$) rats during early postnatal development. Activities per cerebellum ($\blacktriangle$ $\blacklozenge$) and per mg of protein ($\triangle$ $\diamond$). Enzyme activity was measured in cerebellar H$_2$O homogenates (0.5 mg of protein/ml) by following ^{32}P released from ^{32}P-ATP (for the ATPase) or from ^{32}P-5'-AMP (for 5'-nucleotidase) according to modifications of the techniques of Blostein (1968), Widnell (1972), and Wheeler (1975).

Na$^+$,K$^+$-ATPase and 5'-nucleotidase increase, as other biochemical parameters during cerebellar ontogeny, according to a sigmoid curve (Fig. 1).

Food deficit produces a marked reduction in the activity on a per cerebellum basis of Na$^+$,K$^+$-ATPase and 5'-nucleotidase by the end of the second week (that is, during the rapid growth phase). Between PD 20 and PD 40, only Na$^+$,K$^+$-ATPase recovers, and at PD 40 its deficit is only 10% while the deficit of 5' nucleotidase still is about 30%. In terms of specific activity (per mg protein), Na$^+$,K$^+$-ATPase is lower than normal during the

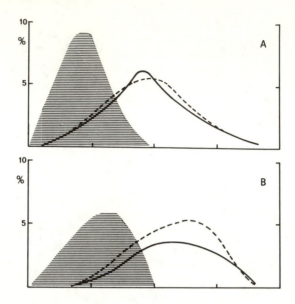

Fig. 2. Daily rate of percentage accumulation of Na^+,K^+-stimulated, ouabain-inhibited ATPase (———), 5'-nucleotidase (— — —), and DNA (shaded curve) in cerebellum during early postnatal development in undernourished (B) rats compared with controls (A).

phase of rapid cerebellar growth, but then becomes normal by PD 40. In contrast, 5'-nucleotidase remains lower than controls from PD 20 onward. This could be a further indication of the reduced oligodendrocyte population and decreased myelin.

We have expressed these results as daily rate of accumulation. Values at each age were first calculated as a percentage of the adult value (= 100%); the rate of daily accumulation was then calculated from these percentage values. In this mode of expression, each sigmoid curve of accumulation shown in Figure 1 is transformed into a peak, the ascending part of which corresponds to the increasing rate of accumulation, the descending part to the decreasing rate of accumulation, and the summit corresponds to the maximal accumulation rate. If maximal accumulation rate persists for a long time, the summit becomes a plateau. Base line values correspond to zero accumulation (i.e., to constant values at different ages). The surface delimited by each peak is proportional to the total amount of each compound. This mode of expression of the data clearly demonstrates the sequential accumulation of DNA (index of cell formation) followed by that of Na^+,K^+-ATPase (index of plasma membrane formation). The period of maximal accumulation rate for DNA is at PD 10 ± 2, while that of the two enzymes is during the third postnatal week. The chronology of accumulation of the two enzymes is slightly altered in undernourished animals. The rapid growth phase of Na^+,K^+-ATPase is delayed by 4–6 days and that of 5′-nucleotidase by 6–8 days, but the major effect in undernourished animals is the flattening of the peaks of daily accumulation (Fig. 2).

Gangliosides. Although gangliosides are present on the surface of virtually all cells, polysialogangliosides are particularly important in the biochemistry and physiology of neuronal plasma membranes (Morgan et al., 1976; Svennerholm, 1980) and accumulate during CNS development at the time when the bulk of the neuronal network is formed (Vanier et al., 1971; Merat and Dickerson, 1973). For this reason, they are often employed as an index of synaptogenesis (Bass, 1981).

In normal rat cerebellum, ganglioside sialic acid accumulates rapidly during the second and third postnatal weeks. Similarly to the other plasma membrane constituents, ganglioside sialic acid concentration expressed on a per DNA (e.g., on a per cell) basis decreases during the first week (a period of moderate but exclusive cell proliferation during which newly formed cells do not grow in size nor develop many processes). After the first week, ganglioside sialic acid concentration per mg DNA increases until postnatal day 40.

Conflicting results have been reported on the effects of food deprivation on CNS ganglioside sialic acid. Some reports indicate a delay of the peak value of maximal concentration on cerebral cortex (Bass, 1981); others indicate either changes (Merat and Dickerson, 1974) or no changes (Geison and Waisman, 1970; Karlsson, 1978) in whole brain concentration or a slight reduction in cerebellar concentration (Ghittoni and Faryna de Raveglia, 1972). In our laboratory (Vitiello et al., in press) we have found that: 1) the cerebellar content of ganglioside sialic acid shows a normal developmental chronology, but the amount of ganglioside sialic acid per cerebellum is lower at each age, and at 40 days the values are about 80% of controls; 2) ganglioside sialic acid concentration (both on a per cell and on a per mg protein basis) is normal at all ages except in the very early postnatal period following prenatal malnutrition, when higher than control concentrations are detected.

These data indicate that the decrease of ganglioside sialic acid content in the cerebellum of undernourished animals is roughly proportional to the decrease in cellularity (whether the undernutrition is imposed pre- and postnatally, or only postnatally). The distribution pattern of the individual gangliosides is identical to controls, indicating that ganglioside sialic acid modifications are mainly, if not only, qualitative.

Phospholipids and cholesterol. Phopholipids and cholesterol are the major constituents of all membranes, and during normal cerebellar growth they display a developmental pattern very similar to that of the other plasma membrane markers: a very slow accumulation in the first week and fast and almost linear growth during the following 3 weeks (Vitiello et al., 1985b). The distribution of different phospholipids shows that the only significant change is a decrease in the percentage of choline phosphoglyceride from PD 5 to 21, with a proportional increase of ethanolamine phosphoglyceride (mainly ethanolamine plasmalogen) (Vitiello et al., unpublished observation).

In undernutrition the phase of fast accumulation of both cholesterol and phospholipid is delayed, and by PD 12 the cerebellar levels are lower than in controls (Vitiello et al., 1985b). Furthermore, in contrast to protein and RNA, the average content of cholesterol and phospholipid per cell (per mg of DNA) are similarly reduced by PD 20 and do not recover after nutritional rehabilitation. An effect of undernutrition on fatty acid composition of phospholipids has also been reported (Rao, 1979).

Thus, the effects of food deficiency on phospholipids and cholesterol suggest a reduction in membrane formation paralleled by little or no alteration of membrane composition.

Myelin markers. Myelin is a highly specialized region of the plasma membrane (the so-called trapezoid process) of the oligodendrocyte (in the CNS) or the Schwann cells (in the peripheral nervous system). In myelinated fibers, the integrity of the myelin sheath is necessary for correct nerve conduction (Morell et al., 1981; Norton, 1977; Rogart and Ritchie, 1977).

The formation of brain myelin is subject to many environmental influences, of which the best studied are those associated with postnatal food deficit (for a review see Wiggins, 1982). Myelin formation in the CNS presumably follows the same pattern as that described by Morell (1977) for the peripheral nervous system: proliferation of the precursors of the myelin-making cells, and growth and maturation of the myelin-making cells, which is completed with the formation of the "trapezoid" process associated with the transformation of its plasma membrane into compact myelin resulting from the acquisition of the specific biochemical constituents characteristic of myelin (Norton, 1981). Because of the chronological differences in myelination in different CNS regions, biochemical studies of myelination in whole brain are difficult to interpret. In contrast, the sequence of events during myelin formation is followed much more easily in rodent cerebellum where myelinated fibers are homogeneous in diameter and their myelination occurs at approximately the same time since myelin is almost exclusively present in the afferent (climbing and mossy fibers) and efferent (Pc and DCNN axons) fibers, while the axons of interneurons (including the parallel fibers) are not myelinated or possess very few myeline lamellae (parallel fibers located deep in the molecular layer) (Palay and Chan-Palay, 1974).

Several specific markers of oligodendrocyte maturation and compact myelin formation are available. To study the effect of undernutrition we used: 1) carbonic anhydrase II (CA II), which in rat cerebellum is exclusively detected in oligodendrocytes (Ghandour et al., 1979, 1980a) and accumulates simultaneously with oligodendrocyte maturation (Ghandour et al., 1980b). 2) 2',3'-cyclic nucleotide-3'-phosphohydrolase (CNPase), an enzyme which, in CNS, is most abundant in myelin but also present in oligodendrocytes (Kurihara and Tsukada, 1967; Kim et al., 1984). CNPase is probably identical to the so-called "Wolfgram protein W1" (Drummond and Dean, 1980). 3) galactolipids, which in the CNS are markers of oligodendrocytes and accumulate in myelin (Matthieu et al., 1973).

As shown in Figure 3, CA II, CNPase, and galactolipids in normal cerebellum accumulate in the sigmoid fashion typical of most parameters of cerebellar growth. The phase of rapid accumulation lasts from PD 8 to 30 for CNPase and from PD 12 to 30 for CA II. The concentration of CA II and the specific activity of CNPase increase with a very similar chronology except that the phase of rapid increase of CA II stops earlier (at PD 25) than that of CNPase (Fig. 3).

With our method (Neskovic et al., 1972), galactolipids are not detectable in rat cerebellum before the end of the first postnatal week. On a per cerebellum basis, they accumulate at a moderate rate until PD 25 and then suddenly at a very rapid rate from PD 25 to 40. The galactolipid concentration rapidly increases between PD 25 and 30 (Fig. 3).

In the cerebellum of undernourished rats, the per age cerebellar content and the concentration per mg of protein of CA II, CNPase, and glicolipids are lower than in controls, and the differences become particularly significant during the phase of rapid accumulation. As already reported by Ghittoni and Faryna de Raveglia (1972), the per age galactolipid content and concentration per mg of protein in undernourished animal cerebella are lower than in controls during the whole period studied, the differences being particularly striking after PD 25 (Fig. 3). No recovery was observed even after a 4-month nutritional rehabilitation.

Morphological and biochemical studies demonstrate that undernutrition reduces myelin formation in the brain (Benton et al., 1966; Siassi and Siassi, 1973; Figlewicz et al., 1978). The effect of food deficit, however, appears to greatly depend on the developmental period during which it is imposed. Even a mild food restriction before weaning can cause permanent deficits in brain myelin lipid and protein, while in animals starved after weaning, the deficit is generally transient and a nutritional rehabilitation is followed by complete recovery of CNS myelin (Wiggins, 1982). The most likely explanation for these results is that, in the sequence of events in the myelination process, more than one phase is vulnerable to undernutrition and one of these phases, which occurs early during brain development, must be

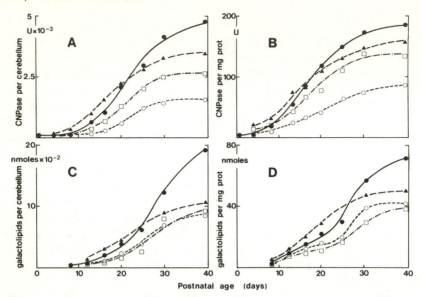

Fig. 3.   Accumulation of two myelin markers, CNPase (A and B) and galactolipids (C and D), during postnatal development of undernourished rats (□) and controls (●). The results obtained in rats made thyroid-deficient (○) and hyperthyroid (▲) by the technique described by Clos et al. (1982) are shown for further comparison. Each point represents the mean of at least three individual values obtained from different pools of cerebella. Depending on the age, the number of cerebella per pool varied from 30 (newborn) to 3 (40-day-old). Single or pooled cerebella were homogenized in water. 2',3'-Cyclic nucleotide 3'-phosphohydrolase (CNPase) was measured on homogenate aliquots (100–200 μg/ml) according to the method of Zanetta et al. (1972). One unit corresponds to one μmole of substrate hydrolyzed/mg protein/hr. Lipids were extracted from cerebellar homogenates and partitioned according to the method of Folch-Pi et al. (1957) as modified by Suzuki (1964). Galactose in the lipid extract was measured according to Neskovic et al. (1972). The average molecular weight of galactolipid was assumed to be 810 and thus the amount of galactose determined was multiplied by a factor of 4.5 to obtain the molar amount of galactolipids.

so vulnerable that the structures established during this period are irreversibly damaged.

A reduced deposition of myelin during development could be due to glial alterations of different type; e.g., either a decreased number of oligodendrocytes or altered oligodendrocyte maturation or formation of myelin deficient in certain constituents. As reported in the section on cell proliferation and final cell composition of cerebellum, cell counts around fissure E have shown a 30% decrease in oligodendrocyte number at PD 35 which does not recover after rehabilitation (Clos et al., 1982). The formation of oligodendrocyte precursor (and, in general, that of glial cell precursors) appears to be more reduced than that of neuroblasts. Since in cerebellum, both glial cells and more than 80% of neurons are formed during the first three postnatal weeks, the preferential effect of undernutrition on glia could be due to a different vulnerability to food deficiency of the two cell populations. However, not only the multiplication of oligodendrocyte precursor cells but also the maturation of oligodendrocytes appears to be affected by undernutrition. In fact, the cerebellar content of CA II at PD 35 is reduced by 44% (significantly more than the oligodendrocyte number). This indicates decreased cellular concentration of the enzyme. Hence, oligodendrocytes are either immature or of smaller size. The same considerations apply to CNPase and galactolipids, the levels of which are also reduced (-43 and -48%, respectively) more than the oligodendrocyte number, indicating that less membranes are formed by each oligodendrocyte or that these membranes have an abnormal composition.

A good comparison of the chronology of cerebellar myelin formation in normal and undernourished animals can be obtained by calculating the daily rate of accumulation of CA II, CNPase, and galactolipids (Fig. 4). This mode of expression of the data clearly demonstrates the sequential accumulation during myelination of oligodendrocyte and myelin markers (CNPase followed by CA II, followed by galactolipids) in cerebella of normal and undernourished rats. In normal cerebellum the maximum accumulation rate of CNPase is around PD 16–18 and that of CA II is around PD 20–22, while galactolipids attain a maximum at approximately PD 28. In undernutrition the peaks of maximum accumulation of CAII and galactolipid are smaller than controls but occur at the same age as in controls. In contrast, the CNPase appears as a plateau with a small peak occurring 8–9 days later than in controls. This would agree with the retarded oligodendrocyte maturation reported by Robain and Ponsot (1978), Lai et al. (1980), and Pasquini et al. (1983).

Thus, it appears that the effects of undernutrition imposed during the lactation on cerebellar myelin are mainly a consequence of the irreversibly reduced number of oligodendrocytes but also of retarded oligodendrocyte maturation, though the latter is of lesser importance.

Data in the literature indicate that in undernutrition the myelin wrapping around peripheral nerves is thinner than that which should be expected from the axonal diameter (Clos and Legrand, 1970), indicating that the axonal-glial equilibrium is altered and that the glial deficit predominates. However, effects on myelination secondary to axonal alteration cannot be excluded. Lai and Lewis (1980) have suggested that in corpus callosum undernutrition has a more marked long-term effect on axonal growth than on oligodendrocyte maturation. This could be also the case for cerebellum, where, in undernourished rats, hypoplasia of Pc, hence possibly also of their axons, has been described (McConnell and Berry, 1978a,b). Also the myelinated mossy fibers and their terminals could be hypoplastic, since they could be

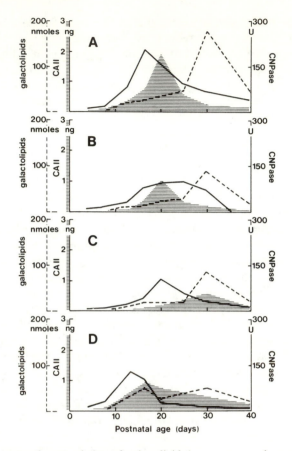

Fig. 4. Daily rate of accumulation of galactolipid (— — —; nmole per day), CNPase (_____; units per day), and CAII (shaded curve; ng per day) in the cerebellum of controls (A), undernourished (B), thyroid-deficient (C), and hyperthyroid (D) rats. The galactolipid and CNPase data were the same as in Figure 2; the CAII data were taken from Ghandour et al. (1980b) and from Clos et al. (1982). Note that in undernutrition the prevalent alteration is the reduced size and the flattening of the peaks, in contrast with the prevalent alterations of chronology observed in rats with thyroid hormone deficit or excess.

functionally less active and/or reduced in number because of the reduced number of granule cells, their postsynaptic partner.

CONCLUSIONS

At the morphological level, it appears that malnutrition essentially affects cell multiplication of neurons and glial cells. The most pronounced lesions are those of glial cells and particularly those of oligodendrocytes.

It also appears that the influence of undernutrition on the rate and extent of cell maturation is either small or nil, but the influence on the extent of growth of cells which remain hypotrophic is greater. This clearly differentiates undernutrition from alteration of CNS development due to hormonal imbalance (i.e., thyroid states, excess of glucocorticoids) which affects rate and extent of cell maturation and thus excludes the possibility that some hormones are major elements in the mechanism of action of the effects of undernutrition on CNS development. The results of undernutrition on cell growth can be long-lasting, as is the case for oligodendrocyte number (the main cause of hypomyelination) and for the alteration of Purkinje cell dendrites.

The absence of increased cellular death and greatly retarded cellular maturation are an indication that undernutrition does not affect to a great extent the synthesis of growth factors and/or factors which stimulate differentiation and maintain the survival of neurons and glial cells.

In undernutrition, the morphological alterations observed at the neuron level and principal cerebellar circuits are moderate. A reduction in the ratio between synapse number and neuron number in the granular layer has been described, but it disappears after nutritional rehabilitation (Bedi et al., 1980a). However the reduction of the number of interneurons such as basket cells which are present in only small numbers in ''normal'' cerebellum could have major long-lasting consequences since these cells are strategically located in a major inhibitory circuit. Unfortunately, no data exist on the functional consequences of such basket cell reduction. There are also no reports in the literature on the formation of heterotopic or heterologous synapses in the cerebella of undernourished animals or on the presence of synapses and circuits due to the persistence of an immature situation (i.e., redundant Purkinje cell recurrent fibers, redundant climbing fibers, and axosomatic synapses between climbing fibers and Purkinje cells). Such alterations have been described in several situations of hypo- or agranularity (due to X-ray treatment, mutations, virus infections, and anti-mitotic drugs). In all these conditions, the effects on the granule cell population are much greater, by far, than in undernutrition.

Evidently these data do not exclude the presence of other, finer, undetected alterations (i.e., the molecular structure of synapses) which may be detected at the biochemical level, but so far there are no reports concerning these fine alterations. Some alterations of neurotransmitter amino acid levels (Rathbun and Druse, 1985) and the developmental pattern of enzymes of neurotransmitter synthesis, like glutamate decarboxylase and choline acetyltransferase (Patel et al., 1978), have been reported. In all cases the alteration was completely restored by nutritional rehabilitation, indicating that the disturbance of cerebellar neurotransmitter systems produced by undernutrition was temporary. Also we should not disregard the possibility of alterations of nerve conduction due to the reduction of the thickness of the myelin sheath around axons and of alteration of neurotransmission due to modification of the recycling of neurotransmitters by astrocytes because of the reduced astrocyte number.

Morphological studies indicate that cell (neurons and oligodendrocytes) number is not restored to normal by nutritional rehabilitation (Clos et al., 1982). Also myelin thickness and total amounts (see Wiggins, 1982) are not restored, but the dendritic field of Purkinje cells is partially restored (McConnell and Berry, 1978a).

The amount literature dealing with alteration of cerebellar function in undernourished rats and with its possible restoration after rehabilitation is small since this function is not easy to study in rodents, and the tests used are either inadequate or insensitive. Available data are limited to reports on the deficit of motor coordination found in adult animals undernourished during early postnatal life (Lynch et al., 1975; Jordan et al., 1979) and on the retarded development of spontaneous motor activity and a variety of reflexes (see Balàzs et al., 1986). These motor alterations have been tentatively correlated with cerebellar lesions selectively produced by postnatal undernutrition, but more recent studies (Smart and Bedi, 1982) cast some doubts on such conclusions. In animals undernourished during early postnatal life, cerebellar function in possibly less efficient but not fundamentally modified probably because of the redundance of cerebellar cells and circuits and the absence of abnormal circuits. Thus cerebellum, which is an excellent model for localizing morphological alterations and for correlating them with biochemical modifications, does not appear to be an ideal model for establishing correlation between these alterations and function in malnourished animals.

ACKNOWLEDGMENTS

We thank Mrs. Simone Boyle-Boiseaux for typing the manuscript and Dr. O.K. Langley for critically reading it. The technical help of Mrs. Y. Schladenhaufen is gratefully acknowledged. This work was partially supported by a Projet de Collaboration Bilatérale, France (Strasbourg and Montpellier)-Italy (Bari), CNR grant 82.2091, and by MPI.

REFERENCES

Altman J (1972a): Postnatal development of the cerebellar cortex in the rat. I. The external germinal layer and the transitional molecular layer. J Comp Neurol 145:353–398.
Altman J (1972b): Postnatal development of the cerebellar cortex in the rat. II. Phases in the maturation of the Purkinje cells and of the molecular layer. J Comp Neurol 145:399–464.

Altman J (1972c): Postnatal development of the cerebellar cortex in the rat. III. Maturation of the components of the granular layer. J Comp Neurol 145:465–514.

Altman J (1982): Morphological development of the rat cerebellum and some of its mechanisms. In Palay SL, Chan-Palay V (eds): "The Cerebellum—New Vistas." Berlin: Springer-Verlag, pp 8–46.

Altman J, Anderson WJ (1971): Irradiation of the cerebellum in infant rats with low-level X-rays: Histological and cytological effects during infancy and adulthood. Exp Neurol 30:492–509.

Altman J, Das GD, Sudarshan K, Anderson JB (1971): The influence of nutrition on neural and behavioral development. II. Growth of body and brain in infant rats using different techniques of undernutrition. Dev Psychobiol 4:55–70.

Anderson WA, Flumerfelt BA (1985): Purkinje cell growth beyond the twenty-third postnatal day. Dev Brain Res 17:195–200.

Balàzs R, Kovàcs S, Cocks WA, Johnson AL, Eayrs JT (1971): Effect of thyroid hormone on the biochemical maturation of rat brain: Postnatal cell formation. Brain Res 25:555–570.

Balàzs R, Lewis PD, Patel AJ (1979): Nutritional deficiencies and brain development. In Falkner F, Tanner JM (eds): "Human Growth." Vol. 3. New York: Plenum Press, pp 415–480.

Balàzs R, Jordan T, Lewis PD, Patel AJ (1986): Undernutrition and brain development. In Falkner F, Tanner JM (eds): "Human Growth." Vol. 3, 2nd Ed. New York: Plenum Publishing, pp 415–473.

Barnes D, Altman J (1973a): Effects of different schedules of early undernutrition on the preweaning growth of the rat cerebellum. Exp Neurol 38:406–419.

Barnes D, Altman J (1973b): Effects of two levels of gestational-lactational undernutrition on the postweaning growth of the rat cerebellum. Exp Neurol 38:420–428.

Bass NH (1981): Ganglioside sialic acid as a quantitative neurochemical index of the integrity of synaptic function in cognitive disorders of development and aging. In Rapport MM, Gorio A (eds): "Gangliosides in Neurological and Neuromuscular Function, Development and Repair." New York: Raven Press, pp 29–43.

Bedi KS, Thomas YM, Davies CA, Dobbing J (1980a): Synapse to neuron ratios of the frontal and cerebellar cortex of 30 day old and adult rats undernourished during early postnatal life. J Comp Neurol 193:49–56.

Bedi KS, Hall R, Davies CA, Dobbing J (1980b): A stereological analysis of the cerebellar granule and Purkinje cells of 30 day old and adult rats undernourished during early postnatal life. J Comp Neurol 193:863–870.

Benton JW, Moser HW, Dodge PR, Carr S (1966): Modification of the schedule of myelination in rat by early nutritional deprivation. Pediatrics 38:155–173.

Berry M, Bradley PM (1976): Growth of Purkinje cell dendrites in the X-irradiated, agranular cerebellar cortex of the rat. Brain Res 116:361–388.

Berry M, Hollingworth T, Anderson EM, Flinn M (1975): The application of network analysis to the study of the branching patterns of dendritic fields. In Kreuzberg GW (ed): "Advances in Neurology." Vol. 12, "Physiology and Pathology of Dendrites." New York: Raven Press, pp 217–245.

Bloom FE, Hoffer BJ, Siggins GR (1971): Studies on norepinephrine-containing afferents to Purkinje cells of rat cerebellum. I. Localization of the fibers and their synapses. Brain Res 25:501–523.

Blostein R (1968): Relationship between erythrocyte membrane phosphorylation and adenosine triphosphate hydrolysis. J Biol Chem 243:1957–1965.

Bradley PM, Berry M (1976): The effects of reduced climbing and parallel fiber input on Purkinje cell dendritic growth. Brain Res 109:133–151.

Bradley PM, Berry M (1978): The effect of neonatal administration of methylazoxymethanol acetate (MAM) on the growth of Purkinje cell dendritic trees in the cerebellum of the rat. Brain Res 143:499–511.

Brizzee KR, Vigt J, Kharetchko X (1964): Postnatal changes in glial neuron index with a comparison of methods of cell enumeration in the white rat. Prog Brain Res 4:136–149.

Brown ML, Guthrie MA (1968): Effect of severe undernutrition in early life upon body and organ weights in adult rats. Growth 32:143–150.

Cammer W, Sacchi R, Kahn S (1985): Immunocytochemical localization of 5'-nucleotidase in oligodendroglia and myelinated fibers in the central nervous system of adult and young rats. Dev Brain Res 20:89–96.

Chase HP, Lindsley WFB Jr, O'Brien D (1969): Undernutrition and cerebellar development. Nature 221:554–555.

Clos J, Favre C, Selme-Matrat M, Legrand J (1977): Effects of undernutrition on cell formation in the rat brain and specially on cellular composition of the cerebellum. Brain Res 123:13–26.

Clos J, Legrand C, Legrand J (1979): Early effects of undernutrition on the development of cerebellar Bergmann glia. Ann Biol Anim Biochem Biophys 19:167–172.

Clos J, Legrand J (1970): Influence de l'insuffisance thyrodienne et de la sous-alimentation sur la croissance et la myélinisation des fibres nerveuses du nerf sciatique chez le jeune rat blanc. Brain Res 22:285–297.

Clos J, Legrand J, Limozin N, Dalmasso C, Laurent G (1982): Effect of abnormal thyroid state and undernutrition on carbonic anhydrase and oligodendroglia development in the rat cerebellum. Dev Neurosci 5:243–251.

Cowan WM (1973): Neuronal death as a regulative mechanism in the control of cell number in the nervous system. In Rockstein M (ed): "Development and Aging in the Nervous System." New York: Academic Press, pp 19–41.

Crnic LA, Chase HP (1978): Models of infantile undernutrition in rats. J Nutr 108:1755–1760.

Debassio WA, Kemper TL (1985): The effects of protein deprivation on neuronal migration in rats. Dev Brain Res 20:191–196.

Del Carro M, Swarz JR (1976): Prenatal development of Bergmann glia fibers in rodent cerebellum. J Neurocytol 5:669–676.

Deo MG, Ramalingaswami V (1965): Reaction of the small intestine to induced protein malnutrition in rhesus monkey: A study of cell population kinetics in the jejunum. Gastroenterology 49:150–157.

Dobbing J (1974): The later development of the central nervous system and its vulnerability. In Davis JA, Dobbing J (eds): "Scientific Foundation of Pediatrics." London: William Heinemann Medical Books, pp 1–17.

Dobbing J, Hopewell JW, Lynch A (1971): Vulnerability of developing brain. VII. Permanent deficit of neurons in cerebral and cerebellar cortex following early mild undernutrition. Exp Neurol 32:439–447.

Dobbing J, Sands J (1973): Quantitative growth and development of human brain. Arch Dis Child 48:757–767.

Drummond RJ, Dean G (1980): Comparison of 2',3'-cyclic nucleotide 3'-phosphodiesterase and the major component of Wolfgram protein W1. J Neurochem 35:1155–1165.

Figlewicz DA, Hofteig JH, Druse MJ (1978): Maternal deficiency of protein or protein and calories during lactation: Effect upon CNS myelin subfraction formation in rat offsprings. Life Sci 23:2163–2172.

Folch-Pi J, Lees M, Sloane-Stanley GH (1957): A simple method for the isolation and purification of total lipids from animal tissues. J Biol Chem 226:497–509.

Friede RL (1973): Dating the development of human cerebellum. Acta Neuropathol 23:48–58.

Fuller GN, Wiggins RC (1984): Differential growth recovery within the brains of postnatally undernourished rats. Dev Brain Res 15:280–282.

Geison RL, Waisman WA (1970): Effects of nutritional status on rat brain maturation measured as lipid composition. J Nutr 100:315–324.

Ghandour MS, Labourdette G, Vincendon G, Gombos G (1981): A biochemical and immunohistological study of S100 protein in developing rat cerebellum. Dev Neurosci 4:98–109.

Ghandour MS, Langley OK, Clos J (1983): Immunohistochemical and biochemical approaches to the development of neuroglia in the CNS, with special reference to cerebellum. Int J Dev Neurosci 1:411–425.

Ghandour MS, Langley OK, Vincendon G, Gombos G (1979): Double labeling immunohistochemical technique provides evidence of the specificity of glial cell markers. J Histochem Cytochem 27:1634–1637.

Ghandour MS, Langley OK, Vincendon G, Gombos G, Filippi D, Limozin N, Dalmasso C, Laurent G (1980a): Immunochemical and immunohistochemical study of carbonic anhydrase II in adult rat cerebellum: A marker for oligodendrocytes. Neuroscience 5:559–571.

Ghandour MS, Vincendon G, Gombos G, Limozin N, Filippi D, Dalmasso C, Laurent G (1980b): Carbonic anhydrase and oligodendroglia in developing rat cerebellum: A biochemical and immunohistological study. Dev Biol 77:73–83.

Ghittoni NE, Faryna de Raveglia I (1972): Influence of neonatal undernutrition on the lipid composition of cerebral cortex and cerebellum of the rat. Neurobiology 2:41–48.

Gombos G, Ghandour MS, Vitiello F, Langley OK, Zanetta J-P, Vincendon G (1980): General outline of biochemical constituents during CNS development. In Di Benedetta C, Balàzs R, Gombos G, Porcellati G (eds): "Multidisciplinary Approach to Brain Development." Amsterdam: Elsevier/North-Holland, pp 15–28.

Gourdon J, Clos J, Costa C, Dainat J, Legrand J (1973): Comparative effects of hypothyroidism, hyperthyroidism and undernutrition on the protein and nucleic acid contents of the cerebellum in the young rat. J Neurochem 21:861–871.

Hàmori J, Somogyi J (1983): Differentiation of cerebellar mossy fiber synapses in the rat: A quantitative electron microscope study. J Comp Neurol 220:365–377.

Hoffer BJ, Siggins GR, Oliver AP, Bloom FE (1973): Activation of the pathway from locus coeruleus to rat cerebellar Purkinje neurons: Pharmacological evidences of noradrenergic central inhibition. J Pharmacol Exp Ther 184:553–569.

Hökfelt T, Fuxe K (1969): Cerebellar monoamine nerve terminals, a new type of afferent fibers to the cortex cerebelli. Exp Brain Res 9:63–72.

Jordan TC, Howells KF, Piggott SM (1979): Effects of early undernutrition on motor coordination in the adult rat. Behav Neurol Biol 25:126–132.

Karlsson I (1978): Effect of malnutrition of ganglioside development. In Neuhoff V (ed): "Proceedings of the European Society for Neurochemistry." Weinheim: Verlag Chemie, pp 189–198.

Kennedy GC (1957): Development with age of hypothalamic restraint upon the appetite of the rat. J Endocrinol 16:9–17.

Kim SU, McMorris A, Sprinkle TJ (1984): Immunofluorescence demonstration of 2',3'-cyclic nucleotide 3'-phosphodiesterase in cultured oligodendrocytes of mouse, rat, calf and human. Brain Res 300:195–199.

Koppel H, Lewis PD, Patel AJ (1983): Cell death in the external granular layer of normal and undernourished rats: Further observations, including estimates of rate of cell loss. Cell Tissue Kinet 16:99–106.

Kornguth SE, Anderson JW, Scott G (1967): Observations on the ultrastructure of the developing cerebellum of the Macaca mulatta. J Comp Neurol 130:1–24.

Kornguth SE, Anderson JW, Scott G (1968): The development of synaptic contacts in the cerebellum of Macaca mulatta. J Comp Neurol 132:531–546.

Kreutzberg GW, Barron KD, Shubert P (1978): Cytochemical localization of 5'-nucleotidase in glial plasma membranes. Brain Res 158:247–257.

Kurihara T, Tsukada Y (1967): The regional and subcellular distribution of 2',3'-cyclic nucleotide 3'-phosphohydrolase in the central nervous system. J Neurochem 14:1167–1174.

Lai M, Lewis PD (1980): Effects of undernutrition on myelination in rat corpus callosum. J Comp Neurol 193:973–982.

Lai M, Lewis PD, Patel AJ (1980): Effects of undernutrition on gliogenesis and glial maturation in rat corpus callosum. J Comp Neurol 193:965–972.

Larramendi LMH (1969): Analysis of synaptogenesis in the cerebellum of the mouse. In Llinas R (ed): ''Neurobiology of Cerebellar Evolution and Development.'' Chicago: AMA ERF, pp 803–843.

Legrand J (1982–1983): Hormones thyroidiennes et maturation du système nerveux. J Physiol (Paris) 78:603–652.

Lewis PD (1975): Cell death in the germinal layers of the postnatal rat brain. Neuropathol Appl Neurobiol 1:1–9.

Lewis PD, Balàzs R, Patel AJ, Johnson AL (1975): The effect of undernutrition in early life on cell generation in the rat brain. Brain Res 83:235–247.

Lewis PD, Patel AJ, Balàzs R (1977): Effect of undernutrition on cell generation in the adult rat brain. Brain Res 138:511–519.

Lewis PD, Patel AJ, Balàzs R (1979): Effect of undernutrition on cell generation in rat hippocampus. Brain Res 168:186–189.

Llinas R (ed) (1969): ''Neurobiology of Cerebellar Evolution and Development.'' Chicago: AMA ERF.

Lynch A, Smart JL, Dobbing J (1975): Motor coordination and cerebellar size in adult rats undernourished in early life. Brain Res 83:249–259.

Matthieu J-M, Widmer S, Herschkowitz N (1973): Biochemical changes in mouse brain composition during myelination. Brain Res 55:391–402.

McConnell P, Berry M (1978a): The effect of refeeding after neonatal starvation on Purkinje cell dendritic growth in the rat. J Comp Neurol 178:759–772.

McConnell P, Berry M (1978b): The effect of undernutrition on Purkinje cell dendritic growth in the rat. J Comp Neurol 177:159–172.

Meller K. Glees P (1969): The development of the mouse cerebellum. A Golgi and EM study. In Llinas R (ed): ''Neurobiology of Cerebellar Evolution and Development.'' Chicago: AMA ERF, pp 783–801.

Merat A, Dickerson JWT (1973): The effect of development on the gangliosides of rat and pig brain. J Neurochem 20:873–880.

Merat A, Dickerson JWT (1974): The effect of the severity and timing of malnutrition on brain gangliosides in the rat. Biol Neonate 25:158–170.

Miale IL, Sidman RL (1961): An autoradiographic analysis of histogenesis in the mouse cerebellum. Exp Neurol 4:277–296.

Morell P (1977): ''Myelin.'' New York: Plenum Press.

Morell P, Bornstein MB, Raine CS (1981): Diseases involving myelin. In Siegel GJ, Albers RW, Agranoff BW, Katzman R (eds): ''Basic Neurochemistry.'' Boston: Little Brown, pp 641–659.

Morgan IG, Tettamanti G, Gombos G (1976): Biochemical evidence on the role of gangliosides in nerve endings. In Porcellati G, Ceccarelli B, Tettamanti G (eds): ''Ganglioside Function: Biochemical and Pharmacological Implications.'' New York: Plenum Press, pp 137–150.

Mueller AJ, Cox WM Jr (1946): The effect of changes in diet on the volume and composition of rat milk. J Nutr 31:249–259.

Mugnaini E, Forströnen PF (1967): Ultrastructural studies on the cerebellar histogenesis. I. Differentiation of granule cells and development of glomeruli in the chick embryo. Z Zellforsch Mikrosk Anat Abt Histochem 77:115–143.

Neskovic N, Sarlieve LL, Nussbaum JL, Kostic D, Mandel P (1972): Quantitative thin-layer chromatography of glycolipids in animal tissues. Clin Chim Acta 38:147–153.

Norton WT (1977): Isolation and characterization of myelin. In Morell P (ed): "Myelin." New York: Plenum Press, pp 161–200.

Norton WT (1981): Formation, structure and biochemistry of myelin. In Siegel GJ, Albers RW, Agranoff BW, Katzman R (eds): "Basic Neurochemistry." Boston: Little Brown, pp 63–92.

Palay SL, Chan-Palay V (1974): "Cerebellar Cortex. Cytology and Organization." Berlin: Springer-Verlag.

Pasquini JM, Bizzozero O, Sato C, Oteiza P, Sato EF (1983): Neonatal hypothyroidism and early undernutrition affect myelin and myelin precursor membrane in a different way. Int J Dev Neurosci 1:105–111.

Patel AJ, Balàzs R, Johnson AL (1973): Effect of undernutrition on cell formation in the rat brain. J Neurochem 20:1151–1165.

Patel AJ, Del Vecchio M, Atkinson DJ (1978): Effect of undernutrition on the regional development of transmitter enzymes: Glutamate decarboxylase and choline acetyl-transferase. Dev Neurosci 1:41–53.

Paula-Barbosa MM, Sobrinho-Simoes MA (1976): An ultrastructural morphogenetic study of mossy fiber endings in pigeon, rat and man. J Comp Neurol 170:365–380.

Privat A (1975): Postnatal gliogenesis in the mammalian brain. Int Rev Cytol 40:281–323.

Purpura DP, Shofer RJ, Housepian EM, Noback CR (1964): Comparative ontogenesis of structure-function relations in cerebral and cerebellar cortex. Prog Brain Res 4:187–221.

Rabié A, Legrand J (1973): Effects of thyroid hormone and undernourishment on the amount of synaptosomal fraction in the cerebellum of the young rat. Brain Res 61:267–278.

Rakic P (1971): Neuron-glia relationship during granule cell migration in developing cerebellar cortex. A Golgi and electron microscopic study in machacus rhesus. J Comp Neurol 141:283–312.

Rakic P, Sidman RL (1970): Histogenesis of cortical layers in human cerebellum, particularly the lamina dissecans. J Comp Neurol 139:473–500.

Ramon y Cajal S (1911): "Histologie du système nerveux de l'homme et des vertébrés." Madrid: Institute Ramon y Cajal, pp 80–106.

Rao PS (1979): Fatty acid composition of cerebrosides and phospholipids in brain of undernourished rats. Nutr Metab 23:136–144.

Rathbun WE, Druse MJ (1985): Maternal undernutrition during lactation: Effect on amino acids in brain regions of offspring. J Neurochem 45:1802–1808.

Robain O, Ponsot G (1978): Effects of undernutrition on glial maturation. Brain Res 149:379–397.

Rogart RB, Ritchie JM (1977): Physiological basis of conduction in myelinated nerve fibers. In Morell P (ed): "Myelin." New York: Plenum Press, pp 117–160.

Shoemaker WJ, Bloom FE (1977): Effect of undernutrition on brain morphology. In Wurtman RJ, Wurtman JJ (eds): "Nutrition and the Brain." New York: Raven Press, pp 147–192.

Siassi F, Siassi B (1973): Differential effects of protein-calorie restriction and subsequent repletion on neuronal and non-neuronal components of cerebral cortex in newborn rats. J Nutr 103:1625–1633.

Smart JL, Bedi KS (1982): Early life undernutrition in rats. 3. Motor performance in adulthood. Br J Nutr 47:439–444.
Smart JL, Dobbing J (1971): Vulnerability of developing brain. II. Effects of early nutritional deprivation on reflex ontogeny and development of behavior in the rat. Brain Res 28:85–95.
Sugita N (1918): Comparative studies on the growth of the cerebral cortex. VII. On the influence of starvation at an early age upon the development of the cerebral cortex in Albino rat. J Comp Neurol 29:177–240.
Suzuki K (1964): A simple and accurate micromethod for quantitative determination of ganglioside patterns. Life Sci 3:1227–1233.
Svennerholm L (1980): Gangliosides and synaptic transmission. In Svennerholm L, Mandel P, Dreyfus H, Urban PF (eds): "Structure and Function of Gangliosides." New York: Plenum Press, pp 533–544.
Swarz JR, Del Cerro M (1977): Lack of evidence for glial cells originating from the external granular layer in mouse cerebellum. J Neurocytol 6:241–250.
Vanier MT, Holm M, Ohman R, Svennerholm L (1971): Developmental profiles of gangliosides in human and rat brain. J Neurochem 18:581–591.
Vaughn JE, Henrikson CK, Grieshaber JA (1974): A quantitative study of synapses on motor neuron dendritic growth cones in developing mouse spinal cord. J Cell Biol 60:664–672.
Vitiello F, Clos J, Vincendon G, Gombos G (1985a): Optimal litter size is required for postnatal developmental studies. Biochem Soc Trans 13:757–758.
Vitiello F, Di Benedetta C, Cioffi LA, Gombos G (1980): Malnutrition and brain development. In Di Benedetta C, Balàzs R, Gombos G, Porcellati G (eds): "Multidisciplinary Approach to Brain Development." Amsterdam: Elsevier/North-Holland, pp 293–309.
Vitiello F, Di Benedetta C, Gombos G (1985b): Preferential effect of early undernutrition on rat cerebellar cholesterol and phospholipids. Biochem Soc Trans 13:758–759.
Vitiello F, Legrand J, Cioffi L, Gombos G (1985c): Comparison of the effect of early undernutrition imposed by two different methods on rat cerebellar development. Biochem Soc Trans 13:759–760.
Wheeler KP (1975): Role of phospholipid in the intermediate steps of the sodium-plus-potassium ion dependent adenosine triphosphatase reaction. Biochem J 146:729–738.
Widnell CC (1972): Cytochemical localization of 5'-nucleotidase in subcellular fractions isolated from rat liver. J Cell Biol 52:542–558.
Wiggins RC (1982): Myelin development and nutritional insufficiency. Brain Res Rev 4:151–175.
Wiggins RC, Benjamins JA, Krigman MR, Morell P (1974): Synthesis of myelin proteins during starvation. Brain Res 80:345–349.
Winick M, Noble A (1966): Cellular response in rats during malnutrition at various ages. J Nutr 89:300–306.
Zacevic N, Rakic P (1976): Differentiation of Purkinje cells and their relationship to other components of developing cerebellar cortex in man. J Comp Neurol 167:27–48.
Zagon IS (1975): Prolonged gestation and cerebellar development in the rat. Exp Neurol 46:69–77.
Zamenhof S, van Marthens E, Grauel L (1971a): DNA (cell number) and proteins in neonatal rat brain: Alteration by timing of maternal dietary protein restriction. J Nutr 101:1265–1270.
Zamenhof S, van Marthens E, Grauel L (1971b): Prenatal cerebral development: Effect of restricted diet, reversal by growth hormone. Science 174:954–955.
Zanetta J-P, Benda P, Gombos G, Morgan IG (1972): The presence of 2',3'-cyclic AMP 3'-phosphohydrolase in glial cells in tissue culture. J Neurochem 19:881–883.

Current Topics in Nutrition and Disease, Volume 16
Basic and Clinical Aspects of Nutrition and Brain Development,
pages 131–155

Current Approaches to the Study of Gene Expression in the Adult and Developing Brain

Barry B. Kaplan

Molecular Neurobiology Program, Department of Psychiatry, Western
Psychiatric Institute and Clinic, University of Pittsburgh School of
Medicine, Pittsburgh, Pennsylvania 15213

INTRODUCTION

During the past decade, the diversity of gene expression in brain has been
examined by RNA-DNA hybridization analysis, in which trace amounts of
radiolabeled single-copy DNA (that portion of the genome coding for the vast
majority of cell protein) is hybridized to excess nuclear or cytoplasmic RNA,
and the fraction of the DNA forming stable hybrids is detected by
hydroxyapatite chromatography or their resistance to hydrolysis by a
single-strand-specific nuclease. This experimental approach facilitates the
detection of gene transcripts present in low copy number (rare RNAs) and
provides a direct estimate of the amount of genetic information expressed in
a given cell type, tissue, or organ. The results of many such investigations
have demonstrated that the brain expresses 2- to 5-fold more genetic
information than other somatic tissues or organs. These findings predict the
existence of thousands of brain-specific polypeptides, the great majority of
which have heretofore gone undetected by conventional protein analysis.
Many of these RNA sequences are developmentally regulated, suggesting
that they play an important role in the elaboration of brain-specific structure
and function. The remarkable diversity of genetic information expressed in
the brain bears on many fundamental issues in neurobiology, including the
ultimate function of this information and the degree to which it participates
in determining the cellular, anatomical, and functional diversity of the organ.

In this chapter, the results of recent molecular biological studies of gene
expression in the brain will be reviewed. Topics to be considered include: the
diversity of gene expression in the adult brain and clonal cell lines of neural
origin, the regional and cellular distribution of gene transcripts, and
alterations in the pattern of gene expression that occur in brain during
postnatal development. The sequence complexity of various RNA popula-

tions in the nervous tissue of lower vertebrate and invertebrate species also will be discussed. Special emphasis will be placed upon the application of RNA-DNA hybridization analysis and recombinant DNA technology to the study of brain development. Details concerning the procedures employed in nucleic acid hybridization and molecular cloning experiments have been discussed extensively and will not be addressed here (see for example, Kaplan, 1982; Glover, 1985; Hames and Higgins, 1985; Kaplan et al., 1985). Also excluded from this chapter will be a discussion of the developmental changes that occur in brain chromatin and chromatin-associated proteins, subjects which have previously been reviewed (Brown, 1983; Serra and Giuffrida, 1986).

DIVERSITY OF GENE EXPRESSION IN BRAIN
Nuclear RNA Sequence Complexity

Results of early RNA-DNA hybridization studies suggested that at least twice as much single-copy DNA was transcribed in brain than in other organs (Brown and Church, 1971, 1972; Hahn and Laird, 1971; Grouse et al., 1972). More recent estimates of brain nuclear RNA complexity, obtained using more efficient RNA extraction techniques and optimal hybridization conditions, revealed even greater complexity than that indicated by those pioneering studies. As shown in Table I, mammalian brain nuclear RNA hybridizes to about 15–20% of the single-copy DNA. Assuming asymmetric transcription, the sequence complexity of this RNA population is approximately $5-8 \times 10^8$ nucleotides, a value 2- to 5-fold greater than that manifest by other somatic tissues or organs. Approximately 65–75% of the total nuclear RNA complexity is found in polyadenylated heterogeneous nuclear RNAs [poly(A)$^+$hnRNA], known precursors to cytoplasmic messengers (see Hahn et al., 1978).

Based on the sequence complexity data, it has been estimated that the brain nuclear RNA population is comprised of as many as 130,000–180,000 different RNA sequences. This initial estimate was obtained by dividing the sequence complexity of the nuclear RNA population by the number average length of the most abundant brain nuclear RNAs, i.e., 4,500 nucleotides (Bantle and Hahn, 1976). However, since the size of the great majority of brain hnRNA (the low abundance complex class) is not established, this value serves only as a first approximation of the diversity of gene transcription in the brain.

Polysomal RNA Sequence Complexity

The sequence complexity of brain total polysomal RNA is given in Table II. At maximum hybridization, mammalian brain polysomal RNA is com-

TABLE I. Base Sequence Complexity of Brain Nuclear RNAs

RNA fraction	Animal species	Single-copy DNA hybridized (%)[a]	Sequence complexity (nt)[b]	Reference
Total hnRNA[c]	Mouse[d]	21.2	8.1×10^8	Bantle and Hahn, 1976
	Mouse[e]	17.2	6.5×10^8	Maxwell et al., 1978
	Mouse[e]	17.8	5.6×10^8	Chaudhari and Hahn, 1983
	Rat[e]	15.6	5.9×10^8	Chikaraishi et al., 1978
	Rat[e]	16.9	6.4×10^8	Grouse et al., 1978
	Rat[e]	13.5	5.1×10^8	Kuroiwa and Natori, 1979
	Sheep[d]	23.8	6.3×10^8	Deeb, 1983
	Goldfish[d]	23.2	1.5×10^8	Kaplan and Gioio, 1986
	Squid[d]	22.8	2.5×10^8	Perrone Capano et al., 1986
Poly(A$^+$)hnRNA	Mouse[d]	13.3	5.0×10^8	Bantle and Hahn, 1976
	Mouse[e]	12.5	4.0×10^8	Chaudhari and Hahn, 1983
	Rat[d]	12.5	4.8×10^8	Kaplan et al., 1978
	Rat[d]	13.0	4.9×10^8	Coleman et al., 1980

[a]Hybridization values given for each study are corrected for the reactivity of the single-copy DNA probe.
[b]Complexity estimates assume that DNA transcription is asymmetric and that the sequence complexity of the mouse, rat, sheep, goldfish, and squid single-copy DNA is 1.7×10^9, 1.9×10^9, 1.33×10^9, 3.3×10^8, and 5.6×10^8 nt, respectively.
[c]hn, Heterogeneous nuclear.
[d]Hybridization values determined by hydroxyapatite chromatography.
[e]Hybridization values determined by S1 nuclease assay.

plementary to approximately 8% of the single-copy DNA. By comparison, liver and kidney polysomal RNA hybridizes to about 2.4 and 1.6% of the single-copy DNA probe, respectively (Chikaraishi, 1979; Hitti and Deeb, 1984). Therefore, consistent with the nuclear RNA data, the complexity of the brain polysomal RNA population is far greater than that of other somatic tissues. In brain, the polysomal RNA complexity is divided equally between polyadenylated [poly(A)$^+$] mRNA sequences and a unique, tissue-specific non-adenylated [poly(A)$^-$] RNA fraction. These subpopulations are considered briefly below.

Poly(A)$^+$mRNA. The sequence complexity of mammalian brain poly(A)$^+$mRNA is approximately 1.5×10^8 nucleotides (Table II), a value sufficient to code for 100,000 different mRNAs averaging 1,500 nucleotides in length. Using recombinant DNA technology, Milner and Sutcliffe (1983) have characterized 191 DNA clones randomly selected from a cDNA library prepared from rat brain poly(A)$^+$mRNA. The tissue distribution, abundance, and size of the corresponding mRNAs was determined by northern blot hybridization. Approximately 18% of the selected cDNAs hybridized equally to poly(A)$^+$mRNA from brain, liver, and kidney (class I mRNAs). The

TABLE II. Base Sequence Complexity of Polysomal RNAs

RNA fraction	Animal species	Single-copy DNA hybridized (%)[a]	Sequence complexity (nt)[b]	Reference
Total polysomal RNA	Mouse[c]	7.7	2.5×10^8	Van Ness et al., 1979
	Mouse[c]	7.4	2.3×10^8	Chaudhari and Hahn, 1983
	Rat[c,d]	8.0	2.9×10^8	Chikaraishi, 1979
	Sheep[d]	5.2	1.4×10^8	Hitti and Deeb, 1984
	Goldfish[d]	6.7	4.4×10^7	Kaplan and Gioio, 1986
	Squid[d]	7.9	8.8×10^7	Perrone Capano et al., 1986
Poly(A)[+]mRNA	Mouse[d]	3.8	1.2×10^8	Bantle and Hahn, 1976
	Mouse[c]	3.6	1.1×10^8	Chaudhari and Hahn, 1983
	Rat[c]	3.2	1.2×10^8	Grouse et al., 1978
	Rat[d]	4.8	1.8×10^8	Chikaraishi et al., 1978
	Rat[c]	3.8	1.4×10^8	Kuroiwa and Natori, 1979
	Rat[d]	4.4	1.7×10^8	Colman et al., 1980
	Rat[d]	4.6	1.7×10^8	Bernstein et al., 1983
Poly(A)[−]mRNA	Mouse[c]	3.6	1.1×10^8	Van Ness et al., 1979
	Rat[c,d]	4.0	1.5×10^8	Chikaraishi, 1979

[a]Hybridization values given for each study are corrected for the reactivity of the single-copy DNA probe.
[b]Complexity estimates assume that DNA transcription is asymmetric and that the sequence complexity of the mouse, rat, sheep, goldfish and squid single-copy DNA is 1.7×10^9, 1.9×10^9, 1.33×10^9, 3.3×10^8 and 5.6×10^8 nt, respectively.
[c]Hybridization values determined by S1 nuclease assay.
[d]Hybridization values determined by hydroxyapatite chromatography.

relative abundance of 26% of the total mRNAs differed widely in the three organs studied and, therefore, were differentially expressed (class II mRNAs). Thirty percent of the cDNA clones examined were expressed only in the brain (class III mRNAs), while an additional 26% of the cDNAs failed to detect their complementary mRNAs at an abundance level of less than 0.01% of the total mRNA population (class IV mRNAs). These cDNA clones are believed to represent low abundance, brain-specific mRNAs expressed in particular cell types or small cell groups located in specific brain regions. These RNA species could be present in many copies per cell type or region but, at the whole brain level, appear very rare. Ten percent of the cDNA clones studied hybridized to multiple mRNAs, some of which may be expressed as members of small multigeneic families. Taken together, approximately 56% of the brain poly(A)[+]mRNA population (classes III and IV) appeared to be tissue-specific, a value consistent with the findings of RNA-DNA hybridization studies.

Interestingly, the rarer mRNA species detected by these cloned cDNA probes were, on average, larger than the more abundant RNAs and tended to be brain-specific. The rarest brain-specific mRNAs averaged 5,000 nucleotides in length, a value two to three times greater than the abundant messages. Based on these findings, it was estimated that the brain contained approximately 30,000 different poly(A)$^+$mRNAs averaging from 4,000 to 5,000 nucleotides, the average length of the rarer, more complex classes of mRNA (Milner and Sutcliffe, 1983). In computing the diversity of the brain mRNA population (see above), previous workers used the number average length of the total mRNA population (1,500 nucleotides), a value which reflects the size of the more abundant mRNAs. However, if these prevalent mRNA species tend to be shorter than the rare mRNAs, the overall number average size of the population could be underestimated (Meyuhas and Perry, 1979). In this instance, earlier workers may have overestimated the diversity of the brain poly(A)$^+$mRNA population. Regardless, however, of the absolute number of RNA species comprising the mRNA population, the data derived from molecular biological studies predict the existence of thousands of brain-specific polypeptides, the functions of which are unknown. Superimposed on this remarkable diversity is the complexity that may arise from differential processing of these mRNAs or their respective polypeptides (for review see Leff et al., 1986).

The reason for the larger size of the rarer brain-specific mRNAs is unknown. It is possible that many of the nucleotides present in these sequences are localized to non-coding regions of the mRNAs. Several recently sequenced brain-specific mRNAs are known to contain long 3' terminal untranslated regions. For example, the rat brain mRNA for the S-100 β subunit contains 276 nucleotides of coding region and 1,092 nucleotides of 3' non-coding sequence (Kuwano et al., 1984). Similarly, the mRNA for rat brain myelin proteolipid protein contains 831 nucleotides of coding region and 2,369 nucleotides of 3' untranslated region (Milner et al., 1985). Whether or not these untranslated regions of the mRNA serve some regulatory function is unknown. Alternatively, the rarer mRNAs could code for proportionately larger proteins, implying that proteins specific to the brain may be larger, on average, than non-specific, "house-keeping" proteins. As suggested by Milner and Sutcliffe (1983), these brain-specific proteins could be synthesized as polyproteins, facilitating the coordinate expression of several individual components of a single system.

Non-adenylated polysomal RNA. In the past it was assumed that, like most eukaryote messengers, brain mRNAs contained a poly(A) sequence at the 3' end. Therefore, early measurements of brain mRNA sequence complexity were derived from the analysis of poly(A)$^+$RNA isolated from polysomes. A unique property of the mammalian brain is that the polysome fraction contains a complex population of non-polyadenylated RNA that does not share sequence homology with polyadenylated messengers (Chikaraishi,

1979; Van Ness et al., 1979). The properties of this RNA population were recently reviewed (Hahn et al., 1986). Polysomal poly(A)$^-$RNA comprises approximately 0.5 to 1.0% of the mass of total polysomal RNA and contains a sequence complexity of approximately 1.4×10^8 nucleotides. The transcription of these sequences and their appearance in the polysome fraction is developmentally regulated, suggesting that poly(A)$^-$RNA plays an important role in brain function (see below). Since polysomal RNAs of high sequence complexity are assumed to be messengers, the non-adenylated RNA fraction has been referred to as poly(A)$^-$mRNA. Consistent with this view, poly(A)$^-$mRNA can function as a template for protein synthesis in a cell-free translation system (Chikaraishi, 1979; Hahn et al., 1983). However, a unique, highly diverse population of poly(A)$^-$mRNA translation products has yet to be identified. Ultimately, definitive proof that polysomal poly(A)$^-$RNAs function as messengers will require the identification of a set of protein products that are not encoded in the poly(A)$^+$mRNA population. This demonstration is especially important as the existence of a complex poly(A)$^-$mRNA population is a marked departure from the dogma of eukaryote cell biology. In this regard, mini cDNA libraries have been constructed (Hahn et al., 1986; Snider and Morrison, 1986), and nucleotide sequence data from select clones can now be obtained. From this information, it should be possible to identify and characterize their respective protein products, as described below.

IDENTIFICATION OF PROTEIN PRODUCTS OF BRAIN-SPECIFIC mRNAs

As mentioned previously, the remarkable complexity of brain mRNA predicts the existence of thousands of organ-specific proteins not yet detected by conventional protein analysis. Ostensibly, these gene products exist in low concentrations, being localized in discrete brain regions and related cell groups. Proteins encoded by these many mRNAs might include enzymes involved in neurotransmitter metabolism, release, and reuptake; neuropeptide, neuromodulator, and hormone precursors and processing enzymes; signal receptor systems; axonal transport systems; ion channels; proteins involved in cell-cell interactions; proteins involved in the establishment of neuronal microheterogeneity and ultrastructure; and the many proteins that might play a role in cognitive brain function.

The identification and characterization of these proteins is now possible using strategies derived from recombinant DNA technology. In this approach, selected brain-specific cDNA clones are analyzed by nucleotide sequencing, providing the partial sequence of the corresponding mRNA and polypeptide. To identify the putative proteins corresponding to these clones, antibodies are raised to synthetic peptides synthesized to small regions of the hypothetical amino acid sequence (see Sutcliffe et al., 1983b). Detection of the putative proteins can then be accomplished by radioimmunoassay or immunoblotting, and their regional and cellular distribution mapped by immunohistochemistry. The efficacy of this experimental approach has been elegantly demonstrated by Sutcliffe and colleagues in the mammalian brain (Sutcliffe et al., 1983a; Bloom et al., 1985; Malfroy et al., 1985) and in the Aplysia nervous system by Scheller and his associates (Nambu et al., 1983; Kreiner et al., 1984).

An excellent example of the successful application of this strategy is the identification of the polypeptide corresponding to the rat brain-specific cDNA clone, p1B236 (Milner, 1986). This cDNA hybridizes to an mRNA species present at an abundance of approximately 0.01% and first appears in the brain 5 to 10 days after birth (Lenoir et al., 1986). Nucleotide sequencing of p1B236 provided the sequence of the carboxy terminal 318 amino acids of the putative polypeptide. A notable feature of the sequence was the presence of several pairs of basic amino acids, i.e., ArgArg, LysLys, and LysArg. These sequences, commonly found in neuropeptide or peptide hormone precursors, are known to be the sites of proteolytic cleavage that produce the requisite bioactive peptides. Peptides were synthesized to regions of the 1B236 protein that corresponded to the most likely products of proteolytic processing, and antibodies to these synthetic peptides were raised in rabbits (Sutcliffe et al., 1983a). Immunocytochemical experiments demonstrated that 1B236 was distributed heterogeneously in the brain, the greatest concentrations located in the olfactory bulbs and peduncle, specific hypothalamic and preoptic nuclei, limbic, and neocortical regions. In colchicine-pretreated rats, large multipolar perikarya were observed within the amygdala, caudate-putamen, cingulate, parietal, and periform cortices, as well as in particular diencephalic and pontine nuclei. The immunocytochemical findings demonstrated that 1B236 was not distributed throughout the nervous system as a general "neural" marker, but was localized to select cell groups within functionally related central systems (Bloom et al., 1985). In electron microscopic studies, a portion of the immunoreactivity in the cortex was found in association with synaptic vesicles.

The various molecular forms of the 1B236 polypeptide have been investigated by radioimmunoassay (Malfroy et al., 1985). The most abundant form is of high molecular weight (approximately 100 kD) and requires detergent for solubilization. In addition, several lower molecular weight species were detected in brain extracts prepared under conditions designed to minimize proteolysis. These molecules corresponded in size to two of the possible products of proteolytic processing predicted from the amino acid sequence of 1B236. These findings, together with the regional distribution, ultrastructural, and electrophysiological properties of 1B236, suggest that this protein may be a prohormone or neuropeptide precursor capable of yielding several transmitter or neuromodulatory products. Regardless of the ultimate functional significance of 1B236, these studies demonstrate the power of this experimental approach in identifying previously undetected gene products that uniquely characterize the brain.

RNA SEQUENCE COMPLEXITY IN CLONAL CELL LINES

The striking diversity of gene expression in the brain is generally interpreted as reflecting the number of different cell types present in the organ. Based on RNA complexity estimates and frequency distribution data, Grouse et al. (1978) speculated that the rat brain could contain as many as 500 different cell types. This prediction is not discordant with the extensive cellular heterogeneity and microdifferentiation manifest by the various cell constituents of the CNS.

Importantly, however, there are data to suggest that neural cells, like the brain itself, may express an unusual fraction of the haploid genome. This possibility derives from a comparison of the nuclear RNA and poly(A)$^+$mRNA sequence complexity of several neural and non-neural cell lines. As shown in Figure 1, poly(A)$^+$mRNA from neuroblastoma and glioma cells hybridizes to 1.5- to 3.0-fold more single-copy DNA than does mRNA from several other somatic cell lines. Identical results were obtained from a comparison of the complexity of total nuclear RNA from these same cell types (Kaplan and Finch, 1982). A similar finding was obtained for poly(A)$^+$RNA isolated from astrocyte primary cell cultures prepared from 3-day-old rat brain (Kaplan et al., 1978). In this study, astrocyte total poly(A)$^+$ RNA hybridized to 7.1% of the single-copy DNA, a value 10% greater than that obtained for liver RNA.

The above observation suggests that the diverse of gene expression in brain is derived from both a marked cellular heterogeneity and the inherent complexity of the cell types that comprise the organ. It should be emphasized that since these findings are from studies of transformed cell lines, the conclusions drawn are necessarily preliminary. Although review of the literature indicates that transformation of cultured cells by either chemical or viral agents does not result in global alterations in gene expression (Getz et al., 1977; Rolton et al., 1977; Williams et al., 1977; Moyzis et al., 1980; Supowit and Rosen, 1980), confirmation of this hypothesis will require the bulk isolation and analysis of specific cell types from brain.

REGIONAL SPECIFICITY OF GENE EXPRESSION

Knowledge of the manner in which gene transcripts are distributed in the brain is essential to understanding the role played by the genome in the

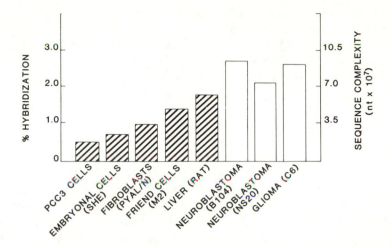

Fig. 1. The sequence complexity of poly(A)$^+$ mRNA from neural and non-neural clonal cell lines. The mRNA complexity of all cell lines was determined by RNA-DNA saturation hybridization using single-copy genomic DNA as a hybridization probe. Hybridization values were determined by hydroxyapatite chromatography and corrected for the reactivity of the DNA probe. The origin of the data is as follows: PCC3 (Jacquet et al., 1978), SHE (Moyzis et al., 1980), PYAL/N (Grady et al., 1978), M2 (Kleiman et al., 1977), liver (Savage et al., 1978), B104 (Kaplan and Finch, 1982), NS20 (Schrier et al., 1978), C6 (Kaplan and Finch, 1982).

elaboration of region-specific structure and function. The rationale for the existence of region-specific mRNAs is derived from the fact that individual brain regions differ widely in their cell composition, connectivity, content of neurotransmitters and neuromodulators, and function. It is conceivable, therefore, that the large diversity of genetic information expressed in the brain evolves from the summation of non-overlapping gene subsets active in a wide variety of highly organized and functionally distinct regions.

At present, an increasing number of molecular biological investigations have addressed this important issue. Results of these studies are somewhat surprising, as they reveal a remarkable homology in the RNA sequences present in the major brain regions. Early RNA-DNA hybridization studies showed little sequence complexity differences in nuclear RNA prepared from several major brain regions (Kaplan et al., 1978; Beckman et al., 1981; Deeb, 1983). Modest differences ($\sim$ 15–30%), however, were reported in the sequence complexity of the regional mRNA populations (Beckman et al., 1981; Kaplan et al., 1982; Hitti and Deeb, 1984). In each of these studies, the cerebellum yielded the lowest RNA complexity values, perhaps reflecting the relatively ''simple'' cytoarchitectonics of this brain region. In view of the uniformity in the diversity of regional nuclear RNA populations, it is possible that post-transcriptional regulatory mechanisms may play an important role in determining the small differences observed in the regional specificity of brain mRNA. Although the expression of many tissue-specific moderately abundant mRNAs is transcriptionally regulated (Derman et al., 1981), there is good evidence to indicate that post-transcriptional mechanisms also are involved in the regulation of organ-specific gene expression (Wold et al., 1978; Shepherd and Flickinger, 1979; Shepherd and Nemer, 1980; Kamalay and Goldberg, 1980; Jefferson et al., 1984; Carneiro and Schibler, 1984).

Using differential colony hybridization, Travis et al. (1986) screened cDNA libraries corresponding to poly(A)$^+$RNA from rat cerebral cortex and hippocampus for RNA sequences showing a region-specific distribution. After screening 2,500 colonies from each of these libraries, these investigators found no cDNA clones that represented region-specific RNAs. From these data, it was concluded that there were probably no RNAs in rat brain with an absolute hippocampus- or neocortex-specific distribution at a relative abundance greater than 0.05%, the limit of sensitivity of the screening procedure employed.

The regional distribution of several anonymous mRNAs has been investigated by in situ hybridization (Branks and Wilson, 1986). The relatively abundant RNA species studied were randomly selected from a cDNA library prepared from mouse brain poly(A)$^+$RNA. Although these mRNAs were expressed in different sets of cells and at different relative abundances within the regions examined, no RNA sequence was limited to a single region. Similar results were obtained by Wood et al. (1986), who used northern blot analysis to compare the distribution of 16 randomly selected cDNA clones in several regions of human brain. These authors concluded that different regions of the brain are not characterized by the expression of unique sets of abundant mRNAs, but rather have distinct patterns of gene expression that depend on the distribution of individual cell types comprising the region.

Recently, Rhyner et al. (1986) described an efficient and sensitive strategy to identify low-abundance, tissue-specific mRNAs that show regional specificity in their expression. In this study, a cDNA library was generated from poly(A)$^+$RNA from rat forebrain after first removing RNA sequences which are expressed in cerebellum by RNA-cDNA solution hybridization (Fig. 2). This procedure is designed to eliminate from the library mRNAs encoding "house-keeping" proteins required by all neurons and glia. The subtracted cDNA library was subsequently screened by differential colony hybridization using cDNA probes generated from various brain regions. Interestingly, no region-specific clones could be identified using total cDNA populations as probes. However, the use of subtracted cDNA probes (specific brain region cDNA minus cerebellar cDNA sequences) greatly

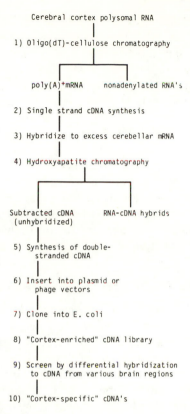

Cerebral cortex polysomal RNA

1) Oligo(dT)-cellulose chromatography

poly(A)⁺mRNA   nonadenylated RNA's

2) Single strand cDNA synthesis

3) Hybridize to excess cerebellar mRNA

4) Hydroxyapatite chromatography

Subtracted cDNA   RNA-cDNA hybrids
(unhybridized)

5) Synthesis of double-
   stranded cDNA

6) Insert into plasmid or
   phage vectors

7) Clone into E. coli

8) "Cortex-enriched" cDNA library

9) Screen by differential hybridization
   to cDNA from various brain regions

10) "Cortex-specific" cDNA's

Fig. 2. Strategy employed in the construction of a subtracted brain "region-specific" cDNA library. Repetition of steps 3 and 4 is recommended to increase the efficiency of the subtraction procedure.

enhanced the sensitivity of the screening procedure; clones corresponding to transcripts present at an abundance as low as 0.0005% could be detected. Under these screening conditions, approximately 5% of the 200 cDNA clones examined revealed regional specificity. These findings clearly show that RNA sequences specific to brain regions are of low abundance and represent only a small fraction of the total RNA population.

The use of neurological mutants may also prove helpful in identifying region- or cell-type-specific mRNAs. In one study, Oberdick et al. (1986) used the Lurcher (Lc) mouse, a mutation that results in the death of nearly all cerebellar Purkinje neurons, to assist in the identification of genes which are either Purkinje cell-specific or regulated by the presence of this cell type. cDNA probes were prepared from Lc and normal brain poly(A)⁺RNA and enriched for "brain-specific" sequences by subtraction hybridization using liver poly(A)$^+$RNA. These cDNAs were cloned into *Escherichia coli* using the λgt10 vector, and the cDNA libraries were screened for clones differentially expressed in Lc and normal brain. One "cerebellar-specific" cDNA clone was identified whose expression was drastically reduced in Lc when compared to the normal cerebellum. Demonstration of the cellular specificity of this clone will require analysis by in situ hybridization.

Taken together, the above findings describe four important features of gene expression in the brain. First, each brain region, regardless of cell composition, structure, or function, utilizes a remarkable amount of genetic information. Second, information necessary for region-specific function is encoded in a minority of the total genes expressed. Third, the majority of these sequences will be present in the specific brain region in relatively low abundance, and may comprise the class IV mRNAs described by Milner and Sutcliffe (1983). Fourth, post-transcriptional mechanisms may play an important role in the regulation of region-specific gene expression.

COMPARATIVE ASPECTS OF GENE EXPRESSION IN BRAIN

An assumption of the above studies is that the unusual amount of genetic information expressed in the brain underlies the organ's wide anatomical and functional diversity. To evaluate the validity of this postulate, a phylogenetic analysis of gene expression in the brain has been initiated (Kaplan et al., 1986). The working hypothesis of this ongoing investigation is that the diversity of gene expression in brain will increase during phylogeny, correlating with the evolutionary development of the organ. It bears mention, however, that there is no a priori reason to believe that evolution of the mammalian brain results directly from the transcription of a large number of new gene "sets." Rather, evolution could occur by alterations in the spatial and temporal pattern of organization of a large number of inherently complex cellular units. In this case, marked increases in the diversity of gene expression in the organ might not be detected during vertebrate evolution.

Figure 3 summarizes the available information on RNA sequence complexity in the brain of various animal species. The data are expressed as the ratio of brain RNA complexity relative to that of a typical non-neural tissue. The comparison suggests that differences in the amount of the haploid genome transcribed in brain relative to other organs is established early in phylogeny, and that these differences tend to increase during evolution. For example, brain nuclear and polysomal RNA of goldfish, a typical teleost, hybridized to 23.2 and 6.7% of the single-copy DNA, respectively (Tables I and II). In contrast, kidney nuclear and polysomal RNA was complementary to 16.1 and 3.1% of the DNA probe, respectively (Kaplan and Gioio, 1986).

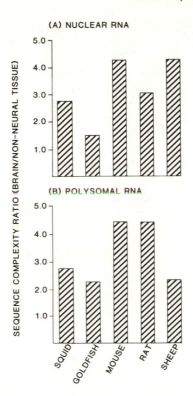

Fig. 3. Phylogenetic comparison of the sequence complexity of brain nuclear and polysomal poly(A)$^+$RNAs. Data are expressed as the ratio of brain RNA complexity relative to the complexity of RNA obtained from a non-neural tissue. Kidney served as the organ of comparison in all animal species except squid and sheep, where the somatic standard was gill and liver, respectively. Origin of the data is as follows: squid (Perrone Capano et al., 1986), goldfish (Kaplan and Gioio, 1986), mouse (Bantle and Hahn, 1976; Van Ness et al., 1979), rat (Chikaraishi et al., 1978; Chikaraishi, 1979), sheep (Deeb, 1983; Hitti and Deeb, 1984). (Reproduced with permission from Kaplan et al., 1986. Copyright 1986, Martinus Nijhoff Publishing.)

Thus, the amount of genetic information expressed in the goldfish brain was 1.5- to 2.2-fold greater than in kidney, a difference that is approximately half that observed in mammalian species. A comparison of the diversity of identical RNA populations obtained from the CNS and gill of squid, a highly evolved cephalopod mollusk, yielded similar results (Perrone Capano et al., 1986). It is noteworthy that in the two non-mammalian species studied, i.e., goldfish and squid, nuclear RNA hybridized to approximately 20–25% of the single-copy DNA (Table I), a value similar to that obtained in mammals.

This observation raises the possibility that the brain transcribes the maximal amount of genetic information available, regardless of species differences in the size of the single-copy genome.

Additionally, there is some evidence to suggest that brain-specific mRNAs may ultimately prove to be conserved during evolution, at least in mammalian brain (Sutcliffe et al., 1986). In this study, ten cDNA clones from rat brain class III mRNAs were hybridized to mRNA from mouse and monkey brain under conditions of high stringency. Nine of these cDNAs hybridized to mouse RNA and half of them showed close sequence homology to monkey brain mRNA.

Combined, the available comparative data support the hypothesis that the striking amount of genetic information expressed in the brain is indicative of the organ's structure and functional heterogeneity.

GENE EXPRESSION IN THE DEVELOPING BRAIN

In comparison to other organs, the brain undergoes profound morphological and biochemical differentiation after birth. Major events typifying postnatal development include neuronal and glial proliferation, cell migration, cell growth and differentiation, synaptogenesis, and myelination, phenomena which are still poorly understood. Ultimately, a detailed understanding of the ontogenesis of the brain will require knowledge of the temporal and spatial pattern of gene expression in the various brain regions and component cells. Recently, some progress has been made toward this goal.

Whole Brain Polyadenylated RNAs

The sequence complexity of rat brain poly(A)$^+$RNA at various ages is shown in Figure 4. A small but significant increase in complexity ($\sim$ 15%) was observed during the first 2 weeks after birth. Once attained, the adult values remained constant for up to 24 months, the average life span of the species (see also Colman et al., 1980). Although modest, the age-dependent increase in the sequence complexity of the poly(A)$^+$RNA population (5.0 $\times$ 10^7 nucleotides) is sufficient to code for 11,000 nuclear RNA sequences averaging 4,500 nucleotides in length.

Using northern blot hybridization, Sutcliffe et al. (1986) investigated the expression of several rat brain-specific class III poly(A)$^+$mRNAs. Four of ten of these individual mRNA species were developmentally regulated, appearing during the first week after birth. From these data, the authors predict that the number of poly(A)$^+$mRNA species that have a postnatal onset may be between 5,000 and 10,000, a value consistent with the results of RNA-DNA hybridization analysis (Kaplan and Finch, 1982).

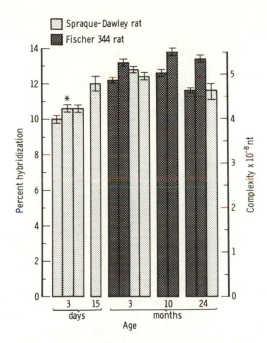

Fig. 4. Effect of age on brain poly(A)$^+$RNA sequence complexity. Poly(A)$^+$RNA from rats of various ages was hybridized to saturation with trace amounts of radiolabeled single-copy DNA and hybridization values determined by hydroxyapatite chromatography. Each bar represents the hybridization values ($\pm$ SEM) from an independent RNA preparation. Complexity estimates were made assuming that transcription is asymmetric and the complexity of the rat single-copy genome is 2.0×10^9 nucleotides. *P < 0.01. (Reproduced with permission from Kaplan and Finch, 1982. Copyright 1982, Academic Press.)

A somewhat different developmental pattern was reported in the brain poly(A)$^+$RNA population of the Swiss Webster mouse (Chaudhari and Hahn, 1983). These investigators observed no difference in the complexity of nuclear or polysomal poly(A)$^+$RNA of newborn and adult animals. Rather, a significant portion ($\sim 20\%$) of the poly(A)$^+$mRNAs present at birth were absent from the 17-day-old fetus. Based on the differences in sequence complexity, it was estimated that about 15,000 different poly(A)$^+$mRNAs of average size (1,500 nucleotides) appeared during the last 3 to 4 days of gestation. At present, reasons for the difference in the ontogenic pattern of gene expression in the rat and mouse is unclear.

Cerebellar Polyadenylated RNAs

Genomic studies. The complexity of nuclear and polysomal poly(A) $^+$RNA also has been examined in the rat cerebellum during postnatal

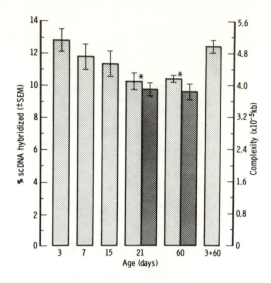

Fig. 5. Sequence complexity and homology of rat cerebellar nuclear poly(A)+RNA during postnatal development. Hybridization values (± SEM) and complexity estimates were obtained as described in Figure 4. Stippled bars at 21 and 60 days are results obtained from a second independent RNA preparation. 3 + 60, addition hybridization reactions containing equal amounts of RNA from 3-day-old and 60-day-old animals. *P < 0.01. (Reproduced with permission from Bernstein et al., 1983. Copyright 1983, Elsevier Publishers.)

development. Surprisingly, the complexity of cerebellar nuclear poly(A)+ RNA (Fig. 5) and poly(A)+mRNA (Fig. 6) decreased after birth. The decrement in the diversity of the nuclear RNA population occurred during the second and third week postpartum, a period when regional cell acquisition and differentiation nears completion. Importantly, cerebellar nucleosome repeat length undergoes a significant lengthening at this time (Jaeger and Kuenzle, 1982), suggesting that changes in chromatin structure may accompany the maturation-dependent alterations in RNA sequence complexity. Interestingly, the changes that occur in cerebellar chromatin are in marked contrast to age-dependent alterations observed in the chromatin of cerebral cortical and hypothalamic neurons (Brown, 1978; Ermini and Kuenzle, 1978; Whatley et al., 1981; Greenwood et al., 1982; Jaeger and Kuenzle, 1982). In these cells, the nucleosome repeat length shortens during postnatal development. The decrease in cortical neuronal DNA repeat length is interpreted to reflect a relative uncoiling (decondensation) of chromatin and is accompanied by an increase in the transcriptional activity of isolated nuclei (Greenwood and Brown, 1982). Based on these observations, one might speculate that concomitant with the reduction in RNA complexity, the transcriptional activity of cerebellar neurons decreases during development.

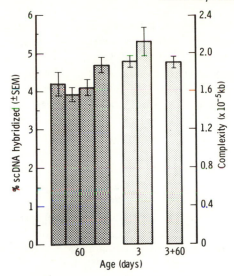

Fig. 6. Complexity and homology of cerebellar poly(A)$^+$mRNA from 3-day-old and 60-day-old rats. All values, determined as described in Figure 4, are given ± SEM. 3 + 60, addition hybridization reactions containing equal amounts of mRNA from 3-day-old and 60-day-old animals. (Reproduced with permission from Bernstein et al., 1983. Copyright 1983, Elsevier Publishers.)

Clearly, the rate of protein synthesis in this brain region declines markedly after birth, the cerebellum showing an exceptionally high rate in the neonate (Dunlop et al., 1977; Shahbazian et al., 1986). Maximal alterations in the pattern of cerebellar mRNA cell-free translation products also take place during the second and third postnatal weeks (Morrison et al., 1981; Soreq et al., 1982). Given these findings, it appears that global changes occur in cerebellar gene expression during postnatal development.

The sequence homology of cerebellar poly(A)$^+$RNA from neonate and adult rats has been investigated using addition hybridization (Bernstein et al., 1983). In this experiment, RNA from neonate and adult was mixed in equal concentrations and hybridized to single-copy DNA. The attainment of hybridization values greater than that achieved with the most complex RNA population alone (i.e., RNA from 3-day-old animals) would be indicative of heterology (non-overlap) in the sequences present in the RNA populations. As seen in Figures 4 and 5, RNA combined from 3-day-old and 60-day-old animals was complementary to the same amount of single-copy DNA as 3-day-old RNA. This result indicates that the majority of RNA sequences transcribed in the adult were already present at birth and that cerebellar maturation is accompanied by a net loss in the amount of genetic information expressed. Comparison of the kinetics of hybridization of poly(A)$^+$mRNA from 3-day-old and 60-day-old animals indicates that the age-related loss in RNA sequences occurs in both the abundant and rare (complex) classes of cerebellar mRNA (Bernstein et al., 1983).

Combined, these findings indicate that cerebellar development is, in part, a function of the conservation of specific sequences, perhaps with a concomitant repression of developmentally significant gene transcripts transiently expressed in the immature (embryonic) tissue. Many of these sequences may be crucially important in establishing the architectonics and specific connections of the region. It bears emphasizing that these findings, obtained at the *genomic* level, do not preclude the possibility that significant age-related differences in gene expression occur at the single gene level or in a subset of genes responsible for region-specific function. Rather, these observations underscore the fact that brain development also encompasses the selective repression of genes expressed in the embryonic tissue, a phenomenon that has received little attention. In addition, cerebellar ontogeny also may include alterations in the relative abundance of specific mRNAs, an aspect of gene regulation that was not addressed in the above study.

Single gene studies. The implementation of recombinant DNA technology has provided additional evidence that selective gene repression plays a central role in the development of the nervous system. Using a subtractive hybridization strategy, Miller et al. (1986) have constructed a cDNA library from embryonic day 16 (ED16) rat brain mRNA. Differential colony screening of this library yielded several cDNA clones that are preferentially expressed in the embryonic brain. One "brain-specific" clone (pDEV02) encodes an mRNA that is transcribed in the external germinal layer of the cerebellum. By postnatal day 22 (PD22), DEV02 mRNA is undetectable in the cerebellum as judged by in situ hybridization. Miller et al. (1986) have described a second clone (2Cl) whose expression follows an interesting developmental pattern. 2Cl mRNA is very abundant in diverse neuronal populations in the embryonic rat nervous system. During embryonic development, 2Cl is most abundant in regions composed of recently differentiated neurons, e.g., the cortical plate and developing spinal ganglion. By PD20, 2Cl is expressed at low levels in some, but not all, of the same groups of neurons. This observation suggests that 2Cl mRNA may be involved in the terminal differentiation and/or maturation of select neuronal subclasses and that its expression is repressed in others.

The above study serves as an excellent first example of the applicability of recombinant DNA technology in the area of developmental neurobiology. Hopefully, this new experimental approach will help to provide much needed insight into the role played by the genome in the development of the nervous system.

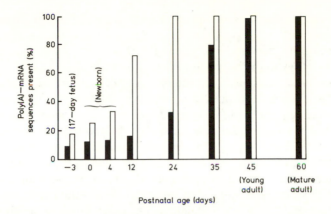

Fig. 7. Appearance of murine brain poly(A)⁻mRNA sequences in nuclear and polysomal RNAs during development. Radiolabeled cDNA, representing the rare (complex) class of poly(A)⁻mRNA of adult brain, was hybridized with polysomal RNA (solid bars) or nuclear RNA (open bars) from mice of the indicated ages. Percentage hybridization was normalized relative to the maximum levels achieved with poly(A)⁻mRNA from adult brain taken as 100% (actual level was 98%). (Reproduced with permission from Chaudhari and Hahn, 1983. Copyright 1983, American Association for the Advancement of Science.)

Non-adenylated RNAs

Measurement of the complexity of murine brain nuclear and polysomal RNA suggests that the genes specifying most of the poly(A)⁻RNA population are not transcriptionally active at birth (Chaudhari and Hahn, 1983). For example, the complexity of brain total polysomal RNA of the newborn was 1.2×10^8 nucleotides, a value approximately half that of the adult. The majority of the complexity (1.0×10^8 nucleotides) was contained in the poly(A)⁺RNA fraction. Similarly, most of the sequence complexity of total nuclear RNA in neonates, unlike that in the adult, was due to polyadenylated RNAs. The complexity of total nuclear RNA reaches adult values by PD21, the increase in complexity being attributable to the addition of a nuclear poly(A)⁻RNA population.

A developmental time course of the appearance of brain polysomal poly(A)⁻RNA is shown in Figure 7. In this experiment, cDNA prepared from the rare (complex) class of poly(A)⁻mRNA of the adult brain was used to probe brain total nuclear and polysomal RNA from animals of various ages. In the neonate, approximately 10% of the adult poly(A)⁻mRNA sequences were present in polysomal RNA. The adult complement of these RNA sequences is attained by PD45. Surprisingly, about 20% of the adult poly(A)⁻mRNA complexity was absent from polysomes even after 35 days of postnatal development. This finding suggests the appearance of several thousand new brain proteins during the transition from "adolescence" to young adult.

The results of Chaudhari and Hahn (1983) also reveal that the appearance of poly(A)$^-$RNA in the polysome fraction is much delayed relative to their appearance in the nucleus. For example, at PD24, all the adult complement of poly(A)$^-$mRNA sequences are present in nuclear RNA, whereas only 30% of these sequences are detected in the polysome. Thus, it appears that a substantial number of the genes encoding polysomal poly(A)$^-$RNAs are transcribed well in advance of their release into the cytoplasm. This observation indicates that post-transcriptional regulatory mechanisms play a crucial role in the expression of this population of brain-specific RNAs. In view of the tissue-specificity and dynamic developmental regulation manifest by the brain poly(A)$^-$RNA population, examination of the anatomical and cellular distribution of specific poly(A)$^-$mRNA sequences during ontogenesis could yield important new information.

CONCLUDING REMARKS

The number of genes transcribed in the mammalian brain, as determined by RNA-DNA hybridization analysis, far exceeds that expressed in other somatic tissues and organs. RNA sequence complexity estimates predict the existence of several thousand brain-specific proteins of unknown function. In one sense, these findings provide an assessment of the enormity of the problem confronting future molecular neurobiologists. It is encouraging that with the advent of recombinant DNA technology it is now possible to identify and characterize a significant number of these putative brain-specific gene products. At the very least, the delineation of the anatomical and cellular distribution of these proteins may facilitate the establishment of new cellular relationships, circuitry, and central systems.

The striking diversity of gene expression in the brain is derived from the remarkable heterogeneity of cell types comprising the organ and, perhaps, from the unusual complexity of the component cells themselves. The regional distribution of gene transcripts in brain suggests that region-specific differences in structure and function may result, in part, from the expression of a small portion (5–10%) of the total number of genes transcribed. Interestingly, a significant portion of these regional differences in gene expression may derive from post-transcriptional regulatory mechanisms. Data obtained from a limited number of phylogenetic studies suggest that differences in the diversity of gene expression in brain, relative to that of non-neural tissue, is established early in vertebrate evolution. Importantly, the differences observed in the complexity of RNA from nervous tissue of lower animal species, relative to non-neural tissue, is significantly less than that observed in mammals. This observation supports the hypothesis that the unusual diversity of gene expression in brain reflects the organ's heterogeneity of structure and function.

At the time of birth, the rodent brain has nearly achieved the adult inventory of polyadenylated nuclear and mRNA sequences. Nevertheless, there exist several thousand mRNAs that first appear during postnatal development. These genes seem to be activated during the first 2 weeks postpartum. The effect of environmental cues and experience on the expression of these developmentally regulated genes is a subject worthy of careful consideration. In this regard, there is some evidence to suggest that environmental factors do affect gene expression in the brain (Grouse et al., 1978, 1979). In contrast to poly$(A)^+$RNA, major developmental changes occur in the non-adenylated RNA population. Few of these RNA sequences are present in the neonate, the adult complement being attained 45 days after birth. Interestingly, the transcription of these genes occurs long before the RNA sequences can be detected in the polysome fraction. This observation suggests that post-transcriptional mechanisms play a critical role in the expression of this unique RNA population that characterizes the brain. Considering the tissue specificity and degree of developmental regulation manifest by this RNA population, the delineation of the function of these gene transcripts seems imperative.

From a developmental viewpoint, the pattern of gene expression observed in the cerebellum raises intriguing questions. This is the first brain region in which the diversity of gene expression decreases during postnatal development. The development of this region is characterized by a selective conservation of RNA sequences already present in the immature tissue. It is possible that many of the genes repressed during development play a transient but critical role in establishing the architectonics and specific connections in the region. At the single gene level, there are specific examples of genes whose transcription is selectively repressed in differentiating neuronal populations. It is now obvious that both the induction and repression of large numbers of genes occur during brain development. Hopefully, the application of new molecular biological technology will provide much needed insight into the role played by the genome in the development of the nervous system.

ACKNOWLEDGMENTS

I am grateful to my colleagues S. Bernstein, A. Gioio, A. Giuditta, and C. Perrone Capano who actively participated in the studies conducted in this laboratory. I thank Ms. J.-L. Knox for assistance in the preparation of this manuscript. The author is grateful to Drs. R.J. Milner and J.G. Sutcliffe

(Research Institute of the Scripps Clinic) for providing unpublished manuscripts and to Dr. W.E. Hahn (University of Colorado School of Medicine) for permission to reproduce previously published findings (Fig. 7). This work was supported by USPHS grants HD11392 and MH00518.

REFERENCES

Bantle JA, Hahn WE (1976): Complexity and characterization of polyadenylated RNA in mouse brain. Cell 8:139–150.

Beckmann SL, Chikaraishi DM, Deeb SS, Sueoka N (1981): Sequence complexity of nuclear and cytoplasmic RNAs from clonal neurotumor cell lines and brain sections of the rat. Biochemistry 20:2684–2692.

Bernstein SL, Gioio AE, Kaplan BB (1983): Changes in gene expression during postnatal development of the rat cerebellum. J Neurogenet 1:71–86.

Bloom FE, Battenberg LF, Milner RJ, Sutcliffe JG (1985): Immunocytochemical mapping of 1B236, a brain-specific neuronal polypeptide deduced from the sequence of a cloned mRNA. J Neurosci 5:1781–1802.

Branks PL, Wilson MC (1986): Patterns of gene expression in the murine brain revealed by in situ hybridization of brain-specific mRNAs. Mol Neurobiol 1:1–16.

Brown IR (1978): Postnatal appearance of a short DNA repeat length in neurons of the rat cerebral cortex. Biochem Biophys Res Commun 84:285–292.

Brown IR (1983): The organization of brain chromatin. In Lajtha A (ed): "Handbook of Neurochemistry," Vol. 5, 2nd Ed. New York: Plenum Press, pp 217–226.

Brown IR, Church RB (1971): RNA transcription from nonrepetitive DNA in the mouse. Biochem Biophys Res Commun 42:850–856.

Brown IR, Church RB (1972): Transcription of nonrepeated DNA during mouse and rabbit development. Dev Biol 29:73–84.

Carneiro M, Schibler U (1984): Accumulation of rare and moderately abundant mRNAs in mouse L-cells is mainly post-transcriptionally regulated. J Mol Biol 178:869–880.

Chaudhari N, Hahn WE (1983): Genetic expression in the developing brain. Science 220:924–928.

Chikaraishi DM (1979): Complexity of cytoplasmic polyadenylated and nonadenylated rat brain ribonucleic acids. Biochemistry 18:3250–3256.

Chikaraishi DM, Deeb SS, Sueoka N (1978): Sequence complexity of nuclear RNAs in adult rat tissues. Cell 13:111–120.

Colman PD, Kaplan BB, Osterburg HH, Finch CE (1980): Brain poly(A)$^+$RNA during aging: Stability of yield and sequence complexity in two rat strains. J Neurochem 34:335–345.

Deeb SS (1983): Sequence complexity of nuclear RNA in brain sections of the sheep. Cell Mol Biol 29:113–119.

Derman E, Krauter K, Walling L, Weinberger C, Ray M, Darnell JE (1981): Transcriptional control in the production of liver-specific mRNAs. Cell 23:731–739.

Dunlop DS, van Elden W, Lajtha A (1977): Developmental effects on protein synthesis rates in regions of the CNS in vivo and in vitro. J Neurochem 29:939–945.

Ermini M, Kuenzle CC (1978): The chromatin repeat length of cortical neurons shortens during early postnatal development. FEBS Lett 90:167–172.

Getz MJ, Reiman HM, Siegel GP, Quinlan TJ, Proper J, Elder PK, Moses HL (1977): Gene expression in chemically transformed mouse embryo cells: Selective enhancement of the expression of C type RNA tumor virus genes. Cell 11:909–921.

Glover DM (1985): "DNA Cloning, A Practical Approach," Vols. 1 and 2. Oxford: IRL Press.

Grady LJ, North AB, Campbell WP (1978): Complexity of poly(A)$^+$ and poly(A)$^-$ polysomal RNA in mouse liver and cultured mouse fibroblasts. Nucleic Acids Res 5:697–712.

Greenwood PD, Brown IR (1982): Developmental changes in DNase I digestibility and RNA template activity of neuronal nuclei relative to the postnatal appearance of a short DNA repeat length. Neurochem Res 7:965–975.

Greenwood PD, Heikkila JJ, Brown IR (1982): Developmental changes in chromatin organization in rat cerebral hemisphere neurons and analysis of DNA reassociation kinetics. Neurochem Res 7:525–539.

Grouse L, Chilton MD, McCarthy BJ (1972): Hybridization of RNA with unique sequences of mouse DNA. Biochemistry 11:798–805.

Grouse LD, Schrier BK, Bennett EL, Rosenzweig MR, Nelson PG (1978): Sequence diversity studies of rat brain RNA: Effects of environmental complexity on rat brain RNA diversity. J Neurochem 30:191–203.

Grouse LD, Schrier BK, Nelson PG (1979): Effect of visual experiences on gene expression during the development of stimulus specificity in cat brain. Exp Neurol 64:354–364.

Hahn WE, Chaudhari N, Beck KW, Pfeffley D (1983): Genetic expression and postnatal development of the brain: Some characteristics of nonpolyadenylated mRNAs. Cold Spring Harbor Symp Quant Biol 48:456–476.

Hahn WE, Chaudhari N, Sikela J, Owens G (1986): Messenger RNA in the brain. In Giuditta A, Kaplan BB, Zomzely-Neurath C (eds): "Role of RNA and DNA in Brain Function." Boston: Martinus Nijhoff, pp 10–22.

Hahn WE, Laird CD (1971): Transcription of nonrepeated DNA in mouse brain. Science 173:158–161.

Hahn WE, Van Ness J, Maxwell IH (1978): Complex population of mRNA sequences in large polyadenylated nuclear RNA molecules. Proc Natl Acad Sci USA 75:5544–5574.

Hames BD, Higgins SJ (1985): "Nucleic Acid Hybridisation, A Practical Approach." Oxford: IRL Press.

Hitti YS, Deeb SS (1984): Complexity of polysomal RNA in sheep brain sections and other organs. Cell Mol Biol 30:169–174.

Jacquet M, Affara NA, Robert B, Jakob H, Jacob F, Gros F (1978): Complexity of nuclear and polysomal polyadenylated RNA in a pluripotent embryonal carcinoma cell line. Biochemistry 17:64–79.

Jaeger AW, Kuenzle CC (1982): The chromatin repeat length of brain cortex and cerebellar neuron changes concomitant with terminal differentiation. EMBO J 1:811–816.

Jefferson DM, Clayton DF, Darnell JE, Reid LM (1984): Post-transcriptional modulation of gene expression in cultured rat hepatocytes. Mol Cell Biol 4:1929–1934.

Kamalay JC, Goldberg RB (1980): Regulation of structural gene expression in tobacco. Cell 19:935–946.

Kaplan BB (1982): RNA-DNA hybridization: analysis of gene expression. In Lajtha A (ed): "The Handbook of Neurochemistry," Vol. 2. New York: Plenum Press, pp 1–26.

Kaplan BB, Finch CE (1982): The sequence complexity of brain ribonucleic acids. In Brown IR (ed): "Molecular Approaches to Neurobiology." New York: Academic Press, pp 71–98.

Kaplan BB, Gioio AE (1986): Diversity of gene expression in goldfish brain. Comp Biochem Physiol 83B:305–308.

Kaplan BB, Gioio AE, Batter DK (1985): The construction and identification of recombinant DNA probes for the study of gene expression in nervous tissue. In Zomzely-Neurath C, Walker WA (eds): "Gene Expression in Brain." New York: John Wiley & Sons, pp 1–22.

Kaplan BB, Gioio AE, Bernstein SL, Batter DK, Perrone Capano C (1982): Analysis of gene expression in brain: Comparative and developmental studies. In Giuffrida Stella AM, Gombos G, Benzi G, Bachelard HS (eds): "Basic and Clinical Aspects of Molecular Neurobiology." Milano: Menarini Press, pp 87–97.

Kaplan BB, Gioio AE, Perrone Capano C, Giuditta A (1986): A comparative study of the diversity of gene expression in brain. In Giuditta A, Kaplan BB, Zomzely-Neurath C (eds): "Role of RNA and DNA in Brain Function." Boston: Martinus Nijhoff Publishing, pp 1–9.

Kaplan BB, Schachter BS, Osterburg HH, de Vellis JS, Finch CE (1978): Sequence complexity of polyadenylated RNA obtained from rat brain regions and cultured rat cells of neural origin. Biochemistry 17:5516–5524.

Kleiman L, Birnie GD, Young BD, Paul J (1977): Comparison of the base-sequence complexities of polysomal and nuclear RNAs in growing Friend erythroleukemia cells. Biochemistry 16:1218–1223.

Kreiner T, Rothbard JB, Schoolnik GK, Scheller RH (1984): Antibodies to synthetic peptides defined by cDNA cloning reveal a network of peptidergic neurons in Aplysia. J Neurosci 4:2581–2589.

Kuwano R, Usui H, Maeda T, Fukui T, Yamanari N, Ohtsuka E, Ikehara M, Takahashi Y (1984): Molecular cloning and the complete nucleotide sequence of cDNA to mRNA for S-100 protein of rat brain. Nucleic Acids Res 12:7455–7465.

Leff SE, Rosenfeld MG, Evans RM (1986): Complex transcriptional units: Diversity in gene expression by alternative RNA processing. Ann Rev Biochem 55:1091–1171.

Lenoir D, Battenberg E, Kiel M, Bloom FE, Milner RJ (1986): The brain-specific gene 1B236 is expressed postnatally in the developing rat brain. J Neurosci 6:522–530.

Malfroy B, Bakhit C, Bloom FE, Sutcliffe JB, Milner RJ (1985): Brain-specific polypeptide 1B236 exists in multiple molecular forms. Proc Natl Acad Sci USA 82:2009–2013.

Maxwell IH, Van Ness J, Hahn WE (1978): Assay of DNA-RNA hybrids by S1 nuclease digestion and adsorption to DEAE-cellulose filters. Nucleic Acids Res 5:2033–2038.

Meyuhas O, Perry RP (1979): Relationship between size, stability, and abundance of the messenger RNA of mouse L cells. Cell 16:139–148.

Miller FD, Naus CCG, Higgins GA, Bloom FE, Milner RJ (1987): Developmentally regulated rat brain mRNAs: Molecular and anatomical characterization. J Neurosci, in press.

Milner RJ (1986): Expression of brain-specific proteins. In Giuditta A, Kaplan BB, Zomzely-Neurath C (eds): "Role of RNA and DNA in Brain Function." Boston: Martinus Nijhoff Publishing, pp 32–41.

Milner RJ, Lai C, Nave K-A, Lenoir D, Ogata J, Sutcliffe JG (1985): Nucleotide sequences of two mRNAs for rat brain myelin proteolipid protein. Cell 42:931–939.

Milner RJ, Sutcliffe JG (1983): Gene expression in rat brain. Nucleic Acids Res 11:5497–5520.

Morrison MR, Pardue S, Griffin WST (1981): Developmental alterations in the levels of translationally active messenger RNAs in the postnatal rat cerebellum. J Biol Chem 256:3550–3556.

Moyzis RK, Grady DL, Li DW, Mirvis SE, Ts'o, POP (1980): Extensive homology of nuclear RNA and polysomal poly (adenylic acid) messenger RNA between normal and neoplastically transformed cells. Biochemistry 19:821–837.

Nambu JR, Taussig R, Mahon C, Scheller RH (1983): Gene isolation with cDNA probes from identified neurons: Neuropeptide modulators of cardiovascular physiology. Cell 35:47–56.

Oberdick J, Levinthal F, Levinthal C (1986): Brain-specific gene expression in the developing cerebellum. Soc Neurosci Abstr 12:215.

Perrone Capano G, Gioio AE, Giuditta A, Kaplan BB (1986): Complexity of nuclear and polysomal RNA from squid optic lobe and gill. J Neurochem 46:1517–1521.

Rhyner TA, Faucon Biguet N, Berrad S, Borbély AA, Mallet J (1986): An efficient approach for the selective isolation of specific transcripts from complex brain mRNA populations. J Neurosci Res 16:167–181.

Rolton HA, Birnie GD, Paul J (1977): The diversity and specificity of nuclear and polysomal poly(A)+RNA populations in normal and MSF-transformed cells. Cell Diff 6:25–39.

Savage MJ, Sala-Trepat JM, Bonner J (1978): Measurement of the complexity and diversity of poly (adenylic acid) containing messenger RNA from rat liver. Biochemistry 17:462–467.

Schrier BK, Zubairi MY, Lettendre CH, Grouse LD (1978): Bromodeoxyuridine effects on the RNA sequence complexity and phenotype in a neuroblastoma clone. Differentiation (Berlin) 12:23–30.

Serra I, Giuffrida AM (1986): Post-translational modifications of chromosomal proteins in neuronal and glial nuclei from developing rat brain. In Giuditta A, Kaplan BB, Zomzely-Neurath C (eds): "Role of RNA and DNA in Brain Function." Boston: Martinus Nijhoff Publishing, pp 182–196.

Shahbazian FM, Jacobs M, Lajtha A (1986): Regional and cellular differences in rat brain protein synthesis in vivo in slices during development. Int J Dev Neurosci 4:209–215.

Shepherd GW, Flickinger R (1979): Post-transcriptional control of messenger RNA diversity in frog embryos. Biochim Biophys Acta 563:413–421.

Shepherd GW, Nemer M (1980): Developmental shifts in the frequency distribution of polysomal mRNA and their post-transcriptional regulation in the sea urchin embryo. Proc Natl Acad Sci USA 77:4653–4656.

Snider BJ, Morrison MR (1986): Cloning and characterization of rat brain polysomal nonadenylated RNAs. Trans Am Soc Neurochem 17:247.

Soreq H, Safran A, Zisling R (1982): Variations in gene expression during development of the rat cerebellum. Dev Brain Res 3:65–79.

Supowit SC, Rosen JM (1980): Gene expression in normal and neoplastic mammary tissue. Biochemistry 19:3452–3460.

Sutcliffe JG, McKinnon RD, Tsou AP (1986): Gene expression in mammalian brain. In Giuditta A, Kaplan BB, Zomzely-Neurath C (eds): "Role of RNA and DNA in Brain Function." Boston: Martinus Nijhoff Publishing, pp 23–31.

Sutcliffe JG, Milner RJ, Shinnick TM, Bloom FE (1983a): Identifying the protein products of brain-specific genes with antibodies to chemically synthesized peptides. Cell 33:671–682.

Sutcliffe JG, Shinnick TM, Green N, Lerner RA (1983b): Antibodies that react with predetermined sites on proteins. Science 219:660–666.

Travis GH, Naus CG, Morrison JH, Bloom FE, Sutcliffe JG (1987): Subtractive cDNA cloning and analysis of primate neocortex mRNAs with regionally-heterogeneous distributions. Neuropharmacology, in press.

Van Ness J, Maxwell IH, Hahn WE (1979): Complex population of nonpolyadenylated messenger RNA in mouse brain. Cell 18:1341–1349.

Whatley SA, Hall C, Lim L (1981): Chromatin organization in the rat hypothalamus during early development. Biochem J 196:115–119.

Williams JG, Hoffman R, Penman S (1977): The extensive homology between mRNA sequences of normal and SV40-transformed human fibroblasts. Cell 11:901–907.

Wold BJ, Klein WH, Hough-Evans BR, Britten RJ, Davidson EH (1978): Sea urchin embryo mRNA sequences in the nuclear RNA of adult tissues. Cell 14:941–950.

Wood TL, Frantz GD, Menkes JH, Tobin AJ (1986): Regional distribution of messenger RNAs in postmortem human brain. J Neurosci Res 16:311–324.

SECTION III: NEUROTRANSMITTERS, NUTRITION, AND BRAIN DEVELOPMENT

Current Topics in Nutrition and Disease, Volume 16
Basic and Clinical Aspects of Nutrition and Brain Development,
pages 159–216
© 1987 Alan R. Liss, Inc.

Dietary Influences on Brain Function: Implications During Periods of Neuronal Maturation

Carol E. Greenwood and Rosemary E.A. Craig

Department of Nutritional Sciences, Faculty of Medicine, University of Toronto, Toronto, Ontario, Canada M5S 1A8

INTRODUCTION

Despite its apparent complexity, the brain is made up of two major types of cells—glia and neurons. The glia are primarily responsible for structure and myelin formation, while neurons are concerned with impulse conduction and the control and coordination of body systems. Metabolic substrates necessary for the development and maintenance of this central nervous systems (CNS) activity are derived from dietary sources. While the optimal nutrient environment for the CNS is unknown, we do know that the brain is dependent on an adequate nutrient supply such that alterations in nutrient supply occurring with nutrient deficiencies, food deprivation, and normal fluctuations in the diet are all circumstances during which nutrition can influence brain metabolism and function. To date, studies have predominantly examined the effects of diet on neuronal function. Much less is known about the responsiveness of glial cells to alterations in nutrient supply in the absence of malnutrition.

The effects of extremes in nutrient availability, such as deficiencies sufficient to affect growth rate and brain cell development in experimental animals, have been well described. For example, both histological and neurochemical abnormalities are observed following protein-calorie malnutrition (for reviews see Burns, 1984, Morgane et al., 1978; Nowak and Munro, 1977). In addition, it is well known that many vitamin or mineral deficiencies in the diet of both man and animals lead to the classical neurological symptoms of their inadequacy. These studies have provided important and fundamental information regarding minimum nutrient requirements for brain growth and development.

In contrast to the well-described effects of severe malnutrition and nutrient deficiencies on the nervous system, much less is known about the effects of normal dietary variations which do not result in malnutrition to either the mother or progeny on neuronal development in the offspring. Extrapolation

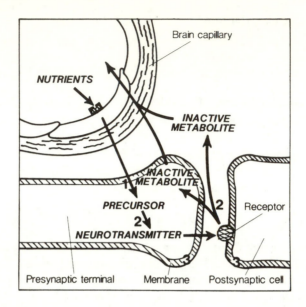

Fig. 1. Three postulated mechanisms whereby diet can modify brain biochemistry and function. 1) Food ingestion causes fluctuations in brain precursor availability and the synthesis of at least five neurotransmitters—serotonin, catecholamines, histamine, glycine, and acetylcholine. 2) Diet is the source of vitamins and minerals serving as cofactors for neurotransmitter synthetic and/or catabolic enzymes. 3) Variations in dietary fats alter nerve cell membrane composition, which in turn may influence neuronal function and/or activity of membrane-bound proteins. Reprinted from Leprohon-Greenwood and Anderson, Food Technology, 1986. 40:132–138 and 149. Copyright by Institute of Food Technologists.

of observations from the malnutrition literature cannot be made because it is impossible to differentiate changes in neuronal function related to neurochemistry from those related to concurrent histological changes resulting from the malnutrition. However, sufficient evidence has accumulated in the last 10 years to show that neuronal function, at least in the developed brain, responds to many characteristics of the normal diet (for reviews see Fernstrom, 1983; Leprohon-Greenwood and Anderson, 1986; Sved, 1983; Young, 1986; Wurtman et al., 1981). There are at least three ways that food modifies brain biochemistry (Leprohon-Greenwood and Anderson, 1986). First, food ingestion causes fluctuations in the availability of the nutrient precursors required for neurotransmitter synthesis. Second, food is the source of those vitamins and minerals that serve as essential co- factors for the enzymes synthesizing neurotransmitters. Third, dietary fats alter nerve cell membrane composition, which in turn influences neuronal function (Fig. 1). Alterations in neuronal function secondary to changes in vitamin and mineral availability and membrane structural changes result from chronic dietary intake and are probably similar in both the developed and developing brain. In contrast, changes in neurotransmitter metabolism resulting from altered precursor availability are observed after the consumption of single meals and are related to the fact that the rate-limiting enzymes necessary for their synthesis are not fully saturated with substrate under normal physiologic conditions. Hence meal-induced fluctuations in brain concentrations of these nutrients can alter neurotransmitter synthesis. Whether this relationship between precursor availability and neurotransmitter synthesis also occurs in the developing brain during periods when enzyme activities have not reached mature levels is presently uncertain. However, evidence suggests that, at least for the neurotransmitter serotonin, this may be so. Therefore, to relate dietary intake to alterations in neurochemistry during development, this chapter will first describe the current knowledge of the effect of composition of food consumed on neurochemical mechanisms in the developed brain and second will relate these observations to the developing brain by examining chronology of neuronal enzyme development and its implications for neuronal metabolism.

BRAIN NUTRIENT METABOLISM

The high metabolic activity of the brain might be taken to provide evidence that the brain is relatively sensitive to fluctuations in the nutrient state of the remainder of the body. Although the brain constitutes only 2% of adult body weight, it receives 15% of the cardiac output and accounts for 20–30% of the body's resting metabolic rate (Siebert et al., 1986; Sokoloff et al., 1977). The reason for the brain's high energy requirement (in humans approximately 17 kcal/100 g brain/min) is uncertain. Protein synthesis, a high-energy-requiring process, is believed to occur in the brain at an overall rate similar to that in muscle (Waelsch and Lajtha, 1961). Alternatively, transmission of nerve impulses via electrical ion gradients and restoration of these gradients through ion pumps requires constant energy utilization and may account for most of the brain's energy consumption (Bachelard et al., 1962; Rang and Ritchie, 1968).

In the developed brain, glucose serves as the major energy source, such that energy requirements of the brain are met almost exclusively through aerobic glucose degradation. This is indicated by the observation that the cerebral respiratory quotient, under normal conditions, is close to 1.0 (Sokoloff et al., 1977). While approximately 7% of glucose taken up by the brain is only degraded to lactic acid, approximately 30% is completely oxidized via the citric acid cycle (Siebert et al., 1986). The remaining 60% of the glucose is converted into amino acids via α-keto acids (Siebert et al., 1986). Since the brain has no stored form of energy, it is dependent upon a constant supply of glucose, which crosses the blood-brain barrier by facilitated transport involving a hexose-specific carrier (Oldendorf, 1971). During prolonged periods of glucose deprivation, the neuronal and glial mitochondria are able to utilize ketone bodies as the major energy source. However, this adaptation to ketone bodies is not complete and the brain still has a mandatory requirement for glucose, probably provided via hepatic conversion of lactic acid to glucose (Sokoloff, 1981).

Like the adult brain, the fetal brain uses glucose supplied by the dam as its major energy source (Jost and Pichon, 1970). When birth interrupts this transfer, glycogen stores accumulated in late fetal life are rapidly exhausted (Jost, 1966). The newborn instead derives energy from β-oxidation of the fats in milk, and the brain relies primarily on ketone bodies for fuel during late lactation (Booth et al., 1980; Drahota et al., 1964; Hawkins et al., 1971; Lockwood and Bailey, 1971; Page et al., 1971). Normal blood glucose levels are maintained by gluconeogenesis from pyruvate, lactate, glycerol, and some amino acids (for review see Girard, 1986). As the suckling period ends and the young animal develops adult feeding patterns, glucose again becomes the important metabolic fuel. Concomitantly, hepatic ketogenic enzymes (Lockwood and Bailey, 1971), use of ketone bodies (Booth et al., 1980; Lockwood and Bailey, 1971; Page et al., 1971), and ketone body transfer across the blood-brain barrier decline (Moore et al., 1976). As developmental changes with respect to ketone body uptake are observed, changes are also seen in the kinetics of glucose transport (Cremer et al., 1979). It has been argued that the underdeveloped blood-brain barrier serves a protective function in the young animal since glucose uptake is less dependent on saturable facilitated transport, and, therefore, during periods of hypoxia, the brain can anaerobically derive ATP via glycolysis and meet its energy requirements (Siebert et al., 1986).

Amino acids play several key roles in the brain. They provide substrate for protein and neurotransmitter synthesis and to a small extent, energy production. The oxidation of amino acids accounts for less than 10% of the total whole-brain energy utilization (Sokoloff et al., 1977). They are taken up by the brain by means of rate-limiting carrier-mediated transport mechanisms (Pardridge, 1977). Generally, free amino acid concentrations in the brain approximate (within a 2-fold range) those in plasma, except that glutamine, taurine, glutamate, aspartate, N-acetylaspartate, and glycine are several orders of magnitude higher in the brain (Glanville and Anderson, 1985; Lajtha et al., 1981). Specific developmental profiles of brain amino acid concentrations are observed. For example, proline, valine, isoleucine, leucine, tyrosine, phenylalanine, lysine, and tryptophan are higher in the immature brain, and their concentrations decline, reaching adult levels by weaning (Agrawal et al. 1966a). While to a certain extent these higher brain amino acid levels during development may represent diffusion across an immature blood-brain barrier, there is evidence suggesting that, at least for the large neutral amino acids, there is a high rate of influx resulting from a very active transport system rather than an incomplete blood-brain barrier (Baños et al., 1978).

Lipid is taken up slowly by diffusion, which is sufficient to provide essential fatty acids to meet the brain's requirement. However, local biosynthesis may be the most important pathway for supplying cerebral fatty acids (Bourre et al., 1978). That is, the brain is capable of de novo synthesis of fatty acids and of elongating and desaturating the essential fatty acids. During early developmental periods when the demand for the long chain polyenoic fatty acids is high, the brain has high enzymatic activity which declines, with time, in a reciprocal manner to liver (Naughton, 1981). The high respiratory quotient of the brain suggests that little fat is catabolized to provide energy under normal circumstances (Sokoloff et al., 1977).

Information on both the mechanism of uptake and factors affecting vitamin and mineral content of the brain is incomplete. Vitamin transport is believed to be by specific, unsaturated transport mechanisms (Ordonez, 1977), which suggests that levels of vitamins in plasma, and hence in the diet, influence the availability of these nutrients to their metabolic sites of action.

Thus, it is clear that support of the dynamic state of brain metabolism, even under conditions of a nutritionally adequate diet, may be influenced by variations in quantitative and qualitative aspects of food consumed. The following sections will examine mechanisms whereby food components, consumed in adequate amounts to prevent severe malnutrition, directly modify brain function. In addition, diet can indirectly influence brain function via afferent vagal signals arising in the periphery and impacting on brain activity. These peripheral events, resulting from food consumption, which modify neuronal activity will not be discussed here; reviews have been published elsewhere (Leprohon-Greenwood and Anderson, 1986; Li and Anderson, 1983).

DIET AND NEUROTRANSMITTER METABOLISM: ROLE OF VITAMINS AND MINERALS

The role of vitamins and minerals in metabolic processes in most body cell types has been well described. However, their role in the nerve cell, particularly in the process of neurotransmission, requires considerable elucidation. Of the fat-soluble vitamins, vitamins A and E are directly involved in neuronal metabolism, whereas the involvement of vitamin D is indirect, due to its effect on calcium metabolism. Vitamin A has an essential role in the visual process of the retina (Kaneko, 1979), whereas vitamin E probably functions as an antioxidant in the brain, as it does in other tissues (Dreyfus and Geel, 1981). In general, water-soluble vitamins function in nerve cells in classes of metabolic reactions which are similar to their function in other cells. For example, vitamin B12 and folate function in transmethylation reactions and in DNA synthesis (Gandy et al., 1973; Dreyfus and Geel, 1981). Thiamin, riboflavin, niacin, pantothenic acid, pyridoxine, and biotin participate as co-enzymes in the metabolism of carbohydrates, fats, and amino acids (Dakshinamurti, 1977; Dreyfus and Geel, 1981). Ascorbic acid functions in hydroxylation reactions in the brain, as it does in other tissues (Sourkes, 1979). It seems logical then that dietary inadequacy of any of the vitamins would alter brain metabolism. However, the point at which neurochemical transmission is affected is undefined.

There are many indications at the biochemical level that neurotransmitter metabolism is altered in nutrient deficiencies and that this may be one of the first aspects of metabolism influenced by nutrient inadequacy. Thiamin, pyridoxine, and ascorbic acid are examples of vitamins which may play a greater role in the control of neurotransmission than is currently appreciated or defined. Thiamin deficiency results in a decrease in the levels of the putative neurotransmitters, glutamate and aspartate, possibly reflecting decreased entry of pyruvate into the Krebs cycle (Hamel et al., 1979). Thiamin has also been postulated to have a direct effect on nerve conduction through thiamin pyrophosphate (Dakshinamurti, 1977). The functional aspects of thiamin deficiency are discussed elsewhere in this volume. In addition to thiamin, both ascorbic acid and pyridoxal phosphate (vitamin B6) are required at points close to neurotransmitter synthesis. Ascorbic acid, which is present in relatively high concentration in the brain, is involved in the conversion of dopamine to norepinephrine by the copper-containing enzyme dopamine-β-hydroxylase (Sourkes, 1979). Pyridoxal phosphate is the coenzyme for aromatic amino acid decarboxylase, which converts dihydroxyphenylalanine to dopamine and 5-hydroxytryptophan to serotonin, but its role in the formation of these two neurotransmitters is not identical. That is, pyridoxal phosphate deficiency in young rats causes a selective deficit in brain serotonin, but not in dopamine or norepinephrine formation (Dakshinamurti, 1982). Thus, the synthesis of these two monoamines by decarboxylation is separately regulated (Siow and Dakshinamurti, 1985), and these authors suggest that pyridoxal phosphate may be more tightly bound to dihydroxyphenylalanine decarboxylase than to 5-hydroxy-tryptophan decarboxylase. The role of folate and vitamin B12 in maintaining CNS transmethylation activity is not fully understood; however, deficiencies of either of these vitamins can affect CNS function. For example, folate coenzymes are required for both the synthesis and degradation of the putative inhibitory neurotransmitter glycine. In addition, 5-methyltetrahydrofolate serves as the methyl donor to homocysteine (Spector et al., 1980) and may function in the maintenance of adequate brain levels of S-adenosyl-methionine (SAM).

SAM is the major methyl donor in many reactions in the brain involving amines, neurotransmitters, proteins, nucleoproteins, and membrane phospholipids. Since brain SAM levels may be compromised in patients receiving L-Dopa for the treatment of Parkinsons disease (Wurtman and Ordonez, 1978), this may be a population particularly at risk with respect to folate deficiency. In addition, a high percentage of depressed patients have poor folate status (Reynolds et al., 1984). Whether the folate deficiency is primary or secondary to depression is unknown, although folate supplementation appears to improve serotonin metabolism, as indicated by an increase in 5- hydroxyindoleacetic acid levels in cerebrospinal fluid in these individuals (Botez et al., 1982). The mechanism whereby folate influences indoleamine metabolism is unknown (methylation reactions are not involved in either the synthesis or degradation of serotonin), but the fact that methylation may be involved is supported by the observation that administration of SAM to humans produces similar changes in 5-hydroxy-indoleacetic acid levels in cerebrospinal fluid (Bottiglieri et al., 1984).

Many minerals are important in nerve function, but there is even less information than for vitamins on the effect of dietary variations in mineral availability on neurotransmission. Calcium is well known to be involved in nerve conduction as the immediate stimulus of depolarization in conduction of nerve impulses. The trace elements iron, copper, and zinc also influence neurotransmitter metabolism, but the mechanisms of these effects are undefined. For example, iron may be a cofactor for tyrosine hydroxylase (Mandell, 1978), as well as for the catecholamine-inactivating enzyme, monoamine oxidase (MAO) (Youdim et al., 1980). In addition, post-synaptically mediated changes may be involved, since brain MAO, tyrosine hydroxylase, and tryptophan hydroxylase activities are unchanged in iron-deficient rats which show inhibition of serotonin and dopamine-mediated behaviors (Youdim et al., 1980, 1982), while the number of D_2-dopamine receptors in brain striatum is reduced (Youdim et al., 1983). Young copper-deficient rats have decreased brain tyrosine hydroxylase activity, which may account for their lowered concentrations of the catecholamines (Morgan and O'Dell, 1977). Zinc status also has a particular impact on the catecholamines, enhancing their concentration in severely (Wallwork et al., 1982), but not in mildly (Halas et al., 1982), deficient young rats by undetermined mechanisms. In addition to its role in neurotransmitter metabolism, zinc may have other important functions in the CNS. As reviewed by Pfeiffer and Braverman (1982), evidence suggests that zinc may be required for histamine storage, axonal transport, neuronal microtubule and tubulin synthesis and assembly, and structural stability of nerve growth factor. Zinc also appears to play an important role in maintenance of hypothalamic-pituitary function (Pfeiffer and Braverman, 1982). For example, physiological concentrations of zinc may inhibit pituitary prolactin secretion (Logan et al., 1983).

In addition to this relative uncertainty of the biochemical role of vitamins and minerals in neurotransmitter metabolism, it is uncertain whether the brain has any special ability, relative to other tissues, to preserve its metabolic and neurochemical activity during nutrient deficiencies. However, folate levels in brain and cerebrospinal fluid are higher than those in the serum, even during periods of folate deficiency (Korevaar et al., 1973). During iron deficiency, brain MAO activity is decreased by only 15%, whereas heart MAO activity is decreased by more than 60%, suggesting some central protection from or resistance to iron deficiency (Youdim et al., 1980). However, this observation cannot be applied to other minerals. Copper-deficient rats show a high correlation between decreased brain tyrosine hydroxylase activity and liver cytochrome oxidase activity, both markers of copper deficiency because of the cofactor role of copper in these enzyme systems (Morgan and O'Dell, 1977).

NEUROTRANSMITTER PRECURSORS AND SYNTHESIS

Studies in the past decade have shown that brain neurotransmitter synthesis is influenced directly by the availability of precursors, which are nutrients, in the diet and blood. The impact of this work has been substantial. First, it has led to the fundamental recognition that brain neurons are vulnerable to normal variations in blood nutrient content. Second, it has led to the exploration of the possible effects that changes in nutrient availability, such as those occurring with variations in meal composition and quantity, have on normal brain function. Third, it has led to the testing of new dietary and pharmacologic approaches to treatment of diseases involving abnormal brain function. Brain neurons use many substances as the chemical link for communication. Such substances, which currently number between 30 and 40, include amino acids, monoamines, and peptides. It had earlier been accepted that the provision of the building blocks for neurotransmitter synthesis was independent of dietary factors. This was based on two assumptions. First, it was thought that the brain could produce sufficient quantities of substrates from internal resources at all times for the synthesis of the neurotransmitters. Second, it was assumed that neurotransmitter synthesis was tied to utilization and not to precursor availability. These assumptions have been supported for many neurotransmitters; however, the dietary provision of substrate for neurotransmitter synthesis has been shown to be important for at least five neurotransmitters.

Serotonin, histamine, and glycine use as precursors the dietary essential amino acids tryptophan (Fernstrom et al., 1973), histidine (Enwonwu and Worthington, 1974); and threonine (Maher and Wurtman, 1980), respectively. The catecholamines use as precursor tyrosine, a dietary semi-essential amino acid available directly from dietary tyrosine and also derived from the essential amino acid phenylalanine (Wurtman et al., 1974; Gibson and Wurtman, 1977). Acetylcholine requires choline as its precursor. Although choline can be synthesized in the brain (Blusztajn and Wurtman, 1981), the precursor availability from diet and plasma also influence the synthesis of acetylcholine (Cohen and Wurtman, 1976).

With the exceptions of tryptophan, tyrosine, histidine, and threonine, fluctuations in brain amino acid concentration over normal ranges have not been shown to influence neurotransmitter synthesis. The amino acids known to function directly as neurotransmitters, such as glutamate, γ-aminobutyric acid, and aspartic acid, are dietary non-essential amino acids, and metabolic controls within the neuron appear to regulate their production and release for neurotransmission purposes (Wurtman et al., 1981).

In order for dietary supply of nutrients (precursors) to influence neurotransmitter synthesis, several criteria must be met (Wurtman et al., 1981). First, changes in circulating concentrations of the precursors must be observed following food consumption. If, for example, intestinal and hepatic mechanisms operate to maintain a constant plasma concentration of these precursors, the brain would be insensitive to altered dietary intake. Second, the transport of the precursor into brain must occur by a non-saturated uptake mechanism in order for plasma precursor levels to be reflected in brain. Third, the rate-limiting enzyme for neurotransmitter synthesis must be unsaturated with substrate under normal physiological conditions. When these three criteria are met, brain neurotransmitter concentrations are altered in response to acute food ingestion. Finally, it must be demonstrated that this increase in neurotransmitter concentration is reflected in the amount of neurotransmitter being released from the neuron and that the increased release of neurotransmitter is influencing neurotransmission and function. While five neurotransmitters have been identified to be under precursor control, this review will focus on only two, serotonin and the catecholamines. Similar mechanisms operate for histamine, glycine, and acetylcholine, especially when precursors are directly administered to experimental animals. The effect of changes in food consumption is less clear for these neurotransmitters, however. In addition, while functional (behavioral) correlates of precursor-induced synthesis of histamine (Sheiner et al., 1985) and acetylcholine (Barbeau et al., 1979) have been demonstrated, the physiological significance of increased glycine synthesis from threonine has not yet been demonstrated.

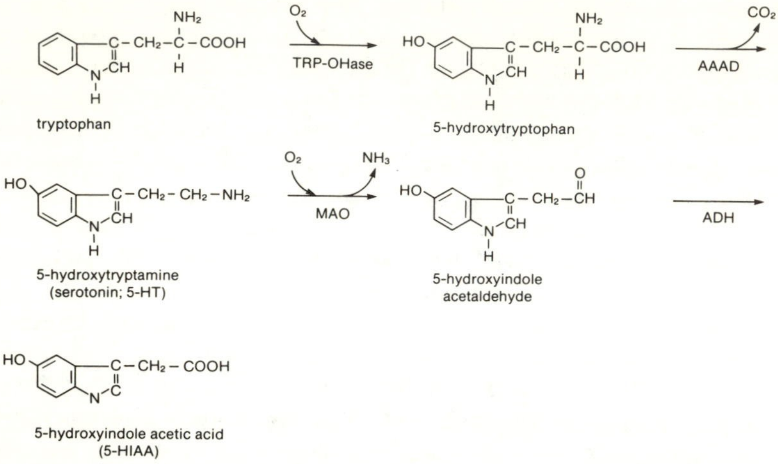

Fig. 2. Serotonin synthesis and degradation. TRP-OHase, tryptophan hydroxylase; AAAD, aromatic amino acid decarboxylase; MAO, monoamine oxidase; ADH, aldehyde dehyrogenase.

Serotonin

Serotonin (5-hydroxytryptamine; 5-HT) is synthesized within neurons from the essential amino acid, tryptophan, by a two-step enzymatic process (Fig. 2). The initial conversion, which involves the hydroxylation of tryptophan to 5-hydroxytryptophan, is catalyzed by the enzyme, tryptophan hydroxylase (TRP-OHase), and requires both molecular oxygen and a reduced pterin as co-factors (Lovenberg et al., 1968). TRP-OHase is highly localized in 5-HT-producing neurons (Aghajanian and Asher, 1971), and its presence within the cell characterizes the neuron as serotonergic. 5-hydroxytryptophan is then decarboxylated (Lovenberg et al., 1962), under the control of L-aromatic amino acid decarboxylase (AAAD), to form 5-HT. AAAD is ubiquitously distributed throughout the brain and is involved in the synthesis of other monoamines, such as the catecholamines. The rate of decarboxylation is relatively fast and exceeds that of tryptophan hydroxylation. Consequently, 5-hydroxytryptophan is not normally found in significant concentrations in the brain. In addition, small amounts of tryptophan can be directly decarboxylated to tryptamine by AAAD (Warsh et al., 1979; Young et al., 1980). The physiologic importance of tryptamine formation in the brain is still controversial.

Once synthesized, 5-HT is stored in the neuron in particulate-bound form (Marchbanks, 1966). There is indirect evidence that intracellular stores of

5-HT may occur in at least two separate compartments (Shields and Eccleston, 1973; Glowinski, 1978) and that newly synthesized 5-HT is preferentially released (Elks et al., 1979). After release into the synapse, 5-HT is retaken up into the presynaptic neuron prior to degradation. The major metabolite of 5-HT, 5-hydroxyindoleacetic acid (5-HIAA) is formed by a two-step enzymatic process. 5-HT is first converted to 5-hydroxyindole acetaldehyde under the control of the mitochondrial enzyme, MAO. 5-Hydroxyindole acetaldehyde is then converted to 5-HIAA, catalyzed by aldehyde dehydrogenase, with small amounts of the aldehyde being reduced to 5-hydroxytryptophol by alcohol reductase (Cheifetz and Warsh; 1980; Diggory et al., 1979). Evidence suggests that little, if any, 5-HT is recompartmentalized after re-uptake into the 5-HT neuron (Glowinski, 1972).

Control of serotonin synthesis. Hydroxylation of tryptophan to 5-hydroxytryptophan is the rate-limiting step in 5-HT synthesis. In vitro studies of partially purified enzyme preparations estimate the Km of TRP-OHase for tryptophan to be approximately 50 μM, when the naturally occurring pterin, tetrahydrobiopterin, is used as a co-factor (Kaufman, 1974). Since brain levels of tryptophan approximate 10–50 μM under normal physiologic conditions, these data suggest that the enzyme is normally only 50% saturated with respect to substrate and that changes in brain tryptophan concentrations could influence the rate of 5-HT formation.

The first indication that brain TRP-OHase is unsaturated in vivo arose from the demonstration that tryptophan administration to rats pretreated with an MAO inhibitor to block catabolism of 5-HT increased brain 5-HT content (Hess and Doepfner, 1961). This led to further studies which showed that large tryptophan loads increased brain content of both 5-HT and 5-HIAA in otherwise untreated animals (Ashcroft et al., 1965), and it is now generally recognized that treatments that elevate brain tryptophan concentrations increase the rate of 5-HT synthesis (for reviews see Fernstrom, 1983; Leprohon-Greenwood and Anderson, 1986; Sved, 1983; Young, 1986; Wurtman et al., 1981) such that a doubling of 5-HT concentrations can be achieved. A dose-dependent increase in brain 5-HT levels is observed after 1 hr with tryptophan loads of up to 50 mg/kg, with higher levels of tryptophan having no further effect on 5-HT synthesis (Fernstrom and Wurtman, 1971). Prolonged feeding of tryptophan to rats results in a similar increase in postprandial levels of brain 5-HT and 5-HIAA (Leprohon and Anderson, 1982; Lasley and Thurmond, 1985), suggesting that significant down-regulation of the enzyme does not occur with time. Obviously direct confirmation of the relationship between brain tryptophan and 5-HT levels cannot be obtained in humans. However, current evidence suggests that the same may be true. In neurologic patients receiving tryptophan, cerebrospinal fluid 5-HIAA concentrations were approximately doubled following a 3-g load of tryptophan, with no further effect of a 6-g load being observed (Young and Gauthier, 1981). While these studies all demonstrate that at high pharmacologic levels tryptophan administration can elevate brain 5-HT concentrations, the precursor effect of tryptophan only took on physiologic significance when it was shown that tryptophan loads as low as 12.5 mg/kg (approximately 5% of the rat's normal dietary tryptophan intake) raised brain 5-HT concentration and that brain 5-HT levels also responded to food ingestion (Fernstrom et al., 1973).

While there is some evidence that end product inhibition of tryptophan hydroxylation may occur (for review see Fernstrom, 1983), this inhibition is obviously not strong enough in vivo to maintain brain 5-HT at a constant level. These data predominantly come from studies in which the rate of 5-HT synthesis was measured either in vitro (Carlsson et al., 1976; Carlsson and Lindqvist, 1972) or in vivo (Hamon et al., 1973) after pretreatment with an MAO inhibitor to elevate neuronal 5-HT levels. While the rate of tryptophan hydroxylation was reduced by approximately 30% after MAO pretreatment, this inhibition was not sufficient to block the rise in 5-hydroxytryptophan formation following tryptophan. Thus the bulk of evidence available to date demonstrates that under normal physiologic conditions brain precursor (tryptophan) availability plays a major role in regulating the rate of 5-HT synthesis. Therefore, factors governing brain tryptophan levels and uptake will in turn influence 5-HT synthesis.

Regulation of brain tryptophan levels. Since tryptophan is an essential amino acid and hence cannot be synthesized de novo, the brain is dependent upon an adequate dietary supply of this amino acid delivered via the plasma. The uptake of tryptophan into brain from plasma, however, is not simply dependent upon circulating concentrations of tryptophan alone. Rather, tryptophan enters the brain via a saturable carrier-mediated system specific for the large neutral amino acids (LNAA; including leucine, isoleucine, valine, tyrosine, phenylalanine, and methionine) located at the blood-brain barrier (Pardridge, 1977). Thus it is the ratio of tryptophan relative to the sum of the competing LNAA that best predicts brain tryptophan concentrations. Two points of interest require clarification with regard to the plasma ratio predicting brain tryptophan levels. First, it has been well established that the affinity (Kd) of the various LNAA for the uptake carrier differ somewhat from one another (Pardridge and Oldendorf, 1975). Hence, prediction of brain tryptophan levels based on circulating plasma amino acid concentrations should correctly take into account the differences in amino acid affinities. Second, while initial studies of the rate of brain amino acid uptake were performed in anesthetized rats, more current data based on conscious, freely moving animals suggest that the actual rate of uptake may have been underestimated in the earlier studies

(Miller et al., 1985). This underestimation of rate of uptake may simply be due to decreased cerebral blood flow in anesthetized animals. This information more accurately allows for the prediction of the kinetics of brain LNAA uptake. However it is probably of little practical relevance to studies examining these relationships among brain tryptophan and plasma amino acid ratios beyond the first pass of the amino acids.

While the value of the plasma tryptophan to LNAA ratio as a predictor of brain tryptophan levels is well recognized, more controversial is the influence of plasma tryptophan binding to albumin. Tryptophan is unique as the only amino acid circulating in the plasma bound to albumin, with only 10–15% of total tryptophan in the free form (McMenamy and Oncley, 1958). Since only free tryptophan can ultimately cross the blood-brain barrier, it was suggested that free rather than total tryptophan determined brain tryptophan levels. To support this hypothesis are data suggesting that displacement of tryptophan from albumin results in increased brain tryptophan levels (Gessa and Tagliamonte, 1974; Knott and Curzon, 1972). For example, a number of experimental treatments, such as increasing the plasma concentration of non-esterified fatty acids or administering drugs such as salicylate or probenecid, will competitively displace tryptophan from albumin and increase brain tryptophan concentrations (Gessa and Tagliamonte, 1974; Knott and Curzon, 1972; Sarna et al., 1985). Conversely it has been argued that since tryptophan binds loosely to albumin (Madras et al., 1974a,b) and has a much higher affinity for the actual uptake carrier than it does for albumin (Yuwiler et al., 1977), that competition for carrier sites is quantitatively more important than albumin binding in determining tryptophan uptake. Taking all available data together, it appears that total tryptophan, albumin binding, and amino acid competition are all important determinants of tryptophan uptake, and that changes in any one of these factors will alter brain tryptophan concentrations and hence brain 5-HT levels.

Dietary control of brain serotonin synthesis. Alterations in dietary tryptophan content can influence both brain tryptophan and 5-HT concentrations. Feeding tryptophan-deficient diets depletes both the tissue pools of tryptophan and brain 5-HT content (Biggio et al., 1974; Culley et al., 1962; Gal and Drewes, 1962; Kantak et al., 1980; Lytle et al., 1975; Wong et al., 1962). Since the concentration of free tryptophan in both the plasma and tissue is lower than most other amino acids (Munro, 1970), reductions in brain 5-HT are seen within relatively short periods of time. Within 4 days of feeding a tryptophan-deficient casein hydrolysate diet, plasma tryptophan concentrations were reduced by 65% resulting in a 35% reduction in brain 5-HT levels (Wong et al., 1962). Conversely, feeding diets supplemented with tryptophan elevate brain 5-HT levels (Lasley and Thurmond, 1985; Leprohon and Anderson, 1982; Wong et al., 1962; Woodger et al., 1979).

The addition of 5% tryptophan to commercial diets increased brain 5-HT concentrations by 50% as compared to rats receiving diets supplemented with 1% tryptophan (Wong et al., 1962). Thus, variations in dietary tryptophan content alter plasma tryptophan concentrations producing changes in brain tryptophan and 5-HT levels.

Alternatively, supplementation of the diet with either leucine (Ramanamurthy and Srikantia, 1970; Yuwiler and Geller, 1965) or phenylalanine (Culley et al., 1962; Green et al., 1962; Yuwiler and Geller, 1966; Yuwiler and Louttit, 1961) reduces brain 5-HT content. Although plasma ratios and brain tryptophan were not measured in many of these studies, it seems reasonable to predict that decreased 5-HT levels result from increased competition for tryptophan uptake into the brain. However, it has also been suggested that these amino acids have direct effects on the 5-HT neuron. Leucine reportedly interferes with serotonergic neurons by affecting either the uptake or release of 5-HT from storage granules (Ramanamurthy and Srikantia, 1970). Phenylalanine, on the other hand, inhibits TRP-OHase activity (Lovenberg et al., 1968) and can thus reduce 5-HT levels.

Research examining the influence of plasma tryptophan to LNAA ratios on 5-HT metabolism has emphasized the role of diet composition, especially the dietary proportion of protein relative to carbohydrate. Protein content of the diet is inversely related to plasma tryptophan to LNAA ratios, while the carbohydrate content of the diet is directly related to plasma tryptophan to LNAA ratios (for reviews see Fernstrom, 1983; Leprohon-Greenwood and Anderson, 1986; Li and Anderson, 1983; Sved, 1983; Wurtman et al., 1981). This relationship between diet and plasma ratios has been most extensively examined in acute, single-meal studies.

Diet-induced changes in plasma amino acid patterns are dependent on insulin release following meal ingestion. Insulin stimulates tissue uptake of all amino acids except tryptophan. Consequently as the carbohydrate content of the diet increases, protein decreases, and insulin secretion is stimulated; plasma tryptophan levels remain constant while the concentrations of the LNAA fall, thus increasing the tryptophan to LNAA ratio (Fernstrom et al., 1975; Glaeser et al., 1983; Li and Anderson, 1982; Møller, 1985; Wurtman and Fernstrom, 1975). Thus, high carbohydrate diets as opposed to high protein diets elevate brain 5-HT concentrations, with this effect of diet on brain neurotransmitter level observed within 20 to 30 min of meal consumption (Li and Anderson, 1982; Wurtman and Fernstrom, 1975). This effect of carbohydrate ingestion can be reproduced by insulin injection (Fernstrom, 1976), demonstrating the involvement of insulin in the relationship between plasma tryptophan to LNAA ratio and diet composition.

The importance of insulin release in diet-induced changes in plasma ratios is supported by observations that plasma tryptophan to LNAA ratios are decreased in diabetic rats (Crandall and Fernstrom, 1980; Glanville and Anderson, 1985; Woodger et al., 1979). Concomitant with low plasma tryptophan to LNAA ratios are decreased brain tryptophan concentrations. Although a reduction in brain 5-HT would be predicted from the lower brain tryptophan, both 5-HT and 5-HIAA levels are maintained at control concentrations in diabetic rats (MacKenzie and Trulson, 1978; Woodger et al., 1979). A compensation for decreased brain tryptophan levels appears to be a result of increased TRP-OHase activity (MacKenzie and Trulson, 1978), although a decreased rate of 5-HT synthesis in the diabetic rat has been reported by other investigators (Crandall et al., 1981). TRP-OHase is also elevated by acute reductions in brain tryptophan due to neutral amino acid loads or a tryptophan-deficient diet (Neckers et al., 1977). Thus it appears that the brain may be capable of compensating for decreased precursor amino acid availability via elevations in TRP-OHase activity.

The fact that brain 5-HT metabolism responds to acute changes in the protein and carbohydrate composition of the diet has been well established and is generally recognized by most investigators. Present evidence suggests that this neurochemical change is an important metabolic cue aiding both experimental animals and man in regulating their intake of carbohydrate and protein (for reviews see Li and Anderson, 1983; Wurtman and Wurtman, 1984). Thus, for example, feeding an animal a pre-meal of carbohydrate causes the animal to subsequently select a high protein meal (Li and Anderson, 1982). To support the hypothesis that this food selection response is mediated by 5-HT are a number of studies showing similar behavioral responses after the administration of either tryptophan or serotonergic drugs (for reviews see Li and Anderson, 1983; Wurtman and Wurtman, 1984). This mechanism appears to be operative in humans as well. Providing young men with either an oral dose (2 g) of tryptophan (Hrboticky et al., 1985) or a mixture of amino acids which either raises or lowers the plasma tryptophan to LNAA ratio (Teff et al., 1985) results in the predicted changes in macronutrient selection during a subsequent meal. Interestingly, females appear to be less responsive to the tryptophan challenge (Hrboticky, 1986). This gender difference may be partially explained by the fact that the metabolic handling of tryptophan is influenced by the stage of the menstrual cycle, with increased kynurenine synthesis being observed during the leuteal stage. Since tryptophan oxidation changes during the menstrual cycle, perhaps influencing tryptophan availability for 5-HT synthesis, it is interesting to speculate that this metabolic change is in part responsible for the changes in carbohydrate and protein selection observed in women over the course of the menstrual cycle (Dalvit-McPhillips, 1983; Hrboticky, 1986).

Since both plasma amino acid patterns and brain 5-HT metabolism respond acutely to either tryptophan supplementation or diet composition, it is appropriate then to ask whether these biochemical changes are observed chronically. Tryptophan itself can induce the hepatic activity of tryptophan pyrrolase, the rate-limiting enzyme in its oxidative degradation. While plasma tryptophan concentrations remain elevated in neuropsychiatric patients receiving tryptophan therapy, the magnitude of change in plasma tryptophan concentration declines with time (Green et al., 1980; Yuwiler et al., 1981). Chronic infusion of a low dose of tryptophan to rats, using a mini-osmotic pump, increased hepatic tryptophan pyrrolase activity to a sufficient extent that no change in plasma tryptophan level was observed after 24 hr (Peters and Buhr, 1984). However, by 96 hr, hepatic tryptophan pyrrolase activity was significantly reduced and plasma tryptophan concentrations elevated in these animals. While these investigators failed to observe changes in brain tryptophan or 5-HT concentrations following the 96-hr infusion, there have been numerous other reports suggesting that 5-HT metabolism remains elevated even after chronic tryptophan supplementation. For example, feeding rats tryptophan-supplemented diets for periods of up to 6 weeks results in elevated brain tryptophan, 5-HT, and 5-HIAA concentrations measured postprandially (Lasley and Thurmond, 1985; Leprohon and Anderson, 1982; Woodger et al., 1979). Similarly increased CSF 5-HIAA levels are observed in neuropsychiatric patients receiving tryptophan chronically (for review see Young, 1986). Thus, it would appear that even under chronic situations, tryptophan administration can enhance brain 5-HT metabolism.

Chronic feeding of single diets with varying protein and carbohydrate concentrations, on the other hand, produces a different profile than that observed in the acute situation. Two to four weeks after feeding rats diets containing from 12 to 40% protein, with carbohydrate content of the diet correspondingly reduced, little or no change in the plasma tryptophan to LNAA ratio or brain tryptophan concentration are observed (Fernstrom et al., 1985; Glanville and Anderson, 1985; Peters and Harper, 1985). In this situation, as the protein content of the diet is increased, both tryptophan and the LNAA are increased such that the absolute amount of each amino acid in the plasma rises, but the actual ratio is unaltered. Thus taking the acute and chronic dietary studies together, it would appear that the body adjusts to defend a certain 5-HT metabolic level. When an animal is allowed to select for both protein and carbohydrate levels as would occur in the wild, it will do so by maintaining a constant proportion of protein and carbohydrate in its diet (Musten et al., 1974). However, when the animal is fed the more unnatural single diet in which it is no longer capable of adjusting its intake of these macronutrients, metabolic adaptation to the new diet works to maintain the plasma tryptophan to LNAA ratio at a constant level. However, while in both situations a constancy of 5-HT metabolism is established, the fixed ratio, single diet feeding paradigm may have profound effects on the animal's response to a tryptophan challenge. For example, in animals preweaned to diets containing either 10 or 39% protein at 17 days of gestation, no change in either the plasma ratio of tryptophan to LNAA ratios, brain tryptophan, or 5-HT turnover was observed at 21 days of age. However, when these animals were challenged with an intraperitoneal injection of tryptophan, a profound effect of diet was observed. Rats consuming the high protein diet had a less dramatic rise in brain tryptophan levels, presumably due to the higher circulating concentrations of the LNAA, and a less marked enhancement of 5-HT synthesis compared to rats consuming the low protein diet (Morris, 1987). Thus, while chronic diet may not influence basal 5-HT metabolism, it will affect the brain's response to an acute challenge.

In summary, it can be seen that dietary treatments which alter brain tryptophan availability influence 5-HT metabolism and that these dietary treatments can have both acute and long-term implications in animals. Since 5-HT metabolism can be altered by dietary means, it is then important to determine whether the neurochemical changes are functionally meaningful.

Functional consequences of altered serotonin synthesis. A substantial amount of evidence has accumulated demonstrating that animal and human behaviors are influenced by alterations in tryptophan availability to the brain (for reviews see Sved, 1983; Young, 1986). Indeed the clinical efficacy of tryptophan in the treatment of a variety of neuropsychiatric disorders has been examined over the last decade (for review see Young, 1986) with promising results in certain circumstances. The underlying hypothesis of these studies is that tryptophan's effectiveness is mediated via enhancement of 5-HT synthesis. Recent neurochemical and electrophysiological data, however, suggest that while 5-HT synthesis may be modulated by tryptophan availability, that the release of 5-HT into the synapse is tightly regulated and independent of intraneuronal 5-HT pool size (Elks et al., 1979; Lookingland et al., 1986; Trulson, 1985). Thus these investigators would argue that the increase in 5-HT synthesis observed following precursor administration or diet-induced alterations in tryptophan availability is of little or no functional significance to the animal (for review see Kuhn et al., 1986). The question arising then is how are behaviors being modulated by tryptophan administration, in an analogous manner to that observed with directly acting serotonergic drugs, if not through 5-HT synthesis and release?

To investigate this controversy, one must first look at the relationship between 5-HT release and nerve activity. Present information suggests that 5-HT release is dependent on nerve firing activity (Hery et al., 1979) and that the activity of 5-HT containing dorsal raphe neurons is regulated, in part, by autoreceptors located on the somato-dendritic region (Aghajanian, 1981; Jacobs et al., 1983; Trulson and Crisp, 1986). Thus, cell bodies in the raphe nucleus show a characteristic slow rhythmic discharge (Aghajanian and Haigler, 1973; Gallagher and Aghajanian, 1976), with this spontaneous activity apparently not being influenced by normal or decreased levels of 5-HT (Trulson and Crisp, 1986). However, administration of either tryptophan or drugs such as LSD or chlorimipramine suppresses the in vivo activity of these cells (Trulson and Jacobs, 1976; Trulson and Crisp, 1986), with autoreceptor occupation apparently mediating this response. This effect of tryptophan on nerve firing activity is dependent on an increase in raphe 5-HT synthesis (Gallagher and Aghajanian, 1976), suggesting direct involvement of 5-HT. Similarly, 5-HT administered iontophoretically onto tissue slices abolishes the in vitro discharge recordings in a time-dependent manner (Trulson and Crisp, 1986). Once the added 5-HT has been catabolized, activity returns to normal. These data suggest that an increase in 5-HT synthesis observed with elevated brain tryptophan levels would decrease neuronal 5-HT firing rate and release and ultimately minimize the functional importance of elevated brain 5-HT levels. For example, an intraperitoneal injection of tryptophan, as well as a long-lasting infusion, gave a transient and moderate elevation in 5-HT release despite the fact that brain 5-HT levels remained elevated for several hours (Ternaux et al., 1976). In addition, the release of ^{3}H-tryptophan administered intraventricularly (measured as ^{3}H-5-HT) was not influenced by diet (varying in tryptophan and LNAA content) fed to cats despite the fact that 5-HT levels responded to the diet manipulation (Trulson, 1985). The interpretation of this latter study, however, has been criticized because the author failed to measure specific activity of the released ^{3}H-5-HT (Anonymous, 1987). Since 5-HT levels responded to the dietary treatments, assuming that the ^{3}H-5-HT freely equilibrated with the releasable pool of 5-HT, these data could be interpreted to suggest that the diet manipulation did indeed influence the actual amount of 5-HT released. That is, the amount of ^{3}H-5-HT released remained constant despite alterations in specific activity.

On the other hand, even if these data are interpreted to suggest that under quiescent circumstances precursor loading would be functionally unimportant, recent data now suggest that the state of arousal of animals undergoing testing is an important variable (Young, 1986). That is, the functional significance of altered brain tryptophan concentrations may only be observed under conditions when the neuron is actively firing. A number of studies support this hypothesis. For example, the release of 5-HT from isolated synaptosomes was found to be independent of intrasynaptosomal tryptophan and 5-HT concentrations under basal circumstances. However when the synaptosomes were depolarized using veratridine, 5-HT release was increased when tryptophan was added to the incubation medium (Wolf and Kuhn, 1986). A similar relationship is observed when in vivo voltammetry is used to measure monoamine activity in the extraneuronal space. Under basal conditions, an intraperitoneal injection of tryptophan to rats did not influence 5-HT release measured in striatum despite elevated striatal 5-HT concentrations. However, when cell bodies (in the dorsal raphe nucleus) were electrically stimulated, 5-HT release was increased in striatum, and, furthermore, this increased release following electrical stimulation was enhanced by pretreating the animals with tryptophan (DeSimoni et al., 1986). While there are concerns that in vivo voltammetry is only measuring extracellular 5-HIAA and not 5-HT and, hence, not a specific method for determining release in vivo (Scatton et al., 1984), these data still suggest that precursor loading may only be effective when neurons are actively firing. Behavioral data also support the hypothesis that arousal state is an important component of functional response to altered brain tryptophan. For example, the behavioral response to diets of differing LNAA composition is greater in aroused than unaroused vervet monkeys (Chamberlain et al., 1987) and similarly the effects of tryptophan supplementation on aggressive behavior in mice is influenced by housing conditions, i.e. single versus group-housed (Lasley and Thurmond, 1985).

If one uses this information to closely examine the findings of Trulson (1985), it is not surprising that he failed to find an effect of diet, and hence brain tryptophan, on 5-HT release. Serotonin release into the lateral ventricle was monitored 3–4 hr postconsumption. However, the increase in electrical activity in the dorsal raphe nucleus following meal consumption had returned to premeal (baseline) levels within 1 hr. Therefore, the release measurements were made during a time when one would not predict effects of precursor loading. Since neurochemical changes associated with meal consumption are observed within 30 min of meal ingestion (Li and Anderson, 1982; Wurtman and Fernstrom, 1975), when firing activity is still enhanced (Trulson, 1985), measurements of release should be made during this period. This relationship between neuronal activity and functional consequences of brain precursor concentrations has previously been documented for the catecholamines (see below, Regulation of Catecholamine Synthesis), and it is not surprising that a similar relationship exists for serotonin. Therefore, experimental paradigms not designed to take this relationship into account are unlikely to observe a positive effect of tryptophan administration or dietary change and hence should not be used to negate the effectiveness of precursor administration. Rather, studies should be designed to examine the dynamic relationship between precursor administration and nerve cell firing rate. This can be easily accomplished by stimulating nerve firing activity pharmacologically or electrically or by taking advantage of arousal states, such as meal ingestion, when nerve activity is increased under more natural circumstances.

Serotonin metabolism during development. The influence of precursor administration and diet-induced alterations in brain tryptophan concentrations on neuronal 5-HT metabolism has been relatively well defined in the adult. Since these relationships were examined under conditions when the enzymes involved in 5-HT metabolism had attained adult levels of activity, the question remains whether similar dietary manipulations result in corresponding alterations in 5-HT metabolism during periods of neuronal development. To address this question, a comparison between developmental profiles of enzyme maturation and brain amino acid concentrations must be made.

The gestational period for the rat is approximately 21 days and brain development begins about gestational day 9 (G9) with the organization of ectodermal cells into a neural plate on the dorsal surface of the embryo. The plate expands and on G10-11 folds in on itself creating a lumen surrounded by a neural tube. The rostral part of the tube develops the three main divisions of the brain (fore-, mid-, and hind-brains), and the caudal portion becomes the spinal cord. The lumen of the neural tube forms the ventricular system of the brain and the central canal of the spinal cord. At this early stage of organogenesis, the brain is acquiring its general adult shape by an orderly process of cell division and migration. The precursors of the two major cell types in the brain differentiate to become neurons and glia. By postnatal day 3 (PN3), neuronal differentiation is essentially complete, and the adult complement of neurons is achieved while glia continue to proliferate (Cowan, 1979; Jacobson, 1978). What follows for the next 3 weeks is a rapid increase in the size of the brain, or growth spurt (Agrawal et al., 1966b), characterized by elaboration of axons, dendrites, and neuronal connections (Eayrs and Goodhead, 1959; Gonatas et al., 1971; Harden et al., 1977; Tissari, 1975), multiplication of glia, and deposition of myelin (Jacobson, 1963); detection of electrical activity (Deza and Eidelberg, 1967); and changes to the adult state of brain metabolism (Booth et al., 1980; Yeung and Oliver, 1967) and behavior (Asano, 1971).

The timetable of cell differentiation for the serotonergic neurons of the raphe nuclei has been established using ^{3}H-thymidine autoradiography. Cell differentiation commences on day 11 postconception and continues through G15. The peak of heavy labeling, i.e., end of cell division, occurs on G14 in the nucleus raphe dorsalis and on G13-14 in the nucleus raphe medianus (Lauder and Bloom, 1974). Axon bundles can be seen projecting from the raphe nuclei as early as G13 and have extended throughout the brain by the 15th day (Lauder and Bloom, 1974). Although well-defined nerve endings can be seen in brain stem by PN1 (Tissari, 1975) and in cerebral cortex by the eighth postnatal day, presynaptic nerve endings and synaptic vesicles continue to increase until relatively late in development, depending upon the brain area examined (Aghajanian and Bloom, 1967; Lauder and Bloom, 1975; Loizou, 1972).

Serotonin can be detected by histochemical techniques as early as G13 (Olson and Seiger, 1972). However, whole brain concentrations of 5-HT are only 25–50% of adult levels at birth (Bennett and Giarman, 1965; Bourgoin et al., 1974; 1977a; Karki et al., 1962; Loizou, 1972; Nair et al., 1976; Tissari, 1973; Tyce et al., 1963). The pattern of regional localization of 5-HT content in the brain of the neonate is similar to that of the adult rat (Nomura et al., 1976), but the postnatal concentrations increase at different rates in the various brain regions (Bourgoin et al., 1977a; Tissari, 1973). For example, 5-HT concentrations in the brain stem were one-third adult levels at birth. A rapid increase in 5-HT content occurred so that adult levels were attained during the third to fourth postnatal week. In contrast, forebrain 5-HT levels were 20% of adult concentration at birth. The rate of increase in 5-HT was much slower than that observed in the brain stem, with adult levels only being reached during the fifth week of life (Bourgoin et al., 1977a). Similarly, Tissari (1973) reported significant differences in neonate 5-HT brainstem concentrations from adult levels only during the first week postweaning, whereas 5-HT content of the hemispheres was only 72% of adult levels at 5 weeks of age. It has been suggested that this progression in 5-HT levels is a result of axons and terminals from 5-HT cell bodies propagating rostrally during the first 5 weeks after birth (Tissari, 1973, 1975). In general, whole brain 5-HT concentrations remain relatively stable for the first 10 days of life and then begin to increase, reaching 80% of adult levels at weaning (Tissari, 1973, Tyce et al., 1963). Adult levels are attained by the sixth postnatal week (Tissari, 1973).

In contrast to low 5-HT, tryptophan concentrations are three to ten times greater in the brains of newborns than in the adult rat (Bourgoin et al., 1974; Kalyanasundaram, 1976; Tyce et al., 1963). Tryptophan levels fall rapidly during the first 3 postnatal days (Bourgoin et al., 1974; Tyce et al., 1963) and then decrease more slowly, reaching adult levels by weaning (Bourgoin et al., 1974; Kalyanasundaram, 1976; Tyce et al., 1963). These high levels of tryptophan in the newborn have been attributed to both age-related differences in amino acid uptake (Bourgoin et al., 1974) and/or increases in the ratio of free/bound tryptophan in the plasma (Bourgoin et al., 1974; Kalyanasundaram, 1976). Specifically, the uptake process for tryptophan has a higher affinity (lower Km) for tryptophan in the 7-day-old rat than in the adult brain (Vahvelainen and Oja, 1972). Unfortunately the affinity for tryptophan was not measured prior to day 7 in this study. While tryptophan per se was not monitored, Baños et al. (1978) demonstrated a high rate of influx for leucine during the first week of life, which then decreased steadily over the period from 1 to 7 weeks of age, reaching adult levels by the seventh postnatal week. This high rate of brain influx appeared to be a result of a very active transport system rather than an incomplete blood-brain barrier. Since tryptophan shares the same transport system for brain uptake with leucine (Pardridge, 1977), it would seem reasonable to predict that the high level of tryptophan at birth is in part due to this active transport system.

An additional factor which may be influencing tryptophan uptake at birth is the plasma ratio of free/bound tryptophan. Since the concentration of free tryptophan in the plasma influences brain tryptophan concentration (see above, Regulation of Brain Tryptophan Levels), increasing plasma-free tryptophan is predicted to elevate brain tryptophan levels. Thus, high brain tryptophan levels in the neonate are consistent with the observation that almost all the plasma tryptophan in the neonate is in the free form (Bourgoin et al., 1977b; Morgane et al., 1978).

Surprisingly, levels of brain 5-HIAA at birth are similar to or greater than adult levels (Nair et al., 1976; Tissari, 1973; Tyce et al., 1963). The concentration of 5-HIAA increases during the suckling period and then falls back to adult levels (Tissari, 1973; Tyce et al., 1963). Although the appearance of 5-HIAA provides evidence for 5-HT turnover in the newborn rat, this high concentration is not attributable to an increased turnover, as a similar turnover time of 1.5 hr was determined in 1-day-old and adult brains (Tissari, 1973). It was originally suggested that the high levels of 5-HIAA were a result of immaturity of the efflux mechanism (Tissari, 1973); this has been refuted. While the carrier-mediated transport system for elimination of organic acids from the brain was not found in the 5-day-old rat, an equally rapid efflux of the organic acid, para-aminohippuric acid, occurred as a result of diffusion through relatively undifferentiated cerebral capillaries (Bass and Lundborg, 1973).

Developmental regulation of serotonin metabolism. The low levels of 5-HT at birth may represent decreased capacity to synthesize, store, and/or take up the neurotransmitter. Of the two anabolic enzymes, the activity of AAAD approximates adult levels at birth (Bennett and Giarman, 1965; Karki et al., 1962), while the activity of TRP-OHase appears to be rate-limiting (Bennett and Giarman, 1965; Deguchi and Barchas, 1972; Schmidt and Sanders-Bush, 1971). At birth, TRP-OHase activity is 20–30% of adult levels. Postnatally, enzyme activity does not begin to increase for the first 8 to 10 days and then increases rapidly, reaching adult levels by weaning (Deguchi and Barchas, 1972; Schmidt and Sanders-Bush, 1971). To support the suggestion that the activity of TRP-OHase is rate-limiting in the early neonatal synthesis of 5-HT are studies demonstrating that the ability of the rat to synthesize 5-HT from peripherally administered 5-hydroxytryptophan is similar in the neonate and adult rat, while the ability of the newborn to synthesize 5-HT from peripherally administered tryptophan is markedly reduced (Bennett and Giarman, 1965).

Conversely, it has been suggested that the low level of 5-HT observed during brain development may reflect a decreased ability of the serotonergic neurons to store 5-HT, with much of the synthesized 5-HT being directly shunted to the catabolic enzyme, MAO (Karki et al., 1962; Tissari, 1973). However, a reduced storage capacity for 5-HT was not confirmed by Bourgoin et al. (1977a), who provided evidence for increased catabolism of 5-HT and suggested that the high level of 5-HIAA in the brain of the newborn may be related to high MAO activity. Although the developmental pattern for total MAO activity parallels that for TRP-OHase (Bennett and Giarman, 1965; Kurzepa and Bojanek, 1965; Robinson, 1968), MAO A activity, the isozyme involved in 5-HT inactivation, is higher in the brainstem of preweaning animals than in adults and similar to adult levels in the forebrain (Bourgoin et al., 1977a). Thus, the low level of 5-HT at birth may be a result of both decreased synthesis and increased catabolism.

It appears that the rat is born with a very immature 5-HT system. Both 5-HT concentrations and enzyme activities increase rapidly during the suckling period, attaining approximately 80% of adult levels by weaning. Adult activity of the 5-HT system is seen by the postnatal week 6. There are, however, a number of different factors which may affect the normal development of the 5-HT system. Of major importance to the developing brain is the nutritional status of the mother during both gestation and lactation and the availability of tryptophan. The effect of maternal malnutrition on 5-HT metabolism has been extensively examined and reviews have been published (Morgane et al., 1978). Of particular importance are results from studies showing that despite the high levels of brain tryptophan during development, tryptophan administration may enhance 5-HT synthesis.

Changes in brain tryptophan availability. Alterations in brain tryptophan availability during gestation or lactation influence 5-HT metabolism. However, the magnitude of response is much less than that observed in the mature animal. For example, elevated brain 5-HT concentrations are observed in the fetus when tryptophan availability is increased (Howd et al., 1975). Tryptophan injections to either the dam (100 mg/kg) or directly to the fetus (500 μg) raised 5-HT concentrations in the fetal brain on G19. Elevated fetal 5-HT levels were observed as early as G15, with increases of approximately 10% on G15 and G17 and approximately 20% on G19 and G22 (birth) (Howd et al., 1975). Similarly, a 20% increase in brain 5-HT was observed in newborn rat pups injected with 200 mg/kg tryptophan (Bennett and Giarman, 1965; Bourgoin et al., 1974).

These data suggest that even in the prenatal rat, 5-HT synthesis can be affected by precursor availability. However, some degree of protection from fluctuations in tryptophan levels is apparent in the newborn (Bennett and Giarman, 1965; Bourgoin et al., 1974). That is, while a 20% increase in 5-HT is observed in the newborn rat receiving 200 mg/kg tryptophan, elevations of 35–45% are apparent in adult rats receiving a similar dose. This relative degree of protection is believed to be a result of low TRP-OHase activity at birth (Bennett and Giarman, 1965). A similar degree of protection from tryptophan administration may still be apparent at weaning. For example, accumulation of 5-HT after monoamine oxidase inhibition plateaued at a fairly low dose of tryptophan (20 mg/kg) in 21-day-old rats, while increased 5-HT accumulation was observed with dosages of up to 100 mg/kg in the adult animal (Atterwill and Green, 1980).

Chronic maternal diet effects 5-HT metabolism in the offspring. When dams were fed a tryptophan-supplemented (1.68%) diet throughout gestation and lactation, whole brain tryptophan, 5-HT, and 5-HIAA levels were elevated in both the dams and offspring at weaning (Leprohon and Anderson, 1982). While brain 5-HT was lower, and brain tryptophan and 5-HIAA were higher in offspring when compared to their dams, as anticipated by developmental profiles, the magnitude of changes was identical for both age groups, suggesting no protection to the progeny in this more chronic situation. Altered maternal dietary protein concentration also influences 5-HT metabolism in the progeny. When dams were fed diets ranging from 10 to 40% casein, basal concentrations of 5-HT and 5-HIAA were unaltered in the weanling offspring (Leprohon and Anderson, 1982). However, 5-HIAA accumulation, assessed using the brain efflux blocker probenecid, was inversely correlated with maternal dietary protein concentration, measured postprandially. This effect of maternal dietary protein concentration on weanling 5-HT metabolism is not observed in 12-hr fasted rats (PN21) (Morris, 1987), suggesting that a challenge, such as a meal, must be administered for the effect to be observed. While this effect of maternal diet on 5- HT metabolism in weanling (PN21) offspring may be a consequence of the offspring beginning to consume the maternal diet, the data clearly show that the immature brain is responsive to changes in dietary supply of amino acids. Since behavioral changes in feeding are associated with this access to the maternal diet during the weaning period (Leprohon and Anderson, 1980, 1982; Morris and Anderson, 1986), the data highlight the importance of selecting appropriate weaning foods for neurochemical and behavioral development of the offspring.

The effect of tryptophan availability on 5-HT metabolism in the developing brain has not been assessed in humans. However, indirect behavioral measurements suggest that the human brain is responsive to dietary alterations in amino acid availability within the first days of life (Yogman and Zeisel, 1983). Alterations in sleep latencies consistent with altered 5-HT metabolism were observed when these infants were fed glucose solutions supplemented with either tryptophan, to enhance, or valine, to diminish, 5-HT metabolism. Thus, despite the immaturity of the 5-HT system, neurochemical and behavioral data suggest that the brain is sensitive to altered precursor levels, even during developmental stages.

Serotonin and early neurogenesis. The possibility has been raised that 5-HT may play a trophic role during neurogenesis, prior to its functioning as a neurotransmitter (for review see Lauder et al., 1982). Specifically, 5-HT may regulate the onset of differentiation of its ultimate target cells. This hypothesis largely arose from the following two observations. First, serotonergic cells are among the first to stop dividing and to begin differentiation, with differentiation well underway several days prior to their target cells (Lauder and Bloom, 1974). Second, it is apparent from histochemical fluorescent techniques that the neurons are capable of synthesizing their neurotransmitter long before they themselves are innervated (Lauder and Bloom, 1974; Olson and Seiger, 1972).

By measuring the incorporation of labeled thymidine into dividing cells, Lauder and Krebs (1976, 1978a,b) demonstrated that administration of the TRP-OHase inhibitor, para-chlorophenylalanine, to pregnant dams delayed the onset of differentiation of 5-HT target cells by 1 to 2 days in the offspring. Furthermore, postnatal studies provided evidence for interactions of 5-HT axons with proliferating glioblasts in the developing cerebellum and with immature granule cells and their precursors in the hippocampus (Lauder et al., 1982). Interestingly, this epigenetic influence of 5-HT is observed during developmental time periods when 5-HT synthesis can be enhanced by precursor administration (see above, Changes in Tryptophan Availability). Whether these diet-induced alterations in 5-HT metabolism influence the normal time course of neuronal differentiation is presently unknown. However, these data suggest that neuronal maturation may be sensitive to metabolic alterations in 5-HT synthesis.

Catecholamines

The catecholamines, dopamine (DA), norepinephrine (NE), and epinephrine, are synthesized from the precursor amino acid, tyrosine, with the end product of tyrosine metabolism determined by the complement of anabolic enzymes present in the neuron (Fig. 3). In all catecholaminergic cells, tyrosine is converted to DA by a two-step enzymatic process involving initial hydroxylation to form 3,4-dihydroxyphenylalanine (DOPA) followed by decarboxylation to DA. Tyrosine hydroxylase (TYR-OHase) is highly localized in catecholaminergic neurons and, like TRP-OHase, requires molecular oxygen, iron, and reduced pterin (tetrahydrobiopterin) as cofactors (Nagatsu et al., 1964; Udenfriend, 1966). DOPA is then rapidly decarboxylated by AAAD to DA, such that little or no DOPA is normally found in brain tissues (Thiede and Kehr, 1981b). In noradrenergic neurons, DA is further hydroxylated to NE under the action of dopamine-β-hydroxylase located in

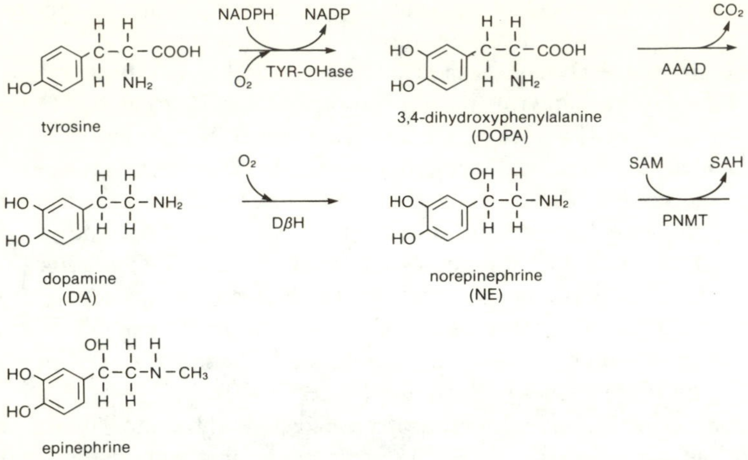

Fig. 3. Catecholamine synthesis. TYR-OHase, tyrosine hydroxylase; AAAD, aromatic amino acid decarboxylase; DβH, dopamine-β-hydroxylase; PNMT, phenylethanolamine-N-methyl transferase; SAM, S-adenosylmethionine; SAH, S-adenosylhomocysteine.

the membrane of storage granules (Goldstein, 1966). Small amounts of NE can be further methylated to form epinephrine in the brain under the action of phenylethanolamine-N-methyltransferase, using S-adenosylmethionine as the methyl donor (Saavedra et al., 1974). The contribution of epinephrine to the total brain content of catecholamines is small.

Two major enzymes are involved in catecholamine degradation: MAO located on the mitochondria of the presynaptic neuron and catechol-O-methyltransferase (COMT) present in the extraneuronal space. Following release, the major metabolic pathway for NE involves reuptake into the presynaptic neuron where it is first deaminated by MAO forming 3,4-dihydroxphenylethyleneglycol aldehyde and then reduced by aldehyde reductase to 3,4-dihydroxyphenylethyleneglycol (DHPG). DHPG then diffuses to the extraneuronal space where it can either be further methylated by COMT to 3-methoxy-4-hydroxyphenylethyleneglycol (MHPG) or directly transported from brain to blood (Fig. 4). NE can also be initially methylated in the synaptic cleft to normetanephrine which is then converted to MHPG in the presynaptic terminal (DeMet and Halaris, 1979; Molinoff and Axelrod, 1971; Thiede and Kehr, 1981a). While this is considered a relatively minor pathway, there is some indication that metabolic clearance of NE is primarily through an initial reuptake in the resting state (Li et al., 1983), but through extraneuronal methylation when the neuron is actively firing (Warsh et al., 1981). Only trace amounts of the acidic metabolites 3,4-dihydroxymandelic acid and 3-methoxy-4-hydroxymandelic acid are observed in brain. In the

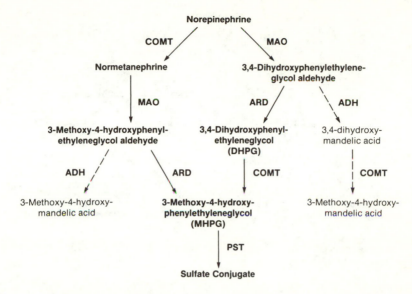

Fig. 4. Norepinephrine catabolism. COMT, catechol-O-methyltransferase; MAO, mono-amine oxidase; ADH, aldehyde dehydrogenase; ARD, aldehyde reductase; PST, phenolsulfotransferase. The dotted arrows indicate minor pathways.

rat, the majority of DHPG and MHPG is sulfated by phenolsulfotransferase prior to efflux (DeMet and Halaris, 1979; Molinoff and Axelrod, 1971; Thiede and Kehr, 1981a).

Similarly, the major catabolic pathway for DA involves an initial reuptake into the presynaptic neuron. However, unlike NE, the acid metabolites predominate (Fig. 5). DA is first deaminated by MAO to 3,4-dihydroxy-phenylacetaldehyde followed by reduction to 3,4-dihydroxyphenylacetic acid (DOPAC) under the action of aldehyde reductase. DOPAC can then be further methylated by COMT to 3-methoxy-4-hydroxyphenylacetic acid (homovanillic acid; HVA) once in the extraneuronal space (Thiede and Kehr, 1981a). While DA can be initially methylated in the synaptic cleft to 3-methoxy-4-hydroxyphenylethylamine and then taken up into the presynaptic terminal and converted to HVA, it would appear that virtually all HVA is derived from methylation of DOPAC and that HVA can be considered a secondary metabolite.

Regulation of catecholamine synthesis. The rate-limiting step for the biosynthesis of the catecholamines is tyrosine hydroxylation. However, unlike 5-HT, the rate of tyrosine hydroxylation is tightly regulated, and precursor dependence is only observed under certain circumstances. Several mechanisms have been proposed as regulating tyrosine hydroxylation, including end product inhibition (Harris and Roth, 1971; Ikeda et al., 1966;

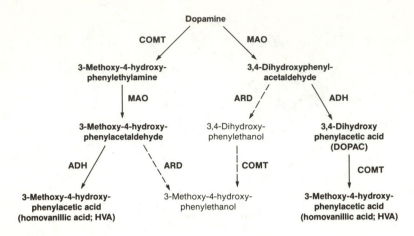

Fig. 5. Dopamine catabolism. Abbreviations are the same as in Figure 4. The dotted arrows indicate minor pathways.

Spector et al., 1967; Udenfriend et al., 1965; Weiner et al., 1972) and autoreceptor occupation (Roth et al., 1975, 1978; Walters and Roth, 1976). While the precise control mechanism is not known, collectively, studies indicate that TYR-OHase activity is tightly regulated such that accumulation of the catecholamines is not observed (for reviews see Fernstrom, 1983; Sved, 1983).

Studies examining precursor dependence of catecholamine synthesis support these observations. In vivo estimates of enzyme kinetics provide evidence that TYR-OHase is 80–100% saturated with tyrosine when neurons are in the resting state (for reviews see Fernstrom, 1983; Sved, 1983). Thus, tyrosine administration to animals has little or no effect on brain catecholamine levels (Carlsson and Lindqvist, 1978; Dairman, 1979; Fernando and Curzon, 1981; Gibson and Wurtman, 1977, 1978; Melamed et al., 1980; Scally et al., 1977; Sved and Fernstrom, 1981). Conversely, administration of LNAA to lower brain tyrosine reduces brain catecholamine synthesis (Carlsson and Lindqvist, 1978; Wurtman et al., 1974), suggesting that the brain is more sensitive to reductions than to elevations in tyrosine levels under quiescent circumstances.

Certain evidence for tyrosine enhancement of catecholamine synthesis is observed, however, when neurons are actively firing and is probably a consequence of phosphorylation-dephosphorylation of TYR-OHase. When neuronal firing activity is increased, either pharmacologically or via electrical stimulation, an increased rate of tyrosine hydroxylation is observed. This acute change in enzyme activity is associated with a calcium- or cyclic-AMP-mediated phosphorylation of TYR-OHase (Joh et al., 1978; Yamauchi and

Fujisawa, 1979) and a resulting increase in the affinity of the enzyme for its cofactor tetrahydrobiopterin (Lovenberg et al., 1975; Murrin et al., 1976; Vulliet et al., 1980; Zivkovic et al., 1975). That is to say, in the unphosphorylated form, TYR-OHase is probably unsaturated with respect to cofactor. However, when phosphorylated, the Km of TYR-OHase for tetrahydrobiopterin decreases such that the enzyme is saturated with co-factor, and tyrosine availability may become rate-limiting (for review see Sved, 1983).

Administration of tyrosine to animals pretreated to enhance neuronal firing rate results in elevated concentrations of the catecholamine metabolites HVA and DOPAC (for DA) and MHPG-SO$_4$ (for NE). For example, increased striatal concentrations of HVA and/or DOPAC were observed following tyrosine administration in rats pretreated with haloperidol (Scalley et al., 1977), reserpine (Oishi and Wurtman, 1982; Sved et al., 1979a), or by partial nigrostriatal lesions (Melamed et al., 1980). A similar effect of tyrosine on DA synthesis and metabolite concentrations was observed in retina following light activation (Fernstrom et al., 1986; Gibson et al., 1983). NE turnover is also enhanced by tyrosine administration (measured as elevated brain MHPG-SO$_4$ concentrations) in rats exposed to cold stress (Gibson and Wurtman, 1977) or treated with probenecid (Gibson and Wurtman, 1978). Reduction of blood pressure in spontaneously hypertensive rats by tyrosine is accompanied by increased brain MHPG-SO$_4$ concentra-tions (Sved et al., 1979b; Yamori et al., 1980), suggesting that central noradrenergic neurons were actively firing and precursor-dependent in these animals.

Not only does it appear that tyrosine concentration becomes rate-limiting when TYR-OHase is in its phosphorylated form, but there is some indication that catecholaminergic neurons become precursor-depleted during periods of increased firing activity. For example, decreased tyrosine levels were observed following drug-induced increases in DA synthesis (Westerink and Wirix, 1983). A similar depletion of tyrosine and dopamine was observed following repeated electrical stimulation of striatal slices in vitro (Milner and Wurtman, 1985) which could be restored by adding tyrosine to the incubation medium. Furthermore, stress-induced depletion of NE in locus ceruleus neurons can be prevented or reversed by tyrosine administration (Lehnert et al., 1984).

Dietary control of catecholamine synthesis. The preceding section indi-cates that brain catecholamine synthesis becomes precursor-dependent when neurons are actively firing. The major source of brain tyrosine is provided by dietary consumption of proteins containing tyrosine and phenylalanine; the latter is rapidly hydroxylated to tyrosine by hepatic phenylalanine hydroxylase (Elwyn, 1970). Therefore, diet-induced alterations in aromatic amino acid availability can influence brain tyrosine levels.

Tyrosine uptake into the brain is dependent on the same LNAA uptake carrier described for tryptophan (see above, Regulation of Brain Tryptophan Levels). Thus, it is the tyrosine to LNAA ratio, rather than plasma tyrosine level alone, that best predicts brain tyrosine levels (Pardridge, 1977). The plasma ratio, and hence its consequences for catecholamine synthesis, is dependent on the relative proportion of protein and carbohydrate in the diet and duration of exposure to the diet.

In the context of single meals, increasing protein (0–40%) and decreasing carbohydrate concentration elevates plasma tyrosine to LNAA ratio and brain tyrosine concentrations (Fernstrom and Faller, 1978; Glaeser et al., 1983). This occurs because the level of tyrosine in the plasma increases relatively more than the competing LNAA due to the combined effect of insulin-induced uptake of the branch chain amino acids into muscle and hepatic conversion of phenylalanine to tyrosine. Catecholamine synthesis responds to this meal-induced alteration in brain tyrosine levels, such that brain DOPA accumulation (measured after administratin of an AAAD inhibitor) and catecholamine metabolite concentrations were enhanced by high protein meals in cold-stressed animals (Gibson and Wurtman, 1977; 1978). Retinal DA metabolism responds in a similar fashion to meal-induced alterations in tyrosine availability. That is, a high protein meal increased retinal tyrosine concentration and DOPAC and DOPA accumulation after light activation (Gibson, 1986). While it is well accepted that treatments such as cold stress and light activation of retina increase neuronal firing rate, there is some indication that meal-feeding itself may activate certain populations of neurons and that precursor dependence may be observed during feeding periods (Biggio et al., 1977; Glanville and Anderson, 1986).

While there is a direct association between high protein meals and brain tyrosine levels in the single-meal paradigm, an inverse relationship is observed with chronic feeding of high protein diets. That is, brain tyrosine levels are lower in animals fed high protein diets (40% casein) with catecholamine metabolism relatively unaffected (Agharanya and Wurtman, 1985; Glanville and Anderson, 1985). In this situation plasma tyrosine levels are unchanged, probably due to enhancement of hepatic tyrosine aminotransferase activity, yet the plasma concentrations of the competing LNAA are elevated, thus increasing competition for brain tyrosine uptake. These metabolic responses to high dietary protein are observed within 3 days of feeding a 30% casein diet (Yokogoshi, 1985). In contrast to this effect of high protein diets, supplementing diets with tyrosine results in chronic elevations in plasma and brain tyrosine levels since hepatic tyrosine aminotransferase activity does not appear to respond to this manipulation (Gibson, 1985). The effect of chronic elevations in brain tyrosine concentrations on catecholamine metabolism has not been extensively examined. However, urinary HVA and MHPG levels were elevated in otherwise untreated women receiving oral tyrosine for 2 days (Johnston et al., 1983), suggesting that catecholamine metabolism can be enhanced by providing more precursor and that neurons physiologically undergo periods of precursor dependence.

In summary, the effects of precursor dependence of catecholamine synthesis have not been as extensively examined as those for serotonin. However, studies using treatments designed to enhance neuronal firing activity clearly indicate that catecholamine metabolism is precursor-dependent in this situation. Dietary protein consumption is a key modulator of brain tyrosine availability, yet acute and chronic feeding of high protein diets will have opposing effects. The effectiveness of long-term precursor manipulation of catecholamine metabolism for treatment of disease is presently uncertain (for review see Sved, 1983), yet with our present understanding of these relationships the future is promising.

Catecholamine metabolism during development. The preceding sections have discussed the influence of precursor administration and diet-induced alterations in brain tyrosine concentrations on catecholamine metabolism in adult brain. However, the relationship between brain tyrosine availability and catecholamine metabolism during neuronal development has not been extensively studied. Therefore, this section will examine this relationship from a theoretical standpoint.

The catecholamines are present early in the sequence of brain organogenesis (Olson and Seiger, 1972), with neuronal division and differentiation occurring within a similar time frame as that previously described for 5-HT. Fluorescence histochemical and ^{3}H-thymidine autoradiographic techniques demonstrate that norepinephrine cell bodies in the locus ceruleus begin to differentiate on G10 and continue until G13, with peak activity on G12 and detection of norepinephrine on G14. Similarly, dopamine cell bodies in the substantia nigra begin differentiation on G11 and continue until G15, with peak differentiation and detection of dopamine on G13 (Olson and Seiger, 1972; Lauder and Bloom, 1974).

As in the adult brain, dopamine and norepinephrine share a common biosynthetic pathway which begins with the conversion of tyrosine to DOPA by TYR-OHase (Nagatsu et al., 1964; Udenfriend, 1966). DOPA is detectable in the brainstem at G14.5 (David, 1984) and at G15 in whole brain (Coyle and Axelrod, 1972b). The specific activity of TYR-OHase increases during late gestation to about 25% of adult values by birth and to adult levels by postnatal week 4 (McGeer et al., 1971; Coyle and Axelrod, 1972b). AAAD converts DOPA to DA (Sourkes, 1966); this enzyme is detectable in brain stem and hypothalamus at G13 (David, 1984) and in whole brain at

G15 (Lamprecht and Coyle, 1972). At birth, the activity of the decarboxylase is similar to that of the adult (Bennett and Giarman, 1965; Karki et al., 1962). The final step in this pathway, DA conversion to NE, is catalyzed by dopamine-β-hydroxylase, and, like AAAD, it is present in brain stem and hypothalamus at G13 (David, 1984) and in whole brain on G15 (Coyle and Axelrod, 1972a). About 35% of adult activity is evident at birth, and adult levels of activity are achieved about 4 weeks postweaning (Coyle and Axelrod, 1972a). The concentrations of tyrosine and its immediate precursor phenylalanine are at least 2–5-fold higher in fetal plasma and brain than in corresponding adult tissues (Agrawal et al., 1966a; Brass et al., 1982). Despite the non-limiting availability of these amino acids, DA and NE concentrations are only 15–30% of adult levels at birth (Karki et al., 1960; Agrawal et al., 1966b; Coyle and Axelrod, 1971; Coyle and Henry, 1973) and take at least 5–7 weeks to rise to adult values (Karki et al., 1962; Loizou, 1969; Coyle and Henry, 1973).

Factors other than precursor availability influencing the amounts of monoamines in the fetal brain include the relative activities of synthetic and catabolic enzymes, neuronal uptake and storage capacities, and axonal maturation. TYR-OHase is the rate-limiting enzyme for catecholamine synthesis in adult rats (Udenfriend, 1966); the same is also true in young animals. Blocking NE synthesis at the level of TYR-OHase or dopamine-β-hydroxylase results in a similar reduction in brain NE (Coyle and Henry, 1973; Coyle, 1977), and suggests that the enzymes are regulated such that once DOPA is formed it is rapidly converted to either DA or NE without accumulation of intermediates. Indeed, regulation of catecholamine synthesis at the level of tyrosine hydroxylation in the immature animal is further suggested by the elevations of fetal brain NE and DA resulting from injections of DOPA, but not tyrosine, to the dam (Lundborg and Kellogg, 1971; Kellogg and Lundborg, 1972). MAO catalyzes the conversion of the monoamines to their respective metabolites and is detected in fetal brain at G15. Since MAO activity is about 30% of adult values (Nachmias, 1960; Saavedra et al., 1974), it is unlikely that overactive catabolism of the monoamines accounts for their lower concentrations in immature brains. The mechanism for active NE uptake can be demonstrated in fetal brain at G18 and shares kinetic and pharmacologic characteristics with the adult uptake system. The Km for NE uptake was similar to that of the adult, while the V_{max} was 20% of adult values at G18 and rose to 100% by 28 days postnatally (Coyle and Axelrod, 1971). Although storage vesicles containing the catecholamines can be visualized before birth (Olson and Seiger, 1972), fewer vesicles are available for NE storage, as suggested by studies with reserpine, a drug that inhibits intraneuronal storage of NE. Sensitivity to the effect of reserpine increases with age (Coyle and Axelrod, 1971). That the immature brain has reduced storage capacity relative to the adult parallels the development of storage sites in the axons. Proliferation of axonal terminals is largely a postnatal event (Loizou, 1972) and taken together with the rate-limiting effect of TYR-OHase and immaturity of storage mechanisms appears to account for lower catecholamine levels in young animals.

The dependence of catecholamine synthesis on precursor availability and the influence of fluctuations in precursor availability on brain development have received less attention than the influence of altered precursor availability on parameters such as plasma amino acids (Isaacs and Greengard, 1980; Dienel, 1981; Brass et al., 1982), myelin (Chase and O'Brien, 1970; Figlewicz and Druse, 1980; Johnson and Shah, 1980), cortical development (Cunningham and Nigam, 1979), cerebellar development (Prensky et al., 1974; Huether and Neuhoff, 1981), behavior (Kaplan et al., 1981), and serotonin metabolism (Lane et al., 1979, Brass et al., 1982, Huether, 1986). Although the paucity of evidence regarding precursor dependence of catecholamine synthesis in the neonatal period precludes definitive conclusions, the lower activity of TYR-OHase (Coyle and Axelrod, 1972b; McGeer et al., 1971), coupled with elevated precursor levels in the plasma and brain (Carver et al., 1965; Agrawal et al., 1966a; Brass et al., 1982) suggests that the enzyme is likely to be more saturated with substrate than is the case with the adult. This is substantiated by a study in which tyrosine was injected into the dam and NE and DA measured in fetal brain 1 and 4 hr later. No changes in NE and DA were apparent (Lundborg and Kellogg, 1971). It would appear that the immature animal is no more dependent on precursors for catecholamine synthesis than is the adult, although the reasons are somewhat different. Further studies examining the relationship between development of adult neuronal electrical activity and precursor availability are necessary prior to making any definite statements with regard to precursor amino acid effects during neuronal maturation.

DIETARY FAT AND NEURONAL FUNCTION

The proceeding sections have discussed mechanisms whereby diet can influence neurochemistry via alterations in the availability of precursors for neurotransmitter synthesis and/or co-factors (micronutrients) for maintenance of enzyme activities. Fat, another dietary constituent, may also have a marked effect on CNS function, mediated via alterations in neuronal membrane composition. These membrane compositional changes may then in turn modify neuronal function by one of several mechanisms.

Certain membrane-intrinsic proteins and membrane-bound enzymes have specific requirements for the annular lipids surrounding them (for review see Sandermann, 1978), which allow the protein or enzyme to achieve its most active conformation. Hence, changes in these boundary lipids may influence enzyme activity.

Changes in the overall physiochemical characteristics of the membrane may influence protein mobility and availability within the membrane. Since the physiochemical characteristics (e.g., fluidity) of the membrane are mediated through changes in fatty acid composition, cholesterol content, and polar head groups of the phospholipid bilayer (for reviews see Brenner, 1984; Gould and Ginsberg, 1984; Shinitzky, 1984; Stubbs and Smith, 1984;), membrane-bound protein function might change with dietary fat, just as bulk membrane composition does.

The metabolism of certain phospholipids may be directly involved in signal transfer across biological membranes. For example, the methylation of phosphatidylethanolamine (PE) to phosphatidylcholine (PC), which is proposed to function in signal transfer across membranes (Hirata and Axelrod, 1980), is stimulated by dopamine in the CNS (Leprohon et al., 1983). Since PEs containing highly unsaturated fatty acids are preferentially methylated (LeKim et al., 1973), as phospholipid fatty acid profiles change with dietary fat, so does the basal rate of PE methylation (Hargreaves and Clandinin, 1986). Whether the magnitude of receptor-mediated activation of the enzyme differs in response to altered dietary fat intake, thus influencing dopamine signal transfer, is presently unknown.

Membrane glycoprotein content appears to be modified by dietary-induced changes in fatty acid profile, especially during early stages of neuronal development (Morgan et al., 1981). Direct evidence that these membrane compositional changes are of functional significance is unavailable. However, as will be discussed below, altered behavior is observed in tandem with altered membrane composition, implying that these biochemical changes are of functional significance. To further explore the possibility that dietary fat influences brain function, the effect of altering dietary fat intake on membrane composition and function and behavior will be discussed.

Dietary Lipids and Neuronal Membranes

The lipid bilayer of brain membranes differs in composition from that found in peripheral tissues in that it contains a much higher proportion of long chain polyunsaturated fatty acids (Tinoco et al,. 1979; Bernsohl and Cohen, 1972). Metabolites of linoleic (C18:2(ω6)) and alpha-linolenic acid (C18:3(ω3)), C20:4(ω6), C22:4(ω6), C22:5(ω3), and C22:6(ω3), respectively, are extremely abundant. PE is particularly rich in these fatty acids, with notably high (30–50%) levels of C22:6(ω3) (Tinoco et al., 1979; O'Brien et al., 1964; Century et al., 1963). The specific role that these polyenoic fatty acids play in excitable tissue has not been clearly defined. However the association of neurological symptoms with their deficiency

(Lamptey and Walker, 1976; Paoletti and Galli, 1972; Holman et al., 1982) points to their importance.

Maintenance of the physiochemical characteristics of neuronal membranes is paramount for normal neuronal function. Therefore, factors which modify membrane composition can have far-reaching effects on the CNS. Dietary fat has been shown to modify brain membrane composition. Changes in fatty acid composition, phospholipid polar head groups, and membrane cholesterol content are apparent in rats fed diets differing in fat source, both in the presence (Brenneman and Rutledge, 1979; Koblin et al., 1980; Paoletti and Galli, 1972; Sun and Sun, 1974) and absence (Bourre et al., 1984; Foot et al., 1982; Lamptey and Walker, 1976; Samulski and Walker, 1982; Tahin et al., 1981) of linoleic and/or alpha-linolenic acid deficiency. If rats are fed linoleate-deficient diets, brain membranes show the now classical changes in fatty acid profiles associated with linoleate deficiency, i.e., decreased (ω6) fatty acids with corresponding increased (ω9) fatty acids and a highly elevated triene/tetraene ratio (Paoletti and Galli, 1972; Sun and Sun, 1974; Koblin et al., 1980).

Variations in dietary fat source, in the absence of linoleate deficiency, also alter the neuronal fatty acid profile (Foot et al., 1982; Tahin et al., 1981). Saturated, mono-, di-, and poly-enoic membrane fatty acids are all affected to some extent, reflecting the patterns of fatty acids consumed. Changes in the polyenoic fatty acids may be the most important functionally, however, since it has been hypothesized that these fatty acids play a specific role in excitable tissue (Tinoco et al.,1979). When comparing the effects of dietary fats high (soybean oil; SBO) and low (safflower or sunflower oils; SFO) in alpha-linolenate (ω3) content, but with similar linoleate (ω6) levels, the SFO diets decreased (ω3) polyenoic fatty acid content and increased (ω6) polyenoic fatty acid content, and, hence, decreased the overall (ω3)/(ω6) ratio in a large variety of brain structures including the whole brain; mitochondrial, microsomal, and synaptosomal membranes; oligodendrocytes; and myelin and astrocytes (Lamptey and Walker, 1976; Bourre et al., 1984; Foot et al., 1982; Tahin et al., 1981). The pattern of change in membrane fatty acid composition was similar even though fat comprised between 1% (Bourre et al., 1984) and 20% w/w (Foot et al., 1982) of the diet and periods of consumption ranged from 21 days (Foot et al., 1982) to two generations (Lamptey and Walker, 1976). These findings are extended to comparisons of other dietary fats which differ in C18:2(ω6)/C18:3(ω3) ratios (Cocchi et al., 1984; Tarozzi et al., 1984). The relative difference between the (ω3) and (ω6) polyenoic fatty acids observed with differing dietary (ω3/(ω6) ratios is most likely a consequence of the competition between C18:2(ω6) and C18:3(ω3) for the desaturase enzymes (Tahin et al., 1981).

Neuronal membrane alterations with variations in dietary fat also include phospholipid polar head groups and membrane cholesterol content (Foot et al., 1982). Phospholipid polar head group composition changes both as a function of (ω6), (ω3) and monounsaturated fatty acids and choline content of the diet, while membrane cholesterol content varies directly with membrane phosphatidylcholine.

Dietary lipid intake influences membrane composition in brain in a manner analogous to that reported in peripheral tissue, although the extent of change varies between tissues and organelles. Brain membranes are traditionally viewed as more resistant to change than those in peripheral tissues (Tahin et al., 1981). Recent data, however, suggest that the brain is much more sensitive to changes in composition of dietary fat than was previously thought. Altered phospholipid polar head group composition was observed within 72 hr of feeding rats phospholipid-supplemented diets (Heger and Peter, 1979). In addition, changes in the dietary source of fat, not including essential fatty acid deficiency, affected overall neuronal membrane composition in as little as 24 days (Foot et al., 1982). Perhaps some of these discrepancies regarding the plasticity of brain membrane composition are a result of differences in the age of the animal at the time of initiating the dietary manipulations—since the developing brain may be more responsive to dietary influence than the adult brain (Matheson et al., 1981). Certainly changes in fetal neuronal membrane fatty acid profile are apparent within 2 days of switching the maternal diet from an SFO-based to an SBO-based diet (Samulski and Walker, 1982). Since dietary fat influences the composition of brain membranes within short periods of time, the next question is whether these changes are of functional significance.

Dietary Lipid, Membrane Lipid Composition, and Brain Function

Variations in membrane lipid composition, including fatty acid profile, cholesterol content, and phospholipid polar head groups, alter the physical characteristics (fluidity) of the membrane (for reviews see Brenner, 1984; Shinitzky, 1984; Boggs, 1980; Stubs and Smith, 1984; Wahle, 1983). The importance of membrane fluidity in relation to its function has been demonstrated. For example, changes in the phase transition temperature (T_t; characteristic of the physical properties of the membrane) induced by dietary fat is correlated with abrupt discontinuities in Arrhenius plots of membrane-bound enzyme activities and changes in phospholipid composition (Innis and Clandinin, 1981a,b). These relationships have been studied more extensively in peripheral tissues. However dietary-fat-induced changes in neuronal membrane composition are associated with abrupt discontinuities in Arrhenius plots for acetylcholinoesterase activity (Foot et al., 1983).

It has been argued that diet-induced modifications in brain membrane composition are not functionally important, since the cell membrane responds to these fluctuations in fatty acid availability by altering other membrane components to maintain its overall fluidity. There is, however, a small body of evidence to support the hypothesis that these diet-induced alterations do indeed influence brain-membrane-associated events. For example, in rats fed linoleate-deficient diets, changes observed included 1) increased $(Na^+ + K^+)$-dependent ATPase activity (Sun and Sun, 1974), 2) decreased concentrations of gangliosides and glycoproteins in combination with decreased activity of their respective synthetic enzymes (Morgan et al., 1981), 3) delayed myelination (Gozzo and D'Udine, 1977; McKenna and Campagnoni, 1979), 4) delayed attainment of adult electrocorticographic activity (D'Udine and Oliverio, 1976), 5) decreased ethanol tolerance (John et al., 1980), 6) reduced anesthetic requirement (Koblin et al., 1980), and 7) decreased norepinephrine uptake in cerebral cortex (Brenneman and Rutledge, 1979). This response to dietary fat is not only a consequence of linoleate deficiency, since similar changes are observed with nutritionally adequate variations in dietary fat source. Altered synaptic plasma membrane acetylcholinesterase activity is apparent after oral administration of phospholipids for 72 hr (Heger, 1979) or after feeding diets with differing fat content for 24 days (Foot et al., 1983). Similar changes are observed with the mitochondrial enzyme, MAO (Crane and Greenwood, 1987), with V_{max} (velocity) but not Km (affinity) responding to changes in dietary fat source after 28 days. While both these enzymes are involved in neurotransmitter degradation, the magnitude of change in enzyme activity is probably not great enough to influence neurotransmitter metabolism. For example, steady state concentrations of brain stem 5-HT and 5-HIAA were unaltered, despite the change in MAO activity (Crane and Greenwood, 1987). However, these data demonstrate that the neuron responds to alterations in dietary fat source within very short periods of time, i.e., several generations of feeding dietary fat are not required for effects on neuronal membrane-associated protein function to be measurable.

Neuroreceptor availability is also sensitive to changes in membrane composition. When membrane composition is altered in vitro either enzymatically or by fusion with exogenous lipids, the number of binding sites as well as the distribution between high and low affinity states is altered (for review see Gould and Ginsberg, 1984, 1985). It has been suggested that, at least for serotonin, the accessibility of binding sites for ligands represents approximately one-fifth of the potential binding capacity stored in membranes (Heron et al., 1980). Increased receptor number measured after membrane manipulation is felt to represent the unmasking of cryptic binding sites embedded in the membrane. By analogy, it may be hypothesized that neuroreceptor availability may also be sensitive to diet-induced alterations in membrane composition; however this relationship has not been extensively

examined. Short-term feeding (4–6 weeks) of diets high or low in polyunsaturated fatty acids did not influence either the number or affinity of striatal
dopamine binding sites in young or senescent mice (Leprohon-Greenwood
and Cinader, 1987). Whether prolonged feeding of these diets would have
influenced receptor availability is unknown.

The only supporting evidence that in vivo modification of neuronal
membrane composition may influence neuroreceptor availability comes from
studies in which the amino acid, methionine, was administered to rats to
enhance the rate of PE methylation to PC. In these studies, an increased
number of striatal D_2-dopamine binding sites was observed after short-term
methionine administration (LeFur et al., 1983; Leprohon et al., 1985).
Concomitant with the increased number of dopamine binding sites were
alterations in membrane fluidity (LeFur et al., 1983) and elevated brain
levels of S-adenosylmethionine, the methyl donor, up to 6 hr after
methionine injection (Greenwood et al., unpublished data). In addition,
injection of the methylation inhibitor, 3-deazaadenosine, to rats for 1 week
caused a decrease in the number of β-adrenergic receptors in hypothalamus
and brain stem without changing affinity for dihydroalprenolol (F. Hirata,
personal communication). Thus changes in catecholaminergic binding sites
are observed in association with modifications in PE methylation in vivo.
Whether there is an essential requirement for PE methylation for this effect
on dopamine receptor number to be observed is not known.

Despite the accumulating evidence that neuronal metabolism responds to
alterations in dietary fat source, there is still not widespread agreement that
the membrane compositional changes are of physiological importance. To
the contrary, it has been argued that the differences observed in membrane-bound protein function with different dietary fats are of such small
magnitude that they are not functionally important. The most convincing data
affirming the physiological significance of this response come from the
behavioral literature showing functional change associated with dietary fat.

Dietary Lipid and Behavior

Not surprisingly, the morphologic and neurochemical consequences of
essential fatty acid deficiency result in behavioral change in animals and
often outlast the period of nutritional insult if imposed prenatally (for review
see Menon and Dhopeshwarkar, 1982). Delayed appearance of motor
reflexes (D'Udine and Oliverio, 1976) as well as impaired cognitive
performance both at weaning and during adulthood (Borgman et al.,
1975a,b; Caffrey and Patterson, 1971; Galli et al., 1975; Lamptey and
Walker, 1976, 1978a,b; Morgan et al., 1981; Paoletti and Galli, 1972;
Rüthrich et al., 1984) are observed in offspring when dams are fed diets
deficient in essential fatty acids during pregnancy and/or lactation. Indeed,

the results of some of these studies have emphasized the requirement for alpha-linolenate as well as linoleate. In addition, reduced intellectual capacity in children whose mothers consumed a low fat diet during pregnancy due to biliary tract disease (Churchill et al., 1967) and neurologic abnormalities in a child receiving a total parenteral nutrition preparation low in alpha-linolenate (Holman et al., 1982) have all been reported, thus emphasizing the need for an adequate supply of essential fatty acids to maintain normal brain functioning. In contrast to these studies using a malnutrition model, the full impact of nutritionally adequate variations in dietary fat source have not been fully explored. However, data have accumulated to suggest that there are behavioral correlates, with a number of different behaviors being affected.

Pain sensitivity, degree of d-amphetamine-induced hypothermia (Yehuda et al., 1986), feeding behavior (Crane and Greenwood, 1987), and cognitive function (Coscina et al., 1986) are influenced by the source of dietary fat fed to rats. Equally important is the fact that motor activity in an open field (including measurements of rearing and defecation) is not affected, suggesting that these effects are not a non-specific response to dietary fat. In these studies, young, rapidly growing rats (60–80 g BW) were fed 20% (w/w) fat diets, containing either lard or SBO for 24 days prior to behavioral testing and throughout the testing paradigm. Differences in both thermoregulation and pain sensitivity were observed after the dietary treatment (Yehuda et al., 1986). Thermoregulation, measured as the ability of an animal to maintain core body temperature during cold exposure (4°C) when preadministered d-amphetamine, is improved in SBO-fed rats. Since the hypothermic response to d-amphetamine is blocked by either dopamine receptor antagonists or lesions to the nucleus accumbens (Yehuda, 1978), it is hypothesized that this is a dopaminergic-mediated response. Pain sensitivity, measured as the time required for an animal to respond to a heat source (58°C), is significantly lower in animals fed SBO than in those fed lard diets. Pretreatment with naloxone, an opiate antagonist, produced similar reductions in response time (48 and 41% of non-naloxone condition for SBO- and lard-fed animals, respectively; unpublished data), suggesting that the opiate system is unaffected by dietary fat. Pain sensitivity can be manipulated by altering serotonergic neurotransmission (Messing and Lytle, 1977; Seltzer et al., 1982). Hence, the changes observed may be a consequence of altered serotonin (5-HT) neurotransmission.

To further probe the possible effect of dietary fat on 5-HT-mediated behaviors, a second serotonergic-mediated behavior, protein intake regulation (for review see Li and Anderson, 1983), was examined. Rats were fed 25% casein diets containing 20% (w/w) fat as SBO or lard for 24 days. (In these studies, 5% SBO and SFO were added to lard before making the diets to ensure adequacy of linoleate and alpha-linolenate intakes.) Rats were then allowed to select for 2 weeks from diets containing 5 or 55% casein but containing the same composition and levels of fat as they were previously fed. While total caloric intake was unaffected, rats consuming the SBO diets selected significantly less protein and more carbohydrate than rats selecting from the lard diets (Crane and Greenwood, 1987). Both the decreased pain sensitivity and altered macronutrient selection observed in the SBO-fed rats are consistent with alterations in serotonergic function. While the V_{max} of mitochondrial MAO activity was reduced in the SBO-fed rats, the magnitude of change in enzyme activity was not sufficient to affect steady state levels of 5-HT or 5-HIAA measured in brain stem (Crane and Greenwood, 1987). Thus, although these data support the hypothesis that the monoaminergic neurons are influenced by dietary fat, the MAO data in themselves do not explain the behavioral differences observed.

Cognitive function, as assessed in rats using a place navigation tank (Morris, 1981), is also influenced by the source of dietary fat (Coscina et al., 1986). Animals are required to find the position of a platform submerged below opaque-water-level through the use of external cues. Animals fed a diet containing 20% SBO performed significantly better on this task in that they required shorter periods of time to find the submerged platform than animals fed a 20% lard diet. While previous studies demonstrated that essential fatty acid deficiency impairs cognitive performance in rats (Borgman et al., 1975b; Caffrey and Patterson, 1971; Galli et al., 1975; Lamptey and Walker, 1976, 1978a; Morgan et al., 1981; Paoletti and Galli, 1971), this study more importantly shows that changes in cognitive function are measurable within 24 days of feeding the animals the test diets and that a deficiency does not have to be imposed for behavioral change to be observed.

Neither the specific mechanism of action of dietary fat on brain function nor the important characteristic of the fat source, i.e., overall saturation index or ω6/ω3 ratio, mediating the behavioral responses have been identified in these studies. However, the impact of dietary fat is widespread. That is, both higher and lower brain functions and behaviors mediated by different neurotransmitter systems are involved. Therefore the influence of fat source on brain function must be fairly generalized. While small changes in catabolic enzyme activity are observed, the magnitude of change is probably not great enough to influence neurotransmitter metabolism per se (Crane and Greenwood, 1987; Foot et al., 1983). Thus these enzyme activity measurements can serve as markers to demonstrate that the neuron has responded to the dietary treatment imposed, but probably will not, in themselves, address the physiologically important changes. To do so, studies will have to address issues such as vesicle-membrane fusion and neurotransmitter release, receptor availability and generation of second messengers, and membrane potential and conduction velocity to be consistent with the widespread functional changes observed.

Dietary Lipids During Infant Development

Clearly the influence of normal variations in dietary fat intake on neuronal function is poorly understood, and optimal fatty acid intake necessary to produce optimal brain function is unknown. At present, there is no reason to believe that fatty acid profiles in human breast milk are inappropriate for CNS development and function. Therefore, the current policy of attempting to mimic human breast milk fatty acid composition in infant formulas is the most prudent one until these relationships are better understood. Undoubtedly the population at greatest risk for development of essential fatty acid deficiency are infants born prematurely since they have low body fat stores and little reserve of essential fatty acids (Clandinin et al., 1981). In addition, the synthesis of long chain derivatives of the dietary essential fatty acids has not been demonstrated in the preterm infant. Therefore these infants may have a specific requirement for the long-chain polyenoic fatty acids. [During normal pregnancy, these fatty acids are produced in and may be transported via the placenta to meet fetal needs (Zimmerman et al., 1979).] The last trimester of human pregnancy is a period of rapid accumulation of fatty acids in neural tissue, especially of the long chain polyenoic fatty acids (Clandinin et al., 1980). Since long-term cognitive impairment may follow developmental essential fatty acid deficiency, it is imperative that an adequate supply of these nutrients be ensured during the fetal and neonatal periods to support optimal brain development.

SUMMARY

Provision of an adequate dietary supply of nutrients to support brain metabolism is essential for the maintenance of central nervous system function. Unquestionably, diets deficient in essential nutrients will adversely influence neuronal metabolism, and functional consequences will be observed if the deficiency is severe and long-term. However, data now suggest that specific aspects of brain metabolism are sensitive to normal fluctuations in nutrient supply. That is, alterations in neurotransmitter metabolism and membrane composition are observed when macronutrient intakes are manipulated within ranges traditionally viewed as healthful. Furthermore, behavioral correlates of these manipulations are apparent. Our understanding of these metabolic responses and the overall consequences in terms of performance is still incomplete. Nevertheless, meal composition is recognized as an important variable. Current research is investigating the possibility that meal patterning throughout the day (i.e., high versus low protein breakfasts and lunches) impacts on our daily performance levels (Spring, 1986). There is a paucity of information regarding dietary fat intake and neuronal function. Nevertheless preliminary findings indicate that the quality of fat consumed influences brain function, probably mediated via alterations in membrane composition. Therefore, prior to making nutritional recommendations to alter macronutrient intake to reduce the risk of specific diseases, it is essential that the full implications of these changes are understood. For example, current research initiatives are investigating the effects of fish oil and/or (ω3) fatty acid consumption in the prevention of coronary heart disease, yet the consequences of these changes on central nervous system function are largely unknown.

The bulk of information on neurologic consequences of altered macronutrient intake within normal, adequate ranges comes from adult (mature) studies. However, data suggest that the immature, developing brain is also sensitive to fluctuations in nutrient supply. For example, while a certain degree of protection from altered precursor availability is afforded due to the immaturity of regulatory enzyme activities, neurotransmitter synthesis can be enhanced (albeit to a lesser degree) by providing more precursor amino acid, especially for the monoaminergic neurotransmitter serotonin. In addition, the developing brain may be more sensitive than the adult brain to variations in fatty acid supply due to the rapid accretion of fatty acids in neuronal tissue during this period. This information points to the importance of maternal nutrition during gestation and lactation, as well as to careful selection of weaning foods to provide the best nutrient environment for central nervous system development. Clearly our overall understanding of developmental aspects of altered nutrient availability in the absence of malnutrition and its long-term consequences are poorly understood, and further research is warranted before specific recommendations can be made.

LITERATURE CITED

Aghajanian GK (1981): The modulatory role of serotonin and multiple receptors in brain. In Jacobs BL, Gelperin A (eds): "Serotonin Neurotransmission and Behavior." Cambridge: MIT Press, pp 156–185.

Aghajanian GK, Asher IM (1971): Histochemical fluorescence of raphe neurons: Selective enhancement by tryptophan. Science 172:1159–1161.

Aghajanian GK, Bloom FE (1967): The formation of synaptic junctions in developing brain: A quantitative electron microscopic study. Brain Res 6:716–727.

Aghajanian GK, Haigler HJ (1973): Studies on the physiological activity of 5-HT neurons. In Bloom FE, Acheson GH (eds): "Pharmacology and the Future of Man," Vol. 4, "Brain, Nerves, and Synapses." Basel: Karger, pp 269–279.

Agharanya JC, Wurtman RJ (1985): Effect of dietary proteins and carbohydrates on urinary and sympathoadrenal catecholamines. Neurochem Int 7:271–277.

Agrawal HC, Davis JM, Himwich WA (1966a): Postnatal changes in free amino acid pool of rat brain. J Neurochem 13:607–615.

Agrawal HC, Glisson SN, Himwich WA (1966b): Changes in monoamines of rat brain during postnatal ontogeny. Biochim Biophys Acta 130:511–513.

Anonymous (1987): Does tryptophan influence serotonin release from brain neurons? Nutr Rev 45:87–89.

Asano Y (1971): The maturation of the circadian rhythm of brain norepinephrine and serotonin in the rat. Life Sci 10:883–894.

Ashcroft GW, Eccleston D, Crawford RBB (1965): 5-Hydroxyindole metabolism in rat brain. A study of intermediate metabolism using the technique of tryptophan loading-I. J Neurochem 12:483–492.

Atterwill CK, Green AR (1980): Responses of developing rats to L-tryptophan plus an MAOI. 1. Monitoring changes in behaviour, brain 5-HT and tryptophan. Neuropharmacology 19:325–335.

Bachelard HS, Campbell WJ, McIlwain H (1962): The sodium and other ions of mammalian cerebral tissues, maintained and electrically stimulated in vitro. Biochem J 84:225–232.

Baños G, Daniel PM, Pratt OE (1978): The effect of age upon the entry of some amino acids into the brain, and their incorporation into cerebral protein. Dev Med Child Neurol 20:335–346.

Baños G, Daniel PM, Moorhouse SR, Pratt OE (1973): The influx of amino acids into the brain of the rat in vivo: The essential compared with some non-essential amino acids. Proc R Soc Lond 183:59–70.

Barbeau A, Growdon JH, Wurtman RJ (eds) (1979): "Nutrition and the Brain, Vol. 5." New York: Raven Press.

Bass NH, Lundborg P (1973): Postnatal development of mechanisms for the elimination of organic acids from the brain and cerebrospinal fluid system of the rat: Rapid efflux of [^{3}H]para-aminohippuric acid following intrathecal injection. Brain Res 56:285–298.

Bennett DS, Giarman NJ (1965): Schedule of appearance of 5-hydroxytryptamine (serotonin) and associated enzymes in the developing rat brain. J Neurochem 12:911–918.

Bernsohl J, Cohen SR (1972): Polyenoic fatty acid metabolism of phosphoglycerides in developing brain. In Ciba Foundation (eds): "Lipids, Malnutrition and the Developing Brain." New York: Elsevier Excerpta Medica North-Holland, pp 159–178.

Biggio G, Fadda F, Fanni P, Tagliamonte A, Gessa GL (1974): Rapid depletion of serum tryptophan, brain tryptophan, serotonin and 5-hydroxyindoleacetic acid by a tryptophan-free diet. Life Sci 14:1321–1329.

Biggio G, Porceddu ML, Fratta W, Gessa GL (1977): Changes in dopamine metabolism associated with fasting and satiation. Adv Biochem Psychopharmacol 16:377–380

Blusztajn JK, Wurtman RJ (1981): Choline biosynthesis by a preparation enriched in synaptosomes from rat brain. Nature 290:417–418.

Boggs JM (1980): Intermolecular hydrogen bonding between lipids: Influence on organization and function of lipids in membranes. Can J Biochem 58:755–770.

Booth RFS, Patel TB, Clark JB (1980): The development of enzymes of energy metabolism in the brain of a precocial (guinea pig) and non-precocial (rat) species. J Neurochem 34:17–25.

Borgman RF, Bursey RG, Caffrey BC (1975a): Influence of dietary fat upon rat gestation and lactation. Am J Vet Res 36:795–798.

Borgman RF, Bursey RG, Caffrey BC (1975b): Influence of maternal dietary fat upon rat pups. Am J Vet Res 36:799–805.

Botez MI, Young SN, Bachevalier J, Gautheir S (1982): Effect of folic acid and vitamin B$_{12}$ deficiencies on 5-hydroxyindoleacetic acid in human cerebro-spinal fluid. Ann Neurol 12:479–484.

Bottiglieri T, Laundy RM, Martin R, Carney MWP, Nissenbaum H, Toone BK, Johnson AL (1984): S-adenosylmethionine influences monoamine metabolism. Lancet 2:224.

Bourgoin S, Artaud F, Adrien J, Hery F, Glowinski J, Hamon M (1977a): 5-Hydroxytrypta-mine catabolism in the rat brain during ontogenesis. J Neurochem 28:415–422.

Bourgoin S, Faivre-Bauman A, Benda P, Glowinski J, Hamon M (1974): Plasma tryptophan and 5-HT metabolism in the CNS of the newborn rat. J Neurochem 23:319–327.

Bourgoin S, Faivre-Bauman A, Hery F, Ternaus JP, Hamon M (1977b): Characteristics of tryptophan binding in the serum of the newborn rat. Biol Neonate 31:141–154.

Bourre JM, Pascal G, Durand G, Masson M, Dumont O, Piciotti M (1984): Alterations in the fatty acid composition of rat brain cells (neurons, astrocytes, and oligodendrocytes) and of subcellular fractions (myelin and synaptosomes) induced by a diet devoid of n-3 fatty acids. J Neurochem 43:342–348.

Bourre JM, Pollet S, Paturneau-Jollas M, Bauman N (1978): Fatty acid biosynthesis during brain development. In Gatt S, Freysz L, Mandel P (eds): "Enzymes of Lipid Metabolism." New York: Plenum Publishing, pp 17–26.

Brass CA, Isaacs CE, McChesney R, Greengard O (1982): The effects of hyperphenylala-ninemia on fetal development: A new animal model of maternal phenylketonuria. Pediatr Res 16:388–394.

Brenneman DE, Rutledge CO (1979): Alteration of catecholamine uptake in cerebral cortex from rats fed a saturated fat diet. Brain Res 179:295–304.

Brenner RR (1984): Effect of unsaturated acids on membrane structure and enzyme kinetics. Prog Lipid Res 23:69–96.

Burns EM (1984): Some effects of malnutrition on synaptic systems: An integration of morphologic, neurochemical and neurophysiological data. In Jones DG (ed): "Current Topics in Research on Synapses, Volume 2." New York: Alan R. Liss, Inc., pp 59–91.

Caffrey B, Patterson MY (1971): Effects of saturated and unsaturated fats on learning, emotionally, and reaction to stress. Psychol Rep 29:79–86.

Carlsson A, Kehr W, Linqvist M (1976): The role of intraneuronal amine levels in the feedback control of dopamine, noradrenaline and 5-hydroxytryptamine synthesis in rat brain. J Neural Trans 39:1–19.

Carlsson A, Linqvist M (1972): The effect of L-tryptophan and some psychotropic drugs on the formation of 6-hydroxytryptophan in the mouse brain in vivo. J Neural Transm 33:23–43.

Carlsson A, Linqvist M (1978): Dependence of 5-HT and catecholamine synthesis on precursor amino acid levels in rat brain. Naunyn-Schmeideberg's Arch Pharmacol 303:157–164.

Carver MJ, Copenhaver JH, Serpan RA (1965): Free amino acids in foetal rat brain. J Neurochem 12:857–861.

Century B, Witting LA, Harvey CC, Horwitt MK (1963): Interrelationship of dietary lipids upon fatty acid composition of brain mitochondria erythrocytes and heart tissue in chicks. Am J Clin Nutr 13:362–368.

Chamberlain B, Ervin FR, Pihl RO, Young SN (1987): The effect of raising or lowering tryptophan levels on aggression in vervet monkeys. Pharmacol Biochem Behav, in press.

Chase PH, O'Brien D (1970): Effect of excess phenylalanine and of other amino acids on brain development in the infant rat. Pediatr Res 4:96–102.

Cheifetz S, Warsh JJ (1980): Occurrence and distribution of 5-hydroxytryptophol in the rat. J Neurochem 34:1093–1099.

Churchill JA, Ayers MA, Caldwell DF (1967): Intelligence of children whose mothers have biliary tract disease. JAMA 201:222–224.

Clandinin MT, Chappell HE, Heim T, Swyer PR, Chance GW (1981): Fatty acid utilization in perinatal de novo synthesis of tissues. Early Hum Dev 5:355–366.

Clandinin MT, Chappell JE, Leong S, Heim T, Swyer RP, Chance GW (1980): Intrauterine fatty acid accretion rates in human brain: Implications for fatty acid requirements. Early Hum Dev 4:121–129.

Cocchi M, Pignatti C, Carpidiani M, Tarozzi G, Turchetto E (1984): Effect of C18:3 (n-3) dietary supplementation on the fatty acid composition of the rat brain. Acta Vitaminol Enzymol 6:151–156.

Cohen EL, Wurtman RJ (1976): Brain acetylcholine: Control by dietary choline. Science 191:561–562.

Coscina DV, Yehuda S, Dixon LM, Kish SJ, Leprohon-Greenwood CE (1986): Learning is improved by a soybean oil diet in rats. Life Sci 38:1789–1794.

Cowan WM (1979): The development of the brain. Sci Am 241:112–133.

Coyle JT (1977): Biochemical aspects of neurotransmission in the developing brain. Int Rev Neurobiol 20:65–103.

Coyle JT, Axelrod J (1971): Development of the uptake and storage of L-[^{3}H]norepinephrine in the rat brain. J Neurochem 18:2061–2075.

Coyle JT, Axelrod J (1972a): Dopamine-β-hydroxylase in the rat brain: Developmental characteristics. J Neurochem 19:449–459.

Coyle JT, Axelrod J (1972b): Tyrosine hydroxylase in rat brain: Developmental characteristics. J Neurochem 19:1117–1123.

Coyle JF, Henry D (1973): Catecholamines in fetal and newborn rat brain. J Neurochem 21:61–67.

Crandall EA, Fernstrom JD (1980): Acute changes in brain tryptophan and serotonin after carbohydrate or protein ingestion by diabetic rats. Diabetes 29:460–466.

Crandall EA, Gillis MA, Fernstrom JD (1981): Reduction in brain serotonin synthesis rate in streptozotocin-diabetic rats. Endocrinology 109:310–312.

Crane SB, Greenwood CE (1987): Dietary fat source influences neuronal mitochondrial monoamine oxidase activity and macronutrient selection in rats. Pharmacol Biochem Behav 27:1–6.

Cremer JE, Cunningham VJ, Pardridge WM, Braun LD, Oldendorf WH (1979): Kinetics of blood-brain barrier transport of pyruvate, lactate and glucose in suckling, weanling and adult rats. J Neurochem 33:439–445.

Culley WJ, Saunders RN, Mertz ET, Jolly DG (1962): Effect of phenylalanine and its metabolites on brain serotonin and plasma tryptophan level. Proc Soc Exp Biol Med 113:645–648.

Cunningham TJ, Nigam N (1979): Evidence for increased neuronal survival in the cerebral cortex of hyperphenylalanimic rats. Anat Rec 193:515.

Dairman W (1979): Catecholamine concentrations and the activity of tyrosine hydroxylase after an increase in the concentration of tyrosine in rat tissues. Br J Pharmacol 44:307–310.

Dakshinamurti K (1977): B vitamins and nervous system function. In Wurtman RJ, Wurtman JJ (eds): ''Nutrition and the Brain,'' Vol. 1. New York: Raven Press, pp 249–318.

Dakshinamurti K (1982): Neurobiology of pyridoxine. In Draper HH (ed): ''Advances in Nutritional Research,'' Vol. 4. New York: Plenum Publishing, pp 143–179.

Dalvit-McPhillips SP (1983): The effect of the human menstrual cycle on nutrient intake. Physiol Behav 31:209–212.

David JC (1984): Relationship between phenolamines and catecholamines during rat brain embryonic development in vivo and in vitro. J Neurochem 43:668–674.

Deguchi T, Barchas J (1972): Regional distribution and developmental change of tryptophan hydroxylase activity in rat brain. J Neurochem 19:927–929.

DeMet EM, Halaris AE (1979): Origin and distribution of 3-methoxy-4-hydroxyphenylglycol in body fluids. Biochem Pharmacol 28:3043–3050.

De Simoni MG, Sakola A, Fodritto F, Dal Toso G, Algeri S (1986): Tryptophan effect on serotonin metabolism and release studies by in vivo voltammetry. Soc Neurosci 12:120.13.

Deza L, Eidelberg E (1967): Development of cortical electrical activity in the rat. Exp Neurol 17:425–438.

Dienel GA (1981): Chronic hyperphenylalaninemia produces cerebral hyperglycinemia in immature rats. J Neurochem 36:34–43.

Diggory GL, Ceasar PM, Morgan RM (1979): The regional metabolism of 5-hydroxytryptamine in mouse brain in vitro. Life Sci 24:1939–1946.

Drahota Z, Hahn P, Kleinzeller A, Kostolanska A (1964): Acetoacetate formation by liver slices from adult and infant rats. Biochem J 93:61–65.

Dreyfus PM, Geel SE (1981): Vitamin and mineral deficiencies. In Siegel GJ, Albers RW, Agranoff BW, Katzman R (eds): "Basic Neurochemistry." 3rd Ed. Boston: Little, Brown, pp 661–679.

D'Udine B, Oliverio A (1976): Lipid malnutrition and early development: A study of motor reflexes and electrocorticographic activity in the mouse. Behav Processes 1:183–190.

Eayrs JT, Goodhead B (1959): Postnatal development of the cerebral cortex in the rat. J Anat 93:385–402.

Elks ML, Youngblood WW, Kizer JS (1979): Serotonin synthesis and release in brain slices: Independence of tryptophan. Brain Res 172:471–486.

Elwyn DH (1970): The role of the liver in the regulation of amino acid and protein metabolism. In Munro HN (ed): "Mammalian Protein Metabolism," Vol. 4. New York: Academic Press, pp 523–557.

Enwonwu CO, Worthington BS (1974): Concentrations of histamine in brain of guinea pig and rat during protein malnutrition. Biochem J 144:601–603.

Fernando JCR, Curzon G (1981): Behavioral responses to drugs releasing 5-hydroxytryptamine and catecholamines: Effects of treatments altering precursor concentrations in brain. Neuropharmacology 20:115–122.

Fernstrom JD (1976): The effect of nutritional factors on brain amino acid levels and monoamine synthesis. Fed Proc 35:1151–1156.

Fernstrom JD (1983): Role of precursor availability in control of monoamine biosynthesis in brain. Physiol Rev 63:484–546.

Fernstrom JD, Faller DV (1978): Neutral amino acids in the brain: Changes in response to food ingestion. J Neurochem 30:1531–1538.

Fernstrom JD, Faller DV, Shabshelowitz H (1975): Acute reduction of brain serotonin and 5-HIAA following food consumption: Correlation with the ratio of serum tryptophan to the sum of competing neutral amino acids. J Neural Transm 36:113–121.

Fernstrom JD, Fernstrom MH, Grubb PE, Volk EA (1985): Absence of chronic effects of dietary protein content on brain tryptophan concentrations in rats. J Nutr 115:1337–1344.

Fernstrom JD, Larin F, Wurtman RJ (1973): Correlation between brain tryptophan and plasma neutral amino acid levels following food consumption in rats. Life Sci 13:517–524.

Fernstrom JD, Wurtman RJ (1971): Brain serotonin content: Physiological dependence on plasma tryptophan levels. Science 173:149–152.

Fernstrom MH, Volk EA, Fernstrom JD, Iuvone PM (1986): Effect of tyrosine administration on dopa accumulation in light- and dark-adapted retinas from normal and diabetic rats. Life Sci 39:2049–2057.

Figlewicz DA, Druse MJ (1980): Experimental hyperphenylalaninemia: Effect on central nervous system myelin subfractions. Exp Neurol 67:315–329.

Foot M, Cruz TF, Clandinin MT (1982): Influence of dietary fat on the lipid composition of rat brain synaptosomal and microsomal membranes. Biochem J 208:631–640.

Foot M, Cruz TF, Clandinin MT (1983): Effect of dietary lipid on synaptosomal acetylcholinesterase activity. Biochem J 211:507–509.

Gal EM, Drewes PA (1962): Studies on the metabolism of 5-hydroxytryptamine (serotonin). II. Effect of tryptophan deficiency in rat. Proc Soc Exp Biol Med 110:368–371.

Gallagher DW, Aghajanian GK (1976): Inhibition of firing of raphe neurons by tryptophan and 5-hydroxytryptophan: Blockade by inhibiting serotonin synthesis with RO-4-4602. Neuropharmacology 15:149–156.

Galli C, Meseri P, Oliverio A, Paoletti R (1975): Deficiency of essential fatty acids during pregnancy and avoidance learning in the progeny. Pharmacol Res Commun 7:71–80.

Gandy G, Jacobson W, Sidman R (1973): Inhibition of transmethylation reaction in central nervous system: An experimental model for subacute combined degeneration of the cord. J Pathol 109:13–14.

Gessa GL, Tagliamonte A (1974): Possible role of free serum tryptophan in the control of brain tryptophan level and serotonin synthesis. Adv Biochem Psychopharmacol 11:119–1131.

Gibson CJ (1985): Induction of liver tyrosine aminotransferase (TAT) activity by high protein diets but not by tyrosine-supplemented diets. Can Fed Biol Soc 28:PA132.

Gibson CJ (1986): Dietary control of retinal dopamine synthesis. Brain Res 382:195–198.

Gibson CJ, Watkins CJ, Wurtman RJ (1983): Tyrosine administration enhances dopamine synthesis and release in light-activated rat retina. J Neurol Transm 56:153–160.

Gibson CJ, Wurtman RJ (1977): Physiological control of brain catecholamine synthesis by tyrosine concentration. Biochem Pharmacol 26:1137–1142.

Gibson CJ, Wurtman RJ (1978): Physiological control of brain norepinephrine synthesis by brain tyrosine concentration. Life Sci 22:1399–1406.

Girard J (1986): Gluconeogenesis in late fetal and early neonatal life. Biol Neonate 50:237–258.

Glaeser BS, Maher TH, Wurtman RJ (1983): Changes in brain levels of acidic, basic, and neutral amino acids after consumption of single meals containing various proportions of protein. J Neurochem 41:1016–1021.

Glanville NT, Anderson GH (1985): The effect of insulin deficiency, dietary protein intake, and plasma amino acid concentrations on brain amino acid levels in rats. Can J Physiol Pharmacol 63:487–494.

Glanville NT, Anderson GH (1986): Hypothalamic catecholamine metabolism in diabetic rats: The effect of insulin deficiency and meal ingestion. J Neurochem 46:753–759.

Glowinski J (1972): Some new facts about synthesis, storage and release processes of monoamines in the central nervous system. In Snyder SH (ed): "Perspectives in Neuropharmacology." New York: Oxford University Press, pp 349–404.

Glowinski J (1978): Properties and functions on intraneuronal monoamine compartments in central aminergic neurons. In Iversen LL, Iversen SD, Snyder SH (eds): "Handbook of Psychopharmacology." New York: Plenum Press, pp 136–167.

Goldstein M (1966): Inhibition of norepinephrine biosynthesis at the dopamine-β-hydroxylation stage. Pharmacol Rev 18:77–82.

Gonatas NK, Autilio-Gambetti L, Gambetti P, Shafer B (1971): Morphological and biochemical changes in rat synaptosome fractions during neonatal development. J Cell Biol 51:484–498.

Gould RJ, Ginsberg BH (1984): Biochemistry and analysis of membrane phospholipids: Applications to membrane receptors. In Venter JC, Harrison LC (eds): "Membranes, Detergents, and Receptor Solubilization." New York: Alan R. Liss, pp 65–83.

Gould RJ, Ginsberg BH (1985): Membrane fluidity and membrane receptor function. In Aloia RC, Boggs JM (eds): "Membrane Fluidity in Biology." New York: Academic Press, pp 257–280.

Gozzo S, D'Udine B (1977): Diet deprived in essential fatty acids affects brain myelination. Neurosci Lett 7:267–275.

Green AR, Aronson JK, Curzon G, Woods HF (1980): Metabolism of an oral tryptophan load. I. Effects of dose and pretreatment with tryptophan. Br J Clin Pharmacol 10:603–610.

Green H, Greenberg SM, Erickson RW, Sawyer JL, Ellison T (1962): Effect of dietary phenlalanine and tryptophan upon rat brain amine levels. J Pharmacol Exp Ther 136:174–178.

Halas ES, Wallwork JC, Sandstead HH (1982): Milk zinc deficiency and undernutrition during the prenatal and postnatal periods in rats. Effects on weight, food consumption and brain catecholamine concentrations. J Nutr 112:542–551.

Hamel E, Butterworth RF, Barbeau A (1979): Effect of thiamine deficiency on levels of putative amino acid transmitters in affected regions of the rat brain. J Neurochem 33:575–577.

Hamon M, Bourgoin S, Glowinski J (1973): Feedback regulation of 5-HT synthesis in rat striatal slices. J Neurochem 20:1727–1745.

Harden TK, Wolfe BB, Sporn JR, Perkins JP, Molinoff PB (1977): Ontogeny of β-adrenergic receptors in rat cerebral cortex. Brain Res 125:99–108.

Hargreaves KM, Clandinin MT (1986): Phosphocholinetransferase and phosphatidylethano-laminemethyltransferase activity in brain responds to alteration in dietary fat. Can Fed Biol Soc 29:PA45.

Harris JE, Roth RH (1971): Potassium-induced acceleration of catecholamine biosynthesis in brain slices. A study of the mechanism of action. Mol Pharmacol 7:593–604.

Hawkins RA, Williamson DH, Krebs HA (1971): Ketone body utilization by adult and suckling rat brain in vivo. Biochem J 122:13–18.

Heger HW (1979): Effect of dietary phospholipids on acetylcholinesterase activity in the rat brain and on phospholipid composition in liver and brain. Gen Pharmacol 10:427–432.

Heger HW, Peter HW (1979): Influence of a lipid diet on the amounts of phospholipids and polyamines in rat brain. Gen Pharmacol 10:433–435.

Heron DS, Shinitzky M, Herskowitz J, Samuel D (1980): Lipid fluidity markedly modulates the binding of serotonin to mouse brain membranes. Proc Natl Acad Sci USA 77:7463–7467.

Hery F, Simonnet G, Bourgoin S, Soubrie P, Artand F, Hamon M, Glowinski J (1979): Effect of nerve activity on the in vivo release of [^{3}H] serotonin continuously formed from L-[^{3}H]tryptophan in the caudate nucleus of the cat. Brain Res 169:317–334.

Hess SM, Doepfner W (1961): Behavioral effects and brain amine content in rats. Arch Int Pharmacodyn Ther 134:89–99.

Hirata F, Axelrod J (1980): Phospholipid methylation and biological signal transmission. Science 209:1082–1090.

Holman RT, Johnson SB, Hatch TF (1982): A case of human linolenic acid deficiency involving neurological abnormalities. Am J Clin Nutr 35:617–623.

Howd RA, Nelson MF, Lytle LD (1975): L-Tryptophan and fetal brain serotonin. Life Sci 17:803–812.

Hrboticky N (1986): "Effects of Tryptophan on Mealtime Food Intake of Normal Weight Men and Women." Ph.D. thesis, University of Toronto, Toronto.

Hrboticky N, Leiter LA, Anderson GH (1985); Effects of L-tryptophan on short-term food intake in lean men. Nutr Res 5:595–607.

Huether G (1986): The depletion of tryptophan and serotonin in the brain of developing hyperphenylalaninemic rats is abolished by the additional administration of lysine. Neurochem Res 11:1663–1668.

Huether G, Neuhoff V (1981): Use of α-methylphenylalanine for studies of brain development in experimental phenylketonuria. J Inherited Metab Dis 4:67–68.

Ikeda M, Fahien LA, Udenfriend S (1966): A kinetic study of bovine adrenal tyrosine hydroxylase. J Biol Chem 241:4452–4456.

Innis SM, Clandinin MT (1981a): Dynamic modulation of mitochondrial inner-membrane lipids in rat heart by dietary fat. Biochem J 193:155–167.

Innis SM, Clandinin MT (1981b): Dynamic modulation of mitochondrial membrane physical properties and ATPase activity by diet lipid. Biochem J 198:167–175.

Isaacs CE, Greengard O (1980): The effect of hyperphenylalaninemia on glycine metabolism in developing rat brain. Biochem J 192:441–448.

Jacobs BL, Heym J, Rasmussen K (1983): Raphe neurons: Firing rate correlates with size of drug response. Brain Res 90:275–278.

Jacobson M (1978): "Developmental Biology." 2nd ed. New York: Plenum Publishing.

Jacobson S (1963): Sequence of myelination in the brain of the albino rat: Cerebral cortex, thalamus and related structures. J Comp Neurol 121:5–29.

Joh TH, Park DH, Reis DJ (1978): Direct phosphorylation of brain tyrosine hydroxylase by cyclic AMP-dependent protein kinase: Mechanism of enzyme activation. Proc Natl Acad Sci USA 75:4744–4748.

John GR, Littleton JM, Jones PA (1980): Membrane lipids and ethanol tolerance in the mouse. The influence of dietary fatty acid composition. Life Sci 27:545–555.

Johnson RC, Shah SN (1980): Effects of α-methylphenylalanine plus phenylalanine treatment during development on myelin in rat brain. Neurochem Res 5:709–718.

Johnston JL, Warsh JJ, Anderson GH (1983): Obesity and precursor availability affect urinary catecholamine metabolite production in women. Am J Clin Nutr 38:356–368.

Jost A (1966): Problems of fetal endocrinology: The adrenal glands. Rec Prog Hormone Res 22:541–569.

Jost A, Pichon L (1970): Hormonal control of fetal development and metabolism. In Levine R, Luft R (eds): "Advances in Metabolic Disorders," Vol. 4. New York: Academic Press, pp 123–184.

Kalyanasundaram S (1976): Effect of dietary protein and calorie deficiency on tryptophan levels in the developing rat brain. J Neurochem 27:1245–1247.

Kaneko A (1979): Physiology of the retina. Ann Rev Neurosci 2:169–191.

Kantak KM, Hegstrand LR, Whitman J, Eichelman B (1980): Effects of dietary supplements and a tryptophan-free diet on aggressive behavior in rats. Pharmacol Biochem Behav 12:174–179.

Kaplan H, Triano T, Donadio M (1981): Behavioral deficit in phenylketonuric rats: Role of aromatic acid metabolites of phenylalanine. Dev Psychobiol 14:201–207.

Karki N, Kuntzman R, Brodie BB (1960): Norepinephrine and serotonin brain levels at various stages of ontogenetic development. Fed Proc 19:282.

Karki N, Kuntzman R, Brodie BB (1962): Storage, synthesis and metabolism of monoamines in the developing brain. J Neurochem 6:53–58.

Kaufman S (1974): Properties of pterin-dependent aromatic amino acid hydroxylases. In Wolstenholme GEW, Fitzsimons DW (eds): "Aromatic Amino Acids in the Brain." Amsterdam: Elsevier, pp 85–108.

Kellogg C, Lundborg P (1972): Production of [^{3}H]catecholamines in the brain following the peripheral administration of ^{3}H-DOPA during pre- and postnatal development. Brain Res 36:333–342.

Knott PJ, Curzon G (1972): Free tryptophan in plasma and brain tryptophan metabolism. Nature 239:452–453.

Koblin DD, Dong DE, Deady JE, Eger EI (1980): Alteration of synaptic membrane fatty acid composition and anesthetic requirement. J Pharmacol Exp Ther 212:546–552.

Korevaar WC, Geyer MA, Knapp S, Hsu LL, Mandell AJ (1973): Regional distribution of 5-methyl-tetrahydrofolic acid in brain. Nature New Biol 245:244–145.

Kuhn DM, Wolf WA, Youdim MBH (1986): Serotonin neurochemistry revisited: A new look at some old axioms. Neurochem Int 8:141–154.

Kurzepa ST, Bojanek J (1965): The 5-HT level and MAO activity in the rat brain during development. Biol Neonate 8:216–221.

Lajtha AL, Maker HD, Clarke DD (1981): Metabolism and transport of carbohydrate and amino acids. In Seigel GJ, Albers RW, Agranoff BW, Katzman R (eds): "Basic Neurochemistry." 3rd Ed. Boston: Little, Brown, pp 329–353.

Lamprecht F, Coyle JT (1972); Dopa decarboxylase in the developing rat brain. Brain Res 41:503–506.

Lamptey MS, Walker BL (1976): A possible essential role for dietary linolenic acid in the development of the young rat. J Nutr 106:86–93.

Lamptey MS, Walker BL (1978a): Learning behavior and brain lipid composition in rats subjected to essential fatty acid deficiency during gestation, lactation and growth. J Nutr 108:358–367.

Lamptey MS, Walker BL (1978b): Physical and neurological development of the progeny of female rats fed an essential fatty acid-deficient diet during pregnancy and/or lactation. J Nutr 108:351–357.

Lane JC, Schone B, Langenbeck U, Neuhoff V (1979): Characterization of experimental phenylketonuria. In Hommes FA (ed): "Models for the Study of Unborn Errors of Metabolism." New York: Elsevier/North-Holland, pp 141–148.

Lasley SM, Thurmond JB (1985): Interaction of dietary tryptophan and social isolation on territorial aggression, motor activity, and neurochemistry in mice. Psychopharmacology 87:313–321.

Lauder JM, Bloom FE (1974): Ontogeny of monoamine neurons in the locus coeruleus, raphe nuclei and substantia nigra of the rat. I. Cell differentiation. J Comp Neurol 155:469–481.

Lauder JM, Bloom FE (1975): Ontogeny of monoamine neurons in the locus coeruleus, raphe nuclei and substantia nigra of the rat. II. Synaptogenesis. J Comp Neurol 163:251–264.

Lauder JM, Krebs H (1976): Effects of p-chlorophenylalanine on time of neuronal origin during embryogenesis in the rat. Brain Res 107:638–644.

Lauder JM, Krebs H (1978a): Serotonin as a differentiation signal in early neurogenesis. Dev Neurosci 1:15–30.

Lauder JM, Krebs H (1978b): Serotonin and early neurogenesis. In Vernadakis A, Giacobini E, Filogama G (eds): "Maturation of Neurotransmission." Basel: Karger, pp 171–180.

Lauder JM, Wallace JA, Krebs H, Petrusz P, McCarthy K (1982): In vivo and in vitro development of serotonergic neurons. Brain Res Bull 9:605–625.

LeFur G, Phan T, Burgevin MC, Flamier A, Mitrani N, Marguis F, Jozefczak C, Uzan A (1983): A subacute treatment of L-methionine induces an increase in the number of ^{3}H-spiperone binding sites in the striatum of the rat. Life Sci 32:2321–2328.

Lehnert H, Reinstein DK, Strowbridge BQ, Wurtman RJ (1984): Neurochemical and behavioral consequences of acute, uncontrollable stress: Effects of dietary tyrosine. Brain Res 303:215–223.

Leprohon CE, Anderson GH (1980): Maternal diet affects feeding behaviour of self-selecting weanling rats. Physiol Behav 24:553–559.

Leprohon CE, Anderson GH (1982): Relationships among maternal diet, serotonin metabolism at weanling, and protein selection of progeny. J Nutr 112:29–38.

Leprohon CE, Blusztajn JK, Wurtman RJ (1983): Dopamine stimulation of phosphatidyl-choline (lecithin) biosynthesis in rat brain neurons. Proc Natl Acad Sci USA 80:2063–2066.

Leprohon CE, Silvestre-Lontok MT, Dyer JR (1985): Methionine administration increases the number of ^{3}H spiperone binding sites in rat's brain striatum. Can Fed Biol Soc 28:PA62.

Leprohon-Greenwood CE, Anderson GH (1986): An overview of the mechanisms by which diet affects brain function. Food Tech 40:132–138 & 139.

Leprohon-Greenwood CE, Cinader B (1987): Variations in age-related decline in striatal D_2-dopamine receptors in a variety of mouse strains. Mech Ageing Dev 38:199–206.

LeKim D, Betzing H, Stoffel W (1973): Studies in vivo and in vitro on the methylation of phosphatidyl-N,N-dimethylethanolamine to phosphatidylcholine in rat liver. Hoppe-Seyler's Z Physiol Chem 354:437–444.

Li ETS, Anderson GH (1982): Self-selected meal composition, circadian rhythms and meal responses in plasma and brain tryptophan and 5-hydroxytryptamine in rats. J Nutr 112:2001–2010.

Li ETS, Anderson GH (1983): Amino acids in the regulation of food intake. Nutr Abs Rev Clin Nutr 53:171–181.

Li PP, Warsh JJ, Godse DD (1983): Rat brain norepinephrine metabolism: Substantial clearance through 3,4-dihydroxphenylethyleneglycol formation. J Neurochem 41:1065–1071.

Lockwood EA, Bailey E (1971): The course of ketosis and the activity of key enzymes of ketogenesis and ketone body utilization during development of the postnatal rat. Biochem J 124:249–254.

Logan JS, Thorner MD, MacLeod RM (1983): Zinc may have a physiological role in regulating pituitary prolactin secretion. Neuroendocrinology 37:317–320.

Loizou LA (1969): The development of monoamine-containing neurones in the brain of the albino rat. J Anat 104:588.

Loizou LA (1972): The postnatal ontogeny of monoamine-containing neurons in the central nervous system of the albino rat. Brain Res 40:395–418.

Lookingland KJ, Shannon NJ, Chapin DS, Moore KE (1986): Exogenous tryptophan increases synthesis, storage, and intraneuronal metabolism of 5-hydroxytryptamine in the rat hypothalamus. J Neurochem 47:205–212.

Lovenberg W, Bruckinck EA, Hanbauer I (1975): ATP, cyclic AMP and magnesium increase the affinity of rat striatal tyrosine hydroxylase for its cofactor. Proc Natl Acad Sci USA 72:2955–2958.

Lovenberg W, Jequier E, Sjoerdsma A (1968): Tryptophan hydroxylation in mammalian systems. Adv Pharmacol 6a:21–36.

Lovenberg W, Weissbach H, Udenfriend S (1962): Aromatic L-amino acid decarboxylase. J Biol Chem 237:89–92.

Lundborg P, Kellogg C (1971): Formation of [^{3}H]noradrenaline and [^{3}H]dopamine in the brain and heart of the rat foetus. Brain Res 29:387–389.

Lytle LD, Messing RB, Fisher LA, Phebus L (1975): Effects of long-term corn consumption on brain serotonin and the response to electric shock. Science 190:692–694.

MacKenzie RG, Trulson ME (1978): Effects of insulin and streptozotocin-induced diabetes on brain tryptophan and 5-HT metabolism in rats. J Neurochem 30:205–211.

Madras BK, Cohen EL, Messing R, Munro HN, Wurtman RJ (1974a): Relevance of free tryptophan in serum to tissue tryptophan concentrations. Metabolism 23:1107–1116.

Madras BK, Cohen EL, Munro HN, Wurtman RJ (1974b): Elevation of serum free tryptophan but not brain tryptophan, by serum non-esterified fatty acids. Adv Biochem Psychopharmacol 11:143–151.

Maher TJ, Wurtman RJ (1980): L-Threonine administration increases glycine concentrations in the rat central nervous system. Life Sci 26:1283–1286.

Mandell AJ (1978): Redundant mechanisms regulating tyrosine and tryptophan hydroxylases. Ann Rev Pharmacol Toxicol 18:461–493.

Marchbanks RM (1966): Serotonin binding to nerve ending particles and other preparations from rat brain. J Neurochem 13:1481–1493.

Matheson DF, Oei R, Roots BI (1981): Effect of dietary lipid on the acyl group composition of glycerophospholipids of brain endothelial cells in the developing rat. J Neurochem 36:2073–2079.

McKenna MA, Campagnoni AT (1979): Effect of pre- and postnatal essential fatty acid deficiency on brain development and myelination. J Nutr 109:1195–1204.

McGeer EG, Fibiger HC, Wickson V (1971): Differential development of caudate enzymes in the neonatal rat. Brain Res 32:433–440.

McMenamy RH, Oncley JL (1958): Specific binding of tryptophan to serum albumin. J Biol Chem 233:1436–1447.

Melamed E, Hefti F, Wurtman RJ (1980): Tyrosine administration increases striatal dopamine release in rats with partial nigrostriatal lesions. Proc Natl Acad Sci USA 77:4305–4309.

Menon NK, Dhopeshwarkar GA (1982): Essential fatty acid deficiency and brain development. Prog Lipid Res 21:309–326.

Messing RB, Lytle LD (1977): Serotonin-containing neurons: Their possible role in pain and analgesia. Pain 4:1–121.

Miller LP, Pardridge WM, Braun LD, Oldendorf WH (1985): Kinetic constants for blood-brain barrier amino acid transport in conscious rats. J Neurochem 45:1427–1432.

Milner JD, Wurtman RJ (1985): Tyrosine availability determines stimulus-evoked dopamine release from rat striatal slices. Neurosci Lett 59:215–220.

Molinoff DB, Axelrod J (1971): Biochemistry of catecholamines. Ann Rev Biochem 40:465–500.

Møller SE (1985): Effect of various oral protein doses on plasma neutral amino acid levels. J Neural Transm 61:183–191.

Moore TJ, Lione AP, Sugden MC, Regen DM (1976): β-Hydroxylbutyrate transport in rat brain: Developmental and dietary modulations. Am J Physiol 230:619–630.

Morgan BLG, Oppenheimer J, Winick M (1981): Effects of essential fatty acid deficiency during late gestation on brain N-acetylneuraminic acid metabolism and behaviour in the progeny. Br J Nutr 46:223–230.

Morgan RF, O'Dell BL (1977): Effect of copper deficiency on the concentrations of catecholamines and related brain activities. J Neurochem 28:207–213.

Morgane PJ, Miller M, Kemper T, Stern W, Forbes W, Hall R, Bronzino J, Kissane J, Harylewicz E, Resnick O (1978): The effects of protein malnutrition on the developing central nervous system in the rat. Neurosci Biobehav Res 2:137–230.

Morris JPF (1987): "Early Dietary Experience and Subsequent Protein Selection in the Rat." Ph.D. thesis, University of Toronto, Toronto, pp 107–127.

Morris JPF, Anderson GH (1986): The effects of early dietary experience on subsequent protein selection in the rat. Physiol Behav 36:271–276.

Morris RGM (1981): Spatial localization does not require the presence of local cues. Learn Motivat 12:239–260.

Munro HN (1970): Free amino acid pools and their role in regulation. In Munro HN (ed): "Mammalian Protein Metabolism, Vol. 4." New York: Academic Press, pp 299–386.

Murrin LC, Morgenroth VH, Roth RH (1976): Dopaminergic neurons effects of electrical stimulation on tyrosine hydroxylase. Mol Pharmacol 12:1070–1081.

Musten B, Peace D, Anderson GH (1974): Food intake regulation in the weanling rat: Self-selection of protein and energy. J Nutr 104:563–572.

Nachmias VT (1960): Amine oxidase and 5-hydroxytryptamine in developing rat brain. J Neurochem 6:99–104.

Nagatsu T, Levitt M, Udenfriend S (1964): Tyrosine hydroxylase: The initial step in norepinephrine biosynthesis. J Biol Chem 239:2910–2917.

Nair V, Tabakoff B, Ungar R, Alivisatos SGA (1976): Ontogenesis of serotonergic systems in rat brain. Res Commun Chem Pathol Pharmacol 14:63–73.

Naughton JM (1981): Supply of polyenoic fatty acids to the mammalian brain: The ease of conversion of the short-chain essential fatty acids to their longer chain polyunsaturated metabolites in liver, brain, placenta and blood. Int J Biochem 13:21–32.

Neckers LM, Biggio G, Moja G, Meek JL (1977): Modulation of brain tryptophan hydroxylase activity by brain tryptophan content. J Pharmacol Exp Ther 201:110–116.

Nomura Y, Naitoh F, Segawa T (1976): Regional changes in monoamine content and uptake of the rat brain during postnatal development. Brain Res 101:305–315.

Nowak TS Jr, Munro HN (1977): Effects of protein-calorie malnutrition on biochemical aspects of brain development. In Wurtman RJ, Wurtman JJ (eds): "Nutrition and the Brain, Vol. 2." New York: Raven Press, pp 193–260.

O'Brien JS, Fillerup DL, Mead JF (1964): Quantification and fatty acid and fatty aldehyde composition of ethanolamine choline and serine glycerophosphatides in human cerebral grey and white matter. J Lipid Res 5:329–338.

Oishi T, Wurtman RJ (1982): Effect of tyrosine on brain catecholamine turnover in reserpine-treated rats. J Neural Transm 53:101–108.

Oldendorf WH (1971): Brain uptake of radiolabelled amino acids, amines and hexoses after arterial injection. Am J Physiol 221:1629–1639.

Olson L, Seiger A (1972): Early prenatal ontogeny of central monoamine neurons in the rat: Fluorescence histochemical observations. Z Anat Entwickl-Gesch 137:301–316.

Ordonez LA (1977): Control of the availability to the brain of folic acid, vitamin B_{12} and choline. In Wurtman RJ, Wurtman JJ (eds): "Nutrition and the Brain, Vol. 1." New York: Raven Press, pp 205–248.

Page MA, Krebs MA, Williamson DA (1971): Activities of enzymes of ketone body utilization in brain and other tissues of suckling rats. Biochem J 121:49–53.

Paoletti R, Galli C (1972): Effect of essential fatty acid deficiency on the central nervous system in the growing rat. In Ciba Foundation (eds): "Lipids, Malnutrition and the Developing Brain." New York: Elsevier Excerpta Medica North-Holland, pp 121–140.

Pardridge WM (1977): Regulation of amino acid availability to the brain. In Wurtman RJ, Wurtman JJ (eds): "Nutrition and the Brain, Vol. 1." New York: Raven Press, pp 141–204.

Pardridge WM, Oldendorf WH (1975): Kinetic analysis of blood brain barrier transport of amino acid. Biochim Biophys Acta 401:128–136.

Peters JC, Harper AR (1985): Adaptation of rats to diets containing different levels of protein: Effects on food intake, plasma and brain amino acid concentrations and brain neurotransmitter metabolism. J Nutr 115:382–398.

Peters RI, Buhr BR (1984): Tryptophan and serotonin metabolism after sustained tryptophan infusion. Neurochem Int 6:685–691.

Pfeiffer CC, Braverman ER (1982): Zinc, the brain and behavior. Biol Psychiatry 17:513–532.

Prensky AL, Fishman MA, Daftari B (1974): Recovery of rat brain from a brief hyperphenylalaninemic insult early in development. Brain Res 73:51–58.

Ramanamurthy RSV, Srikantia SG (1970): Effects of leucine on brain serotonin. J Neurochem 17:27–32.

Rang HP, Ritchie JM (1968): The dependence on external cations of the oxygen consumption of mammalian nonmyelinated nerve fibers at rest and during activity. J Physiol (Lond) 196:163–181.

Reynolds EH, Carney MWP, Toone BK (1984): Methylation and mood. Lancet 2:196–198.

Robinson N (1968): Histochemistry of rat brain-stem monoamine oxidase during maturation. J Neurochem 15:1151–1159.

Roth RH, Morgenroth III VH, Salzman PM (1975): Tyrosine hydroxylase: Allosteric activation induced by stimulation of central noradrenergic neurons. Naunyn-Schmeideberg's Arch Pharmacol 289:327–343.

Roth RH, Salzman PM, Nowycky M (1978): Impulse flow and short term regulation of transmitter biosynthesis in central catecholaminergic neurons. In Lipton MA, Di Mascio A, Killam KF (eds): "Psychopharmacology: A Generation of Progress." New York: Raven Press, pp 185–198.

Rüthrich HL, Hoffman P, Matthies H, Forster W (1984): Perinatal linoleate deprivation impairs learning and memory in adult rats. Behav Neural Biol 40:205–212.

Saavedra JM, Coyle JT, Axelrod J (1974): Developmental characteristics of phenylethanolamine and octopamine in the rat brain. J Neurochem 23:511–515.

Samulski MA, Walker BL (1982): Maternal dietary fat and polyunsaturated fatty acids in the developing foetal rat brain. J Neurochem 39:1163–1168.

Sandermann H (1978): Regulation of membrane enzymes by lipids. Biochim Biophys Acta 515:209–237.

Sarna GS, Kantamaneni, Curzon G (1985): Variables influencing the effect of a meal on brain tryptophan. J Neurochem 44:1575–1580.

Scally MC, Ulus I, Wurtman RJ (1977): Brain tyrosine level controls striatal dopamine synthesis in haloperidol-treated rats. J Neural Transm 41:1–6.

Scatton B, Serrano A, Rivot JP, Nishikawa T (1984): Inhibitory GABAergic influence on striatal serotonergic transmission exerted in the dorsal raphe as revealed by in vivo voltammetry. Brain Res 305:343–352.

Schmidt MJ, Sanders-Bush E (1971): Tryptophan hydroxylase activity in developing rat brain. J Neurochem 18:2549–2551.

Seltzer S, Stoch R, Marcus R, Jackson E (1982): Alteration of human pain threshold by nutritional manipulation and L-tryptophan supplementation. Pain 13:382–393.

Sheiner JB, Morris P, Anderson GH (1985): Food intake suppression by histidine. Pharmacol Biochem Behav 23:721–726.

Shields JP, Eccleston D (1973): Evidence for the synthesis and storage of 5-hydroxytryptamine in two separate pools in the brain. J Neurochem 20:881–888.

Shinitzky M (1984): Membrane fluidity and cellular functions. In Shinitzky M (ed): "Physiology of Membrane Fluidity, Vol. 1." Boca Raton: CRC Press, pp 1–51.

Siebert G, Gessner B, Klasser M (1986): Energy supply of the central nervous system. In Somogyi JC, Hotzel D (eds): "Nutrition and Neurobiology." Basel: Karger, pp 1–26.

Siow YL, Dakshinamurti K (1985): Aromatic L-amino acid decarboxylase in adult rat brain. Can Fed Biol Soc 28:PA-129.

Sokoloff L (1981): Circulation and energy metabolism of the brain. In Seigel GJ, Albers RW, Agranoff BW, Katzman R (eds): "Basic Neurochemistry." 3rd Ed. Boston: Little, Brown, pp 471–495.

Sokoloff L, FitzGerald GG, Kaufman EE (1977): Cerebral nutrition and energy metabolism. In Wurtman RJ, Wurtman JJ (eds): "Nutrition and the Brain, Vol. 1." New York: Raven Press, pp 87–139.

Sourkes TL (1966): Dopa decarboxylase: Substrates, coenzyme, inhibitors. Pharmacol Rev 18:53–60.

Sourkes TL (1979): Nutrients and the cofactors required for monoamine synthesis in nervous tissue. In Wurtman RJ (ed): "Nutrition and the Brain, Vol. 3." New York: Raven Press, pp 265–299.

Spector R, Coakley G, Blakely R (1980): Methionine recycling in the brain: A role for folates and vitamin B_{12}. J Neurochem 34:132–137.

Spector SR, Gordon R, Sjoerdsma A, Udenfriend S (1967): End-product inhibition of tyrosine hydroxylase as a possible mechanism for regulation of norepinephrine synthesis. Mol Pharmacol 3:549–559.

Spring B (1986): Effects of foods and nutrients on the behavior of normal individuals. In Wurtman RJ, Wurtman JJ (eds): "Nutrition and the Brain, Vol. 7." New York: Raven Press, pp 1–47.

Stubbs CD, Smith AD (1984): The modification of mammalian membrane polyunsaturated fatty acid composition in relation to membrane fluidity and function. Biochim Biophys Acta 779:89–137.

Sun GY, Sun AY (1974): Synaptosomal plasma membranes: Acyl group composition of phosphoglycerides and $(Na^+ + K^+)$-ATPase activity during fatty acid deficiency. J Neurochem 22:15–18.

Sved AF (1983): Precursor control of the function of monoaminergic neurons. In Wurtman RJ, Wurtman JJ (eds): "Nutrition and the Brain, Vol. 6." New York: Raven Press, pp 224–275.

Sved AF, Fernstrom JD (1981): Tyrosine availability and dopamine synthesis in the striatum: Studies with gamma-butyrolactone. Life Sci 29:743–748.

Sved AF, Fernstrom JD, Wurtman RJ (1979a): Tyrosine administration decreases serum prolactin levels in chronically reserpinized rats. Life Sci 25:1293–1300.

Sved AF, Fernstrom JD, Wurtman RJ (1979b): Tyrosine administration reduced blood pressure and enhances brain norepinephrine release in spontaneously hypertensive rats. Proc Natl Acad Sci USA 76:3511–3514.

Tahin QS, Blum M, Carafoli E (1981): The fatty acid composition of subcellular membranes of rat liver, heart, and brain: Diet-induced modifications. Eur J Biochem 121:5–13.

Tarozzi G, Barzenti V, Biagi PL, Cocchi M, Lodi R, Maranesi M, Pignatti C, Turchetto E (1984): Fatty acid composition of single brain structures following different alpha linolenate dietary supplementations. Acta Vitaminol Enzymol 6:157–163.

Teff K, Young SN, Tourjman S, Pihl RO, Ervin FR (1985): The influence of lowering brain 5-hydroxytryptamine levels on food selection in normal human males. Can Fed Biol Soc 28:PA130.

Ternaux JP, Boireau A, Bourgoin S, Hamon M, Hery F, Glowinski J (1976): In vivo release of 5-HT in the lateral ventricle of the rat: Effects of 5-hydroxytryptophan and tryptophan. Brain Res 101:533–548.

Thiede HM, Kehr W (1981a): Catecholamine metabolism in rat brain: The role of neutral and acidic catechol metabolites. Naunyn-Schmeideberg's Arch Pharmacol 318:29–35.

Thiede HM, Kehr W (1981b): Endogenous dopa in rat brain: Occurrence, distribution and relationship to changes in catecholamine synthesis. Naunyn-Schmeideberg's Arch Pharmacol 316:299–303.

Tinoco J, Babcock R, Hincenbergs I, Medwadowski B, Miljanich P, Williams MA (1979): Linolenic acid deficiency. Lipids 14:166–173.

Tissari AH (1973): Serotonergic mechanisms in ontogenesis. In Boreus L (ed): "Fetal Pharmacology." New York: Raven Press, pp 237–257.

Tissari AH (1975): Pharmacological and ultrastructural maturation of serotonergic synapses during ontogeny. Med Biol 53:1–4.

Trulson ME (1985): Dietary tryptophan does not alter the function of brain serotonin neurons. Life Sci 37:1067–1072.

Trulson ME, Crisp T (1986): Do serotonin-containing dorsal raphe neurons possess autoreceptors? Exp Brain Res 62:579–586.

Trulson ME, Jacobs BL (1976): Dose-response relationships between systemically administered L-tryptophan or L-5-hydroxytryptophan and raphe unit activity in the rat. Neuropharmacology 15:339–344.

Tyce GM, Flock EV, Owen CA (1963): Tryptophan metabolism in the brain of the developing rat. Prog Brain Res 9:198–203.

Udenfriend S (1966); Tyrosine hydroxylase. Pharmacol Rev 18:43–51.

Udenfriend S, Zaltzman-Nirenburg P, Nagatsu T (1965): Inhibitors of purified beef adrenal tyrosine hydroxylase. Biochem Pharmacol 14:837–845.

Vahvelainen ML, Oja SS (1972): Kinetics of influx of phenylalanine, tyrosine, tryptophan, histidine, and leucine into slices of brain cortex from adult and 7-day-old rats. Brain Res 40:477–488.

Vulliet PR, Langan TA, Weiner N (1980): Tyrosine hydroxylase: A substrate of cyclic AMP-dependent protein kinase. Proc Natl Acad Sci USA 77:92–96.

Waelsch H, Lajtha A (1961): Protein metabolism in the nervous system. Physiol Rev 41:709–736.

Wahle KWJ (1983): Fatty acid modification and membrane lipids. Proc Nutr Soc 42:273–287.

Wallwork JC, Botnen JH, Sandstead HH (1982): Effect of dietary zinc on rat brain catecholamines. J Nutr 112:514–519.

Walters JR, Roth RH (1976): Dopaminergic neurons—alteration in the sensitivity of tyrosine hydroxylase to inhibition by endogenous dopamine after cessation of impulse flow. Biochem Pharmacol 25:649–654.

Warsh JJ, Coscina DV, Godse DD, Chan PW (1979): Dependence of brain tryptamine formation on tryptophan availability. J Neurochem 32:1191–1196.

Warsh JJ, Li PP, Godse DD, Cheung S (1981): Brain noradrenergic neuronal activity affects 3,4-dihydroxyphenylethyleneglycol (DHPG) levels. Life Sci 29:1303–1307.

Weiner N, Clouthier G, Bjur R, Pfeffer I (1972): Modification of norepinephrine synthesis in intact tissues by drugs and during short-term adrenergic nerve stimulation. Pharmacol Rev 24:203–221.

Westerink BHC, Wirix E (1983): On the significance of tyrosine for the synthesis and catabolism of dopamine in rat brain: Evaluation by HPLC with electrochemical detection. J Neurochem 40:758–764.

Wong HL, Harwalker VH, Waisman HA (1962): Effect of dietary phenylalanine and tryptophan on brain serotonin. Arch Biochem Biophys 96:181–184.

Woodger TL, Sirek A, Anderson GH (1979): Diabetes, dietary tryptophan, and protein intake regulation in weanling rats. Am J Physiol 236:R307–R311.

Wolf WA, Kuhn DM (1986); Uptake and release of tryptophan and serotonin: An HPLC method to study the flux of endogenous 5-hydroxyindoles through synaptosomes. J Neurochem 46:61–67.

Wurtman RJ, Fernstrom JD (1975): Control of brain monoamine synthesis by diet and plasma amino acids. Am J Clin Nutr 28:638–647.

Wurtman RJ, Hefti F, Melamed E (1981): Precursor control of neurotransmitter synthesis. Pharmacol Rev 32:315–335.

Wurtman RJ, Larin F, Mostafapour S, Fernstrom JD (1974): Brain catechol synthesis: Control by brain tyrosine concentration. Science 185:183–184.

Wurtman RJ, Ordonez LA (1978): Effects of exogenous L-Dopa on the metabolism of methionine and S-adenosylmethionine in the brain. In Adreoli V, Agnoli A, Fazio C (eds): "Transmethylation and the Central Nervous System." New York: Springer-Verlag, pp 132–143.

Wurtman RJ, Wurtman JJ (1984): Nutrients, neurotransmitter synthesis, and the control of food intake. In Stunkard AJ, Stellar E (eds): "Eating and Its Disorders." New York: Raven Press, pp 77–86.

Yamauchi T, Fujisawa H (1979): Regulation of bovine adrenal tyrosine 3-monooxygenase by phosphorylation-dephosphorylation reaction catalyzed by adenosine 3',5'-monophosphate-dependent protein kinase and phosphorprotein phosphatase. J Biol Chem 254:6408–6413.

Yamori Y, Fujiwara M, Horie R, Lovenberg W (1980): The hypotensive effect of centrally administered tyrosine. Eur J Pharmacol 68:201–204.

Yehuda S (1978): Effects of d-amphetamine on dopamine regulated mechanisms of behavioral and physiological thermoregulation. In Essman WB, Valzelli L (eds): "Current Developments in Psychopharmacology, Vol. 5." New York: Spectrum, pp 125–175.

Yehuda S, Leprohon-Greenwood CE, Dixon LM, Coscina DV (1986): Effects of dietary fat on pain threshold, thermoregulation and motor activity in rats. Pharmacol Biochem Behav 24:1775–1777.

Yeung D, Oliver IT (1967): Gluconeogenesis from amino acids in neonatal rat liver. Biochem J 103:744–748.

Yogman MW, Zeisel SH (1983): Diet and sleep patterns in new born infants. N Engl J Med 309:1147–1149.

Yokogoshi H (1985): Effect of dietary level of protein or methionine and threonine on the amino acids and catecholamines in brains of rats fed a high tyrosine diet. J Nutr Sci Vitaminol 31:519–531.

Youdim MBH, Ben-Schachar D, Ashkenazi R, Yehuda S (1983): Brain iron and dopamine receptor function. In Mandell P, DeFeudis FV (eds): "Advances in Biochemistry and Psychopharmacology." Vol. 37, "CNS Receptors—From Molecular Pharmacology to Behavior." New York: Raven Press, p 357.

Youdim MBH, Green AR, Bloomfield MR, Mitchell BD, Heal DJ, Grahame-Smith DG (1980): The effects of iron deficiency on brain biogenic monoamine biochemistry and function in rats. Neuropharmacology 19:259–267.

Youdim MBH, Yehuda S, Ben-Schachar D, Ashkenazi R (1982): Behavioral and brain biochemical changes in iron-deficient rats: The involvement of iron in dopamine receptor function. In Pollitt E, Liebel RL (eds): "Iron Deficiency: Brain Biochemistry and Behavior." New York: Raven Press, pp 39–55.

Young SN (1986): The clinical psychopharmacology of tryptophan. In Wurtman RJ, Wurtman JJ (eds): "Nutrition and the Brain, Vol. 7." New York: Raven Press, pp 49–88.

Young SN, Anderson GM, Purdy WC (1980): Indolamine metabolism in rat brain studies through measurements of tryptophan, 5-hydroxyindoleacetic acid, and indoleacetic acid in cerebrospinal fluid. J Neurochem 34:309–315.

Young SN, Gauthier S (1981): Effect of tryptophan administration on tryptophan, 5-hydroxyindoleacetic acid, and indoleacetic acid in human lumbar and cisternal cerebrospinal fluid. J Neurol Neurosurg Psychiatry 44:323–328.

Yuwiler A, Brammer GL, Morley JE, Raleigh MJ, Flannery JW, Geller E (1981): Short-term and repetitive administration of oral tryptophan in normal men. Arch Gen Psychiatry 38:619–626.

Yuwiler A, Geller E (1965): Serotonin depletion by dietary leucine. Nature 208:83–84.

Yuwiler A, Geller E (1966): Brain serotonin changes in phenylalanine fed rats: Synthesis, storage and degradation. J Neurochem 16:999–1005.

Yuwiler A, Louttit RT (1961): Effect of phenylalanine diet on brain serotonin in rat. Science 134:831–832.

Yuwiler A, Oldendorf WH, Geller E, Braun L (1977): Effect of albumin binding and amino acid competition on tryptophan uptake into brain. J Neurochem 28:1015–1023.

Zimmerman T, Winkler L, Moller U, Schubert H, Goetze E (1979): Synthesis of arachidonic acid in the human placenta in vitro. Biol Neonate 35:209–212.

Zivkovic B, Giudotti A, Costa E (1975): The regulation of striatal tyrosine hydroxylase ef fects of gammabutyric acid and haloperidol. Naunyn-Schmeideberg's Arch Pharmacol 291:193–200.

Current Topics in Nutrition and Disease, Volume 16
Basic and Clinical Aspects of Nutrition and Brain Development,
pages 217–243
© 1987 Alan R. Liss, Inc.

Taurine and Zinc in Nutrition and Cellular Development

Herminia Pasantes-Morales, Ricardo López-Escalera, and Julio Morán

Instituto de Fisiología Celular, Universidad Nacional Autónoma de México, Apartado Postal 70–600, 04510, México D.F., México

INTRODUCTION

It is now firmly established that nutritional deprivation produces profound alterations on the normal course of brain development, particularly at the critical periods of cell differentiation and migration and establishment of functional circuits. Some specific nutrients, including vitamins, cofactors, and trace minerals, seem to play a key role in the maturational sequence of biochemical and morphological changes involved in the complex process of cellular migration and differentiation. Among these essential nutrients, taurine and zinc show some peculiarities which make them extremely interesting in terms of nutrition and brain development. The critical role played by taurine and zinc in brain maturation and differentiation has been recently recognized by the dramatic consequences resulting from their deficiency in the events leading to the structural and functional completion of brain physiology. In addition, taurine and zinc are involved in the maintenance of the morphological and physiological integrity of the vertebrate retina, as evidenced by the consequences of their deficiency on the visual process. Further similarities between taurine and zinc are their high concentration in the visual cells—one of the highest in animal tissues—and the protection afforded these cells under experimental deleterious conditions (see below, Interactions of Taurine and Zinc With Cell Membranes as a Possible Protective Mechanism).

From a nutritional viewpoint, taurine and zinc are preferentially concentrated in meat, as compared to food from different origin. The concentration of zinc in plants has been already reported (Table I), but there is a lack of information concerning taurine, for which, although it is generally agreed that it is practically absent in plants (Jacobsen and Smith, 1968; Lahdesmaki, 1986), no systematic study with a nutritional approach has been carried out to analyze its content in plants. Since meat intake (the main source of taurine and zinc for some species, including man) may be considerably restricted in some communities either by cultural or socioeconomic conditions, it is important to investigate possible alternate dietary sources of taurine and zinc. Moreover, in view of the severe detrimental effect of taurine and zinc deficiency on brain development, it is important to evaluate the impact of a reduced intake of meat on the concentration of taurine and zinc in human milk.

Taurine and zinc required for brain development are supplied to the fetus by the mother and to the newborn by milk during lactation. As consequence of a reduced supply of these compounds from external sources, milk taurine and zinc levels may drop; it is also possible that adaptive responses occur, including mobilization from endogenous pools in mother's tissues, thus ensuring an adequate supply to the newborn and preventing the negative consequences of their deficiency. In the present work, we examine the reported consequences of taurine and zinc deficiency in animal tissues. A review of the effects of taurine and zinc protecting cell membranes is then discussed vis-à-vis a possible mechanism associated with the abnormalities observed as consequence of taurine and zinc deficiency. Information available on the relative proportions of taurine externally supplied vs. that endogenously synthesized to taurine brain pools is also examined. A report of the analysis carried out in our laboratory on the taurine content of different organs of edible plants is presented, and preliminary results of the taurine content of human milk, examined in terms of diurnal variations and fluctuations during lactation, are described.

TAURINE AND ZINC DEFICIENCY
Effects on Reproduction

The harmful consequences of zinc deficiency on reproduction in animals are well documented (Underwood, 1977). Zinc deficiency causes malformations in fetus of chicks and rats (Underwood, 1977) and to a lesser extent in pigs and lambs (Hill et al., 1983; Apgar and Fitzgerald, 1985). Zinc deficiency during pregnancy also results in prolonged gestation (Bunce et al., 1983) and severe stress of the female during parturition (Apgar, 1975). Prolonged labor, excessive bleeding, failure to eat the afterbirths, and sometimes death at parturition are among the abnormalities observed in zinc-deficient animals (Apgar, 1975, 1976, 1977; Mutch and Hurley, 1980). In all species examined, zinc deficiency results in low birth weights and/or poor survival of offsprings (Apgar, 1976; Mutch and Hurley, 1980). Large numbers of resorptions are associated with malformation in zinc-deficient females (Hurley and Baly, 1982). In humans, lower levels of zinc have been found in a number of complications of pregnancy, and this condition has also been associated with infant malformation (Jameson, 1976; Buamah and Russell, 1984).

The mechanisms involved are not certain. A higher rate of progesterone to estrogen has been considered the cause of prolonged gestation (Bunce et al., 1983), whereas a failure to make hemodynamic adjustments during pregnancy has been cited as the cause of fetal growth retardation (Ahokas et al., 1983) and stress at parturition (Apgar, 1975, 1976, 1977). A 50% reduction of cardiac input with a 75% reduction in blood flow to the uterus and placenta are seen in zinc-deficient rats (Cunnane et al., 1983).

The effect of taurine deprivation on reproduction has been so far examined only in cats. The deficiency has particularly severe effects on pregnancy and outcome. A greatly increased reproductive loss and a wide range of abnormalities in the offspring have been reported in cats fed a taurine-deficient diet. Fetuses are frequently resorbed or aborted, and kittens have a poor survival rate (see Sturman, following chapter). The mechanisms responsible for these effects of taurine deficiency in reproduction have not been determined.

Effects on Retina and Brain

A deleterious effect associated with taurine deficiency was first described in the cat retina (Hayes et al., 1975; Berson et al., 1976). Cats have a restricted ability to synthesize taurine from endogenous precursors and rely on diet to obtain taurine (Hayes and Sturman, 1981). This is not a major problem for a natural carnivore such as the cat, since meat is one of the most abundant sources of taurine (Jacobsen and Smith, 1968; Hayes and Sturman, 1982). When cats are experimentally fed a taurine-free diet, taurine tissue content gradually decreases to levels 40–60% below the normal concentration (Schmidt et al., 1976; Sturman et al., 1978). Although the retina strongly retains its endogenous taurine and is one of the last tissues to become depleted, eventually taurine levels decrease. A reduction below 50% of the normal concentration results in retinal degeneration characterized first by a decrease in amplitude of the electroretinogram responses (Berson et al., 1976), followed by a severe morphological alteration of the photoreceptor cells (Hayes et al., 1975; Berson et al., 1976). The otherwise highly ordered structure of membranous discs in the outer segments becomes disarranged; the discs appear extremely disoriented, with twisting often extending through the entire length of the segment (Berson et al., 1976) (Fig. 1). Acute swelling of the distal end of the outer segment causes marked distortion. As the pathology progresses, the entire photoreceptor cell population degenerates and eventually blindness occurs. Before a critical point is reached, at which

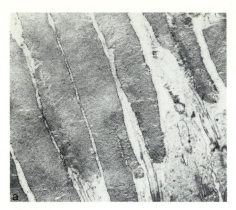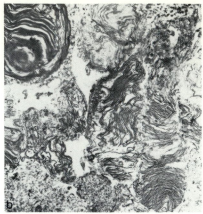

Fig. 1. Photoreceptor degeneration associated with taurine deficiency in cats. Cats fed a taurine-free diet for 25 weeks show a severe disturbance of the photoreceptor outer segments. Disarrangement of the lamellar discs and acute swelling characterize the pathology associated with taurine deficiency. a) Control. × 22,000. b) Taurine-deficient. × 15,000.

irreversible changes have occurred, the structural and functional damage may be prevented by a diet supplemented with taurine (Hayes et al., 1975).

Following these first observations in cats, the retinal pathology associated with taurine deficiency has been described in other species. In rats, which, in general, can synthesize taurine (Pasantes-Morales et al., 1977; Huxtable and Lippincot, 1982b), not all organs in the same animal are able to form taurine to the same extent (Huxtable and Lippincot, 1982a,b). Thus, although liver is able to synthesize taurine actively, the retina, and particularly the photoreceptors, obtain a large proportion of their endogenous taurine from that circulating in plasma (Mathur et al., 1976; Quesada et al., 1984), actively accumulating it through a high-affinity, energy-dependent transport system (Salceda and Pasantes-Morales, 1982; Schmidt, 1981). Therefore, it is possible to decrease retinal taurine levels by interfering with this transport process. Treatment of rats with a structural analog of taurine, guanidino-ethanesulfonate (GES) which blocks taurine transport (Huxtable et al., 1979), leads to a marked decrease of taurine content in the retina (Lake, 1981; Lake, 1982a; Quesada et al., 1984). As consequence of this reduction in endogenous taurine, the characteristic pattern of retinal degeneration appears in rats, with properties identical to those observed in cats, i.e., a reduced electroretinogram (Fig. 2) and a structural degeneration of photoreceptors (Lake, 1982b; Pasantes-Morales et al., 1983).

Retinal dysfunction has been also observed in monkeys fed a taurine-free formula, with similar structural damage associated with abnormal bioelectri-

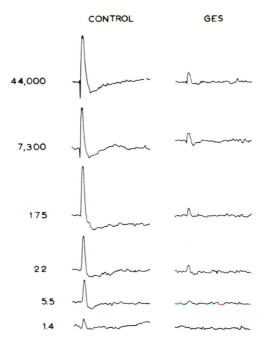

Fig. 2.   Electroretinogram (ERG) abnormalities produced by retinal taurine depletion in rats. The a and b wave amplitudes are markedly reduced. b wave values are 0.58 ± 0.03 mV in controls and 0.16 ± 0.009 in taurine-deficient rats; a wave amplitudes are 0.30 ± 0.002 mV in controls and 0.04 mV in deficient animals. Rats were made taurine-deficient by administration of guanidino-ethanesulfonate (GES) as described in Pasantes-Morales et al. (1983). The ERG recordings were made 8 weeks after treatment, when taurine levels in the retina have decreased from 24.5 μmole/g in control rats and to 14.2 μmole/g in GES-treated rats. The figures on the left are the light intensities used for the ERG recording.

cal responses of the retina (Sturman et al., 1984). Also, in children receiving long-term total parenteral nutrition, a decrease of taurine plasma levels is observed, coincident with some abnormalities in the electroretinogram (Geggel et al., 1985). Both abnormal conditions are corrected by taurine supplementation (Sturman et al., 1984; Geggel et al., 1985). It is important to note that humans, as the cat, have a limited ability to form taurine because of the low activity of the cysteine sulfinate decarboxylase, one of the key enzymes in the biosynthetic pathway of taurine (Jacobsen et al., 1964).

It has been reported that taurine deficiency also produces severe disorganization of the tapetal rods. These cells are used in cats for reflecting light back through the retina and maximizing retinal sensitivity in low-light situations. Tapetal rods in taurine-deficient cats show membrane alterations (see Sturman, following chapter).

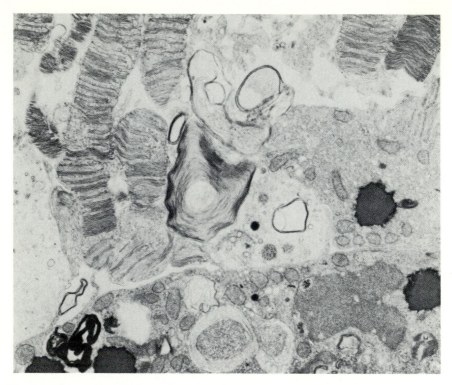

Fig. 3.   Pigmentary epithelium cells and photoreceptors of a zinc-deficient rat maintained on a commercially prepared zinc-deficient pelleted diet and zinc-free deionized water for 7 weeks. × 11,200 (from Leuré-Dupreé and Bridges, 1982, with permission).

Tapetoretinal degeneration is so far the only described effect of taurine deficiency in adult animals. In the developing brain, however, severe alterations, associated with taurine deficiency in the mother, have been described in cats (see Sturman, following chapter).

Remarkable similarities exist in retina and the developing brain with respect to taurine and zinc deficiencies. Similar to taurine, zinc is found concentrated in the retina (Halsted et al., 1974), associated with photoreceptors. Deprivation of zinc also leads to retinal pathology, characterized by an alteration in the structure and organization of the photoreceptor discs, which in many respects resembles the degeneration observed in taurine deficiency (Leure-Dupree and Bridges, 1982). Figure 3 shows the profound alteration in the membranes of the photoreceptor outer segment. The retinal pigment epithelial cells also show severe morphological alterations, accompanied by the presence of irregularly shaped opaque inclusion bodies.

With respect to brain development, there is evidence indicating that severe

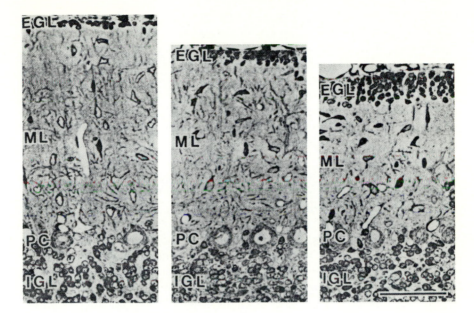

Fig. 4. Effect of zinc deficiency on the maturation of the cerebellar cortex of 21-day-old rats. Left: normal control. Middle: pair-fed group. Right: zinc-deficient group. The pair-fed group was included because zinc-deficient mothers become anorexic. The pair-fed group consists of mothers receiving the same amount of food consumed by mothers in the zinc-deficient group. Sections were obtained from lobule VI along the posteriorsuperior fissure. Bar = 50 μm EGL: external granule layer; ML: molecular layer; Pc: Purkinje cell layer; IGL: internal granule cell layer. Reproduced from Dvergesten et al., 1983, with permission.

zinc deficiency during gestation produces congenital malformations in the brain (Sandstead et al., 1983). As in taurine deficiency, zinc-deficient animals show a reduction in brain size (Dvergesten et al., 1983). Also, one of the most conspicuous effects of zinc deficiency in the cerebellum, the impaired acquisition of granule cells (Fig. 4), is similar to that observed in taurine-deficient cats. A detailed analysis of neuronal changes produced by zinc deficiency has been carried out in the cerebellar cortex of rats. This study showed that cerebellar cortex of zinc-deficient rats is underdeveloped, and, in addition to the persistence of the external granule cells already mentioned, it shows a reduction in the thickness of the molecular layer and a decrease in the area of the internal granule cell layer. A significant decrease in the total number of granule cells and in the ratio of granule cells to Purkinje cells is in comparison to normal rats also observed (Dvergesten et al., 1983).

Zinc deficiency has also a marked effect on the dendritic growth of neurons in the cerebellar cortex. The most striking effect is observed in the size and branching of the Purkinje cell dendritic tree (Dvergesten et al.,

1984b) (Fig. 5). The width of the Purkinje cell dendrites varies from 30 to 100 μm in zinc-deficient rats to a width of 100 to 200 μm in normal pups. In some instances, zinc deficiency not only slows the differentiation of Purkinje cells, but also can cause Purkinje cells to differentiate abnormally. Whether the growth of the Purkinje cells is impaired permanently in these zinc-deficient rats is unknown. These abnormalities in Purkinje cells may be related to the reduction in the number of granule cells, since the formation of parallel fibers may be impaired. This might cause the Purkinje cell dendrites to become misaligned and with smaller dendritic trees, fewer branches, and multiple primary dendrites.

The dendritic arbor of some of the basket and stellate cells also appears immature and reduced in size in zinc-deficient rats (Fig. 6) (Dvergesten et al., 1984b). As suggested for the Purkinje cells, parallel fibers may be influencing the dendritic differentiation of basket and stellate cells (Rakic and Sidman, 1973; Sotelo, 1975). Therefore, a deficit in parallel fibers may cause the dendritic arbor of basket and stellate cells to be disoriented and reduced in size. A note of caution should be made when the effects of zinc deficiency on brain development are analyzed. One of the well-known effects of zinc deprivation is a marked decrease in maternal food consumption. It is therefore important to discriminate between the effects of undernutrition and those which should be adscribed to zinc deficiency. Although some of the effects of malnutrition and zinc deficiency on brain development often develop in the same direction (Griffin et al., 1977; McConnell and Berry, 1981; Pysh et al., 1979; West and Kemper, 1976; Dvergesten et al., 1984b), the quantitative effects of zinc deficiency are clearly more pronounced (Dvergesten et al., 1984a,b).

Interactions of Taurine and Zinc With Cell Membranes as a Possible Protective Mechanism

The degeneration produced by taurine and zinc deficiency in the retina is clearly associated with alterations in membrane structure and organization (Hayes et al., 1975; Leure-Dupree and Bridges, 1982). The failure of the developing brain to attain a normal cytoarchitectural organization in taurine and zinc deficiency (Sturman et al., 1985; Dvergesten et al., 1983) may also be related to derangement of cell membranes, resulting in impaired cell-to-cell communication.

Experimental evidence supports the interaction of taurine and zinc with cell membranes to provide a membrane stabilizing effect. The first suggestion of a stabilizer action of taurine in membranes was derived from the protection afforded by taurine to skeletal muscle sarcoplasmic vesicles during the isolation procedure (Huxtable and Bressler, 1973). Since this early observation, the protective effect of taurine on cell membranes has been

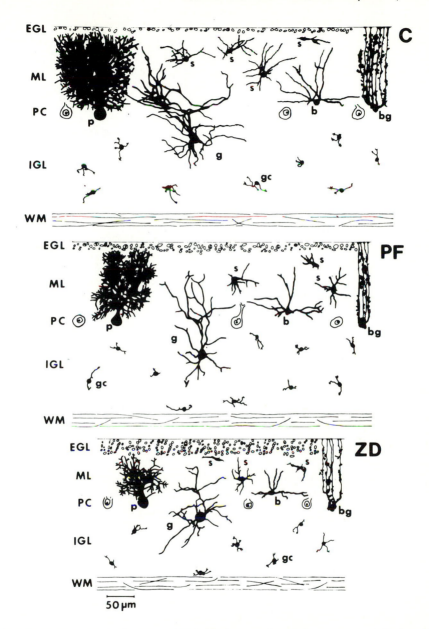

Fig. 5. Camera lucida drawing of Golgi-impregnated cerebellar neurons of 21-day-old zinc-deficient (ZD) pair-fed (PF) and normal control (C) rats. Zinc deficiency produces a decrease in the molecular layer and a reduction in the dendritic tree of Purkinje cells. Basket cells, stellate cells, and Golgi II neurons also have dendritic trees that are reduced in size. EGL: external granule layer; UL: molecular layer; PC: Purkinje cell layer; IGL: internal granule layer; WM: white matter; s: stellate cell; b: basket cell; bg: Bergmann glial fibers; g: Golgi II neurons; gc; granule cells. Reproduced from Dvergesten et al., 1984a, with permission.

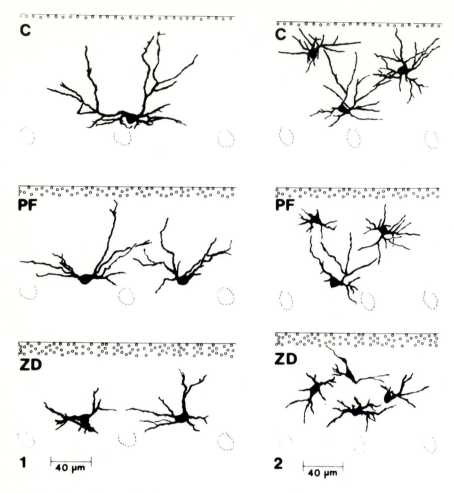

Fig. 6. Alterations produced in cerebellar basket cells (1) and stellate cells (2) by zinc deficiency. In zinc-deficient rats (ZD) the dentritic arbors of the basket cells and stellate cells are immature and reduced in size as compared to pair-fed (PF) and control (C) animals. Reproduced from Dvergesten et al., 1984b, with permission.

extensively documented. This effect is particularly clear in isolated photoreceptor outer segments (Pasantes-Morales, 1986). The outer segments have a structural organization consisting of highly ordered stacks of membranous discs. Biochemically, these membranes are also notable for their unusually high proportion of polyunsaturated fatty acids (Daemen, 1973), which give the membrane a high fluidity (Fig. 7). Apparently such a

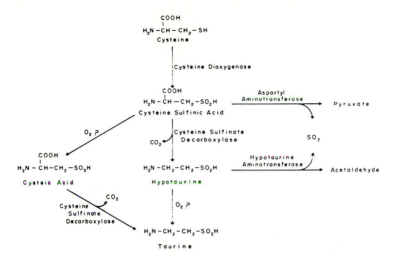

Fig. 7.   Biosynthetic pathway of taurine in vertebrate tissues.

precise lipid composition involving much unsaturation is critical for providing the specific microenvironment required for movement and conformational changes of rhodopsin during phototransduction (Bonting et al., 1977; Cone, 1972). This characteristic, however, makes these membranes particularly vulnerable to damage caused by excessive light (Skyes et al., 1981; Noell et al., 1966) or situations generating free radicals (Wiegand et al., 1983). Also, this peculiarity may increase membrane permeability (Pasantes-Morales et al., 1981; Pasantes-Morales and Cruz, 1984; Chan et al., 1982). When isolated outer segments are exposed to continuous light, an extensive disruption of the outer segment structure is observed, characterized by acute swelling and membrane disorganization (Fig. 8). Taurine, at concentrations ranging from 5 to 25 mM, provides complete protection against the light-induced damage (Fig. 9). Other conditions producing damage to the photoreceptor structure include exposure to ferrous sulfate, a free-radical-generating condition (Fig. 8) (Rapp et al., 1982; Pasantes-Morales and Cruz, 1984); to a Ca-Mg-free medium, which increases ionic permeability; and to urea (Pasantes-Morales, unpublished). Taurine and zinc provide protection under these conditions, maintaining the outer segment structure (Pasantes-Morales and Cruz, 1984). In some cases, taurine and zinc act synergically, increasing the protection provided by each one separately. In all these conditions, damage is prevented when sodium or chloride in the medium are replaced by non-permeant ions. This observation suggests a mechanism for the protective effect of taurine and zinc related to regulation of membrane permeability.

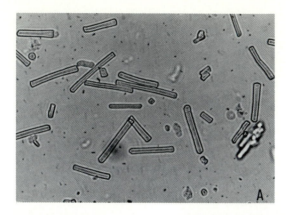

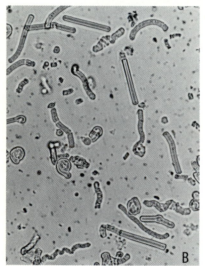

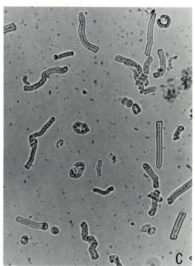

Fig. 8. The structure of photoreceptor outer segments isolated from the frog retina, incubated in physiologic medium (A), and exposed to intense and prolonged light (B) or to ferrous sulfate (C). Outer segments incubated in a physiologic Krebs-bicarbonate medium maintain an organized structure for several hours. Illumination (2,500 lux) for 2 h or exposure to a medium containing 200 μM ferrous sulfate results in profound alteration of the outer segment structure. Swelling and disc protrusion characterize the alteration induced by the indicated experimental conditions.

Protective effects of taurine and zinc, similar to those observed in isolated outer segments, have also been described in human cultured lymphoblastoids exposed to membrane destabilizers (Pasantes-Morales et al., 1984). Retinol, Retinoic acid, and iron ascorbate all produce acute cell swelling and markedly reduce viability (Fig. 10). The presence of taurine and/or zinc

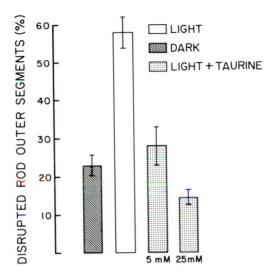

Fig. 9. Protective effect of taurine on the structure of isolated photoreceptor outer segments exposed to light. The experimental conditions are as described in Figure 8. Taurine at the indicated concentrations affords complete protection to the outer segments. Results are the means ± S.E.M. of five to ten separate determinations.

counteracts swelling and preserves cell viability (Pasantes-Morales et al., 1984).

Taurine is able to prevent cell damage in heart preparation perfused with a calcium-free medium and reperfused with a physiological medium containing calcium (Kramer et al., 1981). This treatment, known as the "calcium paradox" (because damage occurs when tissue is exposed to the physiological conditions), induces extensive cellular and functional damage, probably due to massive calcium entry during reperfusion. The cell lesion consists in changes in the regions of the intercalar discs, the splitting of the glycocalyx, and a massive release of intracellular compounds such as potassium and lactate dehydrogenase (Crevey et al., 1978). The presence of taurine during perfusion largely protects the cells from many of the damaging effects of calcium overload (Kramer et al., 1981; Chovan et al., 1980). The effect of zinc in this preparation has not been examined.

Recently, the effects of taurine in a model of liver damage have been investigated (Nakashima et al., 1983). Treatment with CCL_4 induces an increase in lipid peroxides associated with cellular necrosis. Oral administration of taurine decreases membrane lipid peroxidation in hepatocytes and microsomes and protects hepatic cells from the deleterious effect of the solvent. The effects of zinc protecting biological membranes have been demonstrated in a variety of preparations (Chvapil, 1973; Bettger and

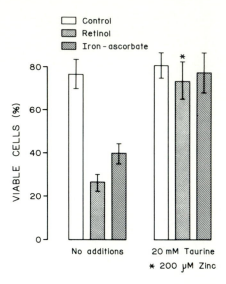

Fig. 10. Protective effect of taurine and zinc on cell viability of human cultured lymphoblastoids exposed to membrane destabilizers. Cells were exposed for 30 min to retinol (10 μm) or to iron-ascorbate (0.2 mM ferrous sulfate, 0.4 mM ascorbate) in the presence or absence of 20 mM taurine and 200 μM zinc chloride. After this time, the number of viable cells was estimated by trypan blue exclusion. Cells exposed to iron-ascorbate and to retinol showed acute swelling in a very low proportion of viable cells. Taurine and zinc counteract swelling and preserve cell viability to values close to control. Results are the means ± S.E.M. of six to eight separate determinations.

O'Dell, 1981). It is well known that addition of zinc to buffers during isolation of membrane fractions promotes cohesiveness and maintains the activity of membrane-bound enzymes. The properties of this action of zinc suggest that it is mediated through an interaction with SH groups of the membrane protein by a non-enzymatic process (Chvapil, 1973). Other effects of zinc also indicate interactions with the lipid components of the membrane particularly on processes of membrane lipid peroxidation (Bettger and O'Dell, 1981; Chvapil, 1973). High concentrations of zinc decrease the osomotic fragility of erythrocytes by a temperature-independent process. It also protects erythrocytes against hemolysis induced by a number of toxins (Bettger and O'Dell, 1981). In vivo, zinc administration protects normal rats against the effect of bacterial toxins and carbon tetrachloride. Excess zinc protects against testicular damage induced by cadmium and against cardiac necrosis induced by isoproterenol (Bettger and O'Dell, 1981; Chvapil, 1973). Other evidence of the involvement of zinc in membrane function include effects on ion permeability. In muscle, zinc alters the permeability to major ions, the contractile force, the transmembrane potential, and the spontaneous activity of muscle cells. The in vitro assembly of microtubules, which are vital structural and functional components of biomembranes, is affected by zinc. Finally, zinc confers increased thermal stability to lipid bilayers (Bettger and O'Dell, 1981; Chvapil, 1973).

From all these observations, Chvapil has proposed the following functions for zinc at the cell surface: 1) interaction with enzymes controlling the integrity of the membrane; 2) interference with macromolecular components of the membrane, changing their conformation or enzyme substrate specificity; and 3) interference with the generation of membrane lipid peroxidation. Many of these effects of zinc in the structure and function of biomembranes may be based on the abnormalities observed in differentiation and organization of neurons in the developing brain.

TAURINE POOLS IN THE BRAIN: BIOSYNTHESIS VS. EXOGENOUS SUPPLY

Taurine biosynthesis in animal tissues is directly linked to the metabolism of sulfur amino acids (see Sturman, following chapter). Several pathways have been described, but the preferred route in most tissues involves cysteine as precursor (Fig. 7). (Jacobsen et al., 1964). Cysteine is oxidized by cysteine dioxigenase, and the product of the reaction, the cysteine sulfinic acid, is decarboxylated by the cysteine sulfinate dacarboxylase forming hypotaurine. Subsequent oxidation of hypotaurine results in taurine formation. The ability of species to form taurine from endogenous precursors greatly varies, and variations are observed among different tissues of the same species (Sturman and Hayes, 1980; Huxtable and Lippincott, 1982a). In general, liver has a great ability to form taurine in many species; brain has a moderate ability, whereas heart, muscle, and lymphocytes obtain most of their endogenous pool of taurine from that synthesized elsewhere and taken up from plasma through active transport mechanisms. Studies of Huxtable and Lippincott (1982a,b) have shown that even in species with a great ability to form taurine, dietary taurine is a substantial source of taurine pools in tissues. Thus, adult rats fed a high taurine diet obtain as much as 60% of their taurine from the diet. The animals fed a taurine-free diet, respond not by increasing biosynthesis but by decreasing the rate of excretion of the amino acid. The adaptive response also considers taurine requirements which are different among species. Taurine demand due to metabolic requirements and digestive physiology, particularly that related to lipid metabolism and the conjugation of bile acids with either taurine or glycine, plays an important role in the possibilities of species to adaptate to dietary taurine restrictions.

Some species, such as the guinea pig, make only glycocholate (Spaeth and Schneider, 1974); others, like the cat, make only taurocholate (Robin et al., 1976); whereas other species normally synthesize both types of bile acid (Hayes and Sturman, 1981).

Conjugation of the acids with taurine is a trait that appears early in evolution, whereas conjugation with glycine is a relatively recent phylogenetic development, most characteristic of herbivorous animals. Conjugating bile acids with glycine provides a mechanism for resisting taurine depletion and the adverse consequences of this deficiency. In cats, the high taurine demand imposed by the bile acid pool precipitates depletion in tissues and leads to alterations caused by taurine deficiency which are not easily seen in other species. In line with this notion, it has been observed that one of the adaptive responses to restriction in dietary taurine in humans is a change in bile acid conjugation from predominantly taurocholate, which is the normal situation, to predominantly glycocholate (Brueton et al., 1978). This mechanism, together with a low rate of excretion of taurine (Gaull et al., 1977), increases resistance to taurine depletion.

The requirement of taurine for normal brain development makes it necessary to evaluate the comparative importance of biosynthesis versus diet as sources of taurine in the developing brain. In most species, the immature brain contains high concentrations of taurine at a time when the activity of the enzymes involved in the major biosynthetic pathways is very low (Sturman and Hayes, 1980). This is an indication of the importance of an exogenous supply to the endogenous brain taurine pools. In a nutritional analysis made by Huxtable and Lippincott (1982a,b, 1983) on the relative contribution of diet and biosynthesis in the adult rat, it was shown that even in this species, with a high capability for synthesizing taurine, a substantial amount is regularly obtained from dietary sources. This is valid for most tissues and particularly for the brain, where the diet contributes more than 50% of the total taurine pool.

In the same study (Huxtable and Lippincott, 1983), the contribution of taurine from the mother to the pups was calculated at birth, midnursing, and immediately prior to weaning. Although pups were able to synthesize some taurine even in utero, the proportion of taurine in brain obtained from the mother was as high as 96% in the newborn. This figure decreased with development to around 35% at weaning. In species such as the cat, with low ability to synthesize taurine, the concentrations of the amino acid in cerebella of kittens born by taurine-deprived mothers was only 30% of that found in kittens of normal mothers (see Sturman et al., following chapter). Therefore, most of the taurine required for optimal brain development proceeds from the mother via milk, particularly in those species with limited endogenous synthesis of taurine.

TABLE I. Zinc Content of Food[a]

	Zinc content (mg/100 g)
Roast beef	6.40
Chicken breast	1.10
Chicken thigh	2.80
Fish	2.50
Cheese	0.30
Milk	0.34
Potatoes	0.29
Rice	0.98
Peas	0.69
Carrots	0.25
Tomatoes	0.20
Green beans	0.21
Pears	0.08
Peaches	0.07
Apricots	0.12
Rye bread	1.34
White bread	0.57
Whole wheat bread	1.04

[a]After Osis et al., 1972.

DIETARY SOURCES OF TAURINE AND ZINC
Concentration of Zinc in Animal and Plant Food

The concentration of zinc in food is shown in Table I. The largest amount is found in food of animal origin, particularly in meat. Lower amounts are found in vegetables or seeds. From a study of the estimated intake of zinc of pregnant and non-pregnant women, it was concluded that serum zinc concentrations of vegetarian women were generally not different from non-vegetarians (King et al., 1981). Daily zinc intake by pregnant women calculated from dietary recollected information was remarkably similar, 9–11 μg for middle income American women (Hambridge et al., 1983), Mexican-American (Hunt et al., 1979), Lebanese (Turnlund et al., 1983) or British (Abraham, 1982). Only one report of 7 μg per day for vegetarian Asian women suggests that meat intake may be important for fulfilling the dietary requirements of zinc (Abraham, 1982). It is known that only a small percentage of ingested zinc is absorbed. The absorption depends on many factors including body size, level of dietary zinc, and presence in the diet of antagonizing substances, such as calcium, phytate, or chelating agents (Evans, 1976). The major inhibitor of zinc absorption is dietary phytic acid which is present in many cereal grains (O'Dell, 1969). All these factors must be considered for accurate estimations of the amount of zinc available for cell function.

Concentration of Taurine in Animal and Plant Food

It is well known that taurine content in animal tissues is much higher than that found in plants (Roe and Weston, 1965; Jacobsen and Smith, 1968; Lahdesmaki, 1986). The large amounts of taurine in muscle makes meat the main natural supply of taurine for humans. However, no systematic study has been carried out so far on the taurine content of food other than meat. Results of our work on the analysis of taurine in food of plant origin are compared to those reported for animal food. The study includes the analysis of more than 40 fruits and vegetables, seeds, grains, and nuts, with particular emphasis on the plants which constitute the main dietary intake of many rural populations in several countries. Taurine in food was measured in perchloric acid extracts, free of lipids, following a modification of the procedure of Garvin (1960). The perchloric acid extracts containing the free amino acids were hydrolyzed with 6 N HCl, evaporated and washed twice, then resuspended in water, pH adjusted to 1.5, and transferred to a column packed with Dowex 50-H$^+$ (6 × 30 mm). Taurine was eluted with water until a 3-ml volume was collected. Under the conditions of this analysis, the recovery of taurine in the 3 ml of eluate after passage through the column was 75%. No other amino acid was found in the eluate as determined by high performance liquid chromatography. The eluate was neutralized, and taurine quantitation was carried out by the fluorometric determination of an ortophtaldialdehyde-taurine derivative. The fluorescent reaction product was measured using excitation and emission wavelengths of 370 and 465 nm, respectively. Fluorescence of the taurine derivative was linear at taurine concentrations of 10 to 200 nmole. A standard curve of taurine was run through the entire procedure, beginning with the hydrolysis step. Table II shows the amount of taurine found in food of animal origin including beef, chicken, lamb, pork, fish, and sea food. Taurine levels in milk and dairy products, chicken eggs, and honey are also shown in Table II. The edible part in each case has been analyzed, and attention has been paid to obtain samples corresponding to different animals. Table III is a list of the fruits and plants analyzed in which no traces of taurine were found. Table IV shows the taurine content in seeds, grains, and nuts. For those seeds which are commonly eaten cooked, the analysis were carried out in the cooked seed, taking care to collect all cooking water. Nuts were blended and weighed before the analysis.

The results of this study show that food of plant origin cannot replace meat as a source of taurine. The daily requirement of taurine has not been determined so far, although indirect data exist (Gaull et al., 1977; Geggel et al., 1985). Sturman et al. (following chapter) report that a daily supplementation of 40 μmole of taurine to taurine-depleted kittens is able to correct consequences of the deficiency in brain. However, it is difficult to extrap-

TABLE II. Taurine Content of Food of Animal Origin

	Taurine concentration (μmole/g of edible tissue)[a]
Beef	6.8 ± 0.4 (4)
Pork	4.1 ± 0.3 (4)
Chicken breast	1.4 ± 0.1 (3)
Chicken leg	8.6 ± 0.4 (3)
Lamb	4.7 ± 0.3 (5)
Fish	11.6 ± 0.5 (5)
Clam	1.7 ± 0.1 (3)
Oyster	2.3 ± 0.2 (3)
Octopus	7.9 ± 0.2 (5)
Shrimp	12.4 ± 0.1 (5)
Ham	N.D.
Lard	N.D.
Egg yolk	N.D.
Egg white	N.D.
Cow milk (commercial)	N.D.
Cow milk (unprocessed)	0.9 ± 0.1 (4)
Yogurt	0.4 ± 0.02 (3)
Cheese	N.D.
Honey	N.D.

[a]Results are the mean ± S.E.M. of the number of separate determinations indicated in parentheses.

olate from this observation the human requirements. The present results of taurine content in food of plant origin will help to obtain this necessary information.

MILK AS SOURCE OF ZINC AND TAURINE FOR POSTNATAL BRAIN DEVELOPMENT

Zinc Concentration

There are many reports in the literature on the zinc content of human milk (see Gaull et al., 1982 for a review). The amount of zinc reported varies, the mean being around 0.9–1.4 mg/l at 6–12 months of lactation. The concentration of zinc in milk is higher at 1 month of lactation or less, with reported values between 2.9–4.7 mg/l (Krebs et al., 1985). A decline of zinc concentration in human milk is observed as lactation progresses. The decrease is about 60% between 1 and 3 months, and decreases further so that between 8 and 12 months, zinc levels have declined to about 20% of the concentration found at 1 month of lactation (Krebs et al., 1985). The mammary gland appears to have homeostatic mechanisms to control milk zinc since milk zinc concentration has been reported not to correlate with maternal zinc status or dietary zinc intake (Vuori and Kuitunen, 1979 ;

TABLE III. Fruits and Vegetables With Detectable Taurine[a]

Roots	Fruits
Carrot	Chili
Radish	Cucumber
Turnip	Tomato
Stems	Pumpkin
Beet	Avocado
Onion	Eggplant
Potato	Apple
Sweet potato	Pear
Leaves	Orange
Brussel sprout	Banana
Lettuce	Strawberry
Spinach	Grape
Cabbage	Flowers
Garlic	Cauliflower
Cactus	Broccoli

[a]Samples of about 1 g (wet weight) were analyzed. The lower limit of the technique for taurine analysis is 5 nmole.

Moser and Reynolds, 1983). However, a recent study of Krebs et al. (1985) on the effect of moderate zinc supplementation, corresponding to the total daily zinc Recommended Dietary Allowance showed that the decline in zinc concentration in milk between 6 and 12 months of lactation is less sharp. The difference observed in this study between the zinc concentration in milk of zinc-supplemented mothers as compared to non-supplemented is only 10% between 1 and 6 months of lactation, but this difference increases to 50% between 7 and 9 months of lactation. This difference may have implications of nutritional importance in countries where older infants typically continue to derive a large percentage of their nutrients from breast milk.

Taurine Concentrations

The subject of taurine concentration in human milk has raised a great deal of interest because cow milk, which has often been used as a replacement for human milk, contains very low amounts of taurine. Commercially prepared formulas, until recently, also contained low amounts of taurine, resembling the composition of cow milk more than that of human milk in this respect. Recently, a number of laboratories have supplemented formulas with taurine concentrations closer to the physiologic amount found in maternal milk.

Still, our knowledge of the handling of taurine by the mammary gland is very poor. The amount of taurine in human milk has been reported, but information about other aspects of taurine handling is still scarce. There is no data about changes with lactation time, about diurnal or within the feed variations or about differences in the amount of taurine at the beginning and

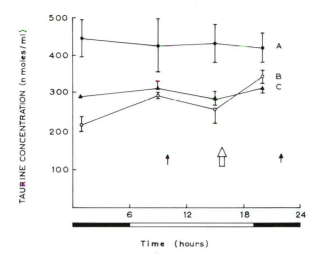

Fig. 11. Taurine concentration in milk samples obtained from three lactating women for 24 h. Samples were collected before nursing at the indicated time for 3 days; results are the means ± S.E.M. of the three samples collected at the same time on each day. A) 27-year-old woman, with 4 children, at 2 weeks of lactation. B) 22-year-old woman at 12 months of lactation. C) 25-year-old woman at 6 months of lactation. Arrows correspond to meal time, the largest arrow corresponding to the largest meal.

the end of nursing. Also, a correlation has yet to be established between the dietary supply of taurine and its concentration in milk.

In this chapter we present preliminary results of a study on the variations of taurine concentration in milk throughout the day and on the amount of taurine present in fractionated samples of milk obtained from serial extractions. These analyses are a necessary antecedent for adequate sample collection for studies on the effect of the dietary intake on the concentration of taurine in human milk.

Figure 11 shows the concentration of taurine in samples of milk collected from three women, four times during a 24-h cycle for 3 days. One of the series (A) corresponds to a 1-week period of lactation and contains higher concentrations of taurine, in agreement with the report of Rassin et al. (1978). The other two series correspond to 12 months of lactation (B) and 6 months of lactation (C). Analysis of serial samples collected from one breast did not show significant differences.

NUTRITIONAL IMPLICATIONS AND CONCLUDING REMARKS

The importance of an adequate supply of taurine and zinc for the optimal development of brain has now strong experimental support. The particular

TABLE IV. Taurine Content of Seeds, Grains, and Nuts

	Taurine concentration (μmole/g dry weight)[a]
Rice	N.D. (3)
Corn	N.D. (4)
Oatmeal	N.D. (3)
Wheat	N.D. (4)
Barley	N.D.
Black bean	.005 (6)
White bean	.003 (6)
Lentil	N.D. (6)
Chick pea	N.D. (6)
Almond	N.D. (4)
Peanut	N.D. (4)
Pistachio	N.D. (4)
Walnut	N.D. (4)
Chestnut	N.D. (4)

[a]Seeds were weighed uncooked, then cooked in a small amount of water, and homogenates were made after addition of the necessary amount of perchloric acid to make a 1.2 M final concentration in the coction water.

aspects of brain maturation where taurine and zinc appear to be involved, i.e., the process of cell migration and the successful organization of neuronal layers, are of extreme importance for the establishment of functional cell circuits and synaptic contacts. These processes, occurring at the late stages of brain maturation, are critical for the adequate performance of both relatively simple somatic functions as well as the most elaborate tasks of integrative and intellecutal work. The injury to these processes by nutritional deficiencies such as those discussed in this chapter have not been appropriately evaluated so far. In countries where the quality of nutrition has considerably declined in recent years, including a severe reduction of meat intake, emphasis should be put on providing those elements which are of particular importance for the optimal brain development. Supplementation of specific nutrients, such as taurine and zinc, as dietary complements during the critical periods of brain maturation may be advised or even provided by health institutions in communities with a risk of deficiency. In socioeconomic terms, such supplementation may be more efficient and feasible than trying to make major changes in the general nutritional scheme of the community. For taurine as well as for zinc, the supplementary amount which should be provided during lactation is easily obtained by means of simple technological devices from animal sources rich in these compounds, such as commercially invaluable fish and sea food.

ACKNOWLEDGMENTS

The authors wish to thank Dr. Ryan J. Huxtable for the analysis of some samples. The assistance of Ms. Y. Diaz de Castro in typing this manuscript is also acknowledged. The experimental work on this chapter was supported by grant no. PCALCNA-050281 from CONACYT.

REFERENCES

Abraham R (1982): Trace element intake by Asians during pregnancy. Proc Nutr Soc 41:261–265.

Ahokas RA, Anderson GD, Lipshitz J (1983): Effect of dietary restriction, during the last week only or throughout gestation on cardiac output and uteroplacental blood flow in pregnant rats. J Nutr 113:1766–1776.

Apgar J (1975): Effects of some nutritional deficiencies on parturition in rats. J Nutr 105:1553–1561.

Apgar J (1976): Zinc requirement for normal parturition in rats. Nutr Rep Int 15:553–559.

Apgar J (1977): Effects of zinc deficiency and zinc repletion during pregnancy on parturition in two strains of rats. J Nutr 107:1399–1403.

Apgar J, Fitzgerald JA (1985): Effect on the ewe and lamb on low zinc intake throughout pregnancy. J Anim Sci 60:1530–1539.

Berson EL, Hayes KC, Robin AR, Schmidt SY, Watson G (1976): Retinal degeneration in cats fed casein. II. Supplementation with methionine, cysteine and taurine. Invest Ophthalmol Vis Sci 15:52–58.

Bettger WJ, O'Dell BL (1981): A critical physiological role of zinc in the structure and function of biomembranes. Life Sci 28:1425–1438.

Bonting SL, Van Breugel PJGM, Daemen FJM (1977); Influence of the lipid environment on the properties of rhodopsin in the photoreceptor membrane. Adv Exp Med Biol 83:175–189.

Brueton MJ, Berger HM, Brown GA, Ablitt L, Iyngkaran N, Wharton BA (1978): Duodenal bile acid conjugation patterns and dietary sulphur amino acids in the newborn. Gut 19:95–98.

Buamah PK, Russell M (1984): Maternal zinc status: A determination of central nervous system malformation. Br J Obstet Gynaecol 91:788–790.

Bunce GE, Wilson GR, Mills CF, Klopper A (1983): Studies on the role of zinc in parturition in the rat. Biochem J 210:761–767.

Chan PH, Yurko M, Fishman RA (1982): Phospholipid degradation and cellular edema induced by free radicals in brain and cortical slices. J Neurochem 38:525–531.

Chaovan JP, Kulakowski EC, Sheakowski S, Schaffer SW (1980): Calcium regulation by the low-affinity taurine binding sites of cardiac sarcolemma. Mol Pharmacol 17:295–300.

Chvapil M (1973): New aspects in the biological role of zinc: A stabilizer of macromolecules and biological membranes. Life Sci 13:1041–1049.

Cone RA (1972): Rotational diffusion of rhodopsin in the visual receptor membrane. Nature 236:39–43.

Crevey BJ, Langer GA, Frank JS (1978): Role of calcium in maintenance of rabbit myocardial cell membrane structural and functional integrity. J Mol Cell Cardiol 10:1081–1100.

Cunnane SC, Majid E, Senior J, Mills CF (1983): Uteroplacental dysfunction and prostaglandin metabolism in zinc deficient pregnant rats. Life Sci 32:2471–2478.

Daemen FJM (1973): Vertebrate rod outer segment membranes. Biochim Biophys Acta 300:255–288.

Dvergesten CL, Fosmire GJ, Ollerich DA, Sandstead HH (1983): Alterations in the postnatal development of the cerebellar cortex due to zinc deficiency. I. Impaired acquisition of granule cells. Brain Res 271:217–226.

Dvergesten CL, Fosmire GJ, Ollerich DA, Sandstead HH (1984a): Alterations in the postnatal development of the cerebellar cortex due to zinc deficiency. II. Impaired maturation of Purkinje cells. Dev Brain Res 16:11–20.

Dvergesten CL, Johnson LA, Sandstead HH (1984b): Alterations in the postnatal development of the cerebellar cortex due to zinc deficiency. III. Impaired dendritic differentiation of basket and stellate cells. Dev Brain Res 16:21–26.

Evans GW (1976): Zinc absorption and transport. In Prasad AD, Oberleas D (eds): ''Trace Elements in Human Health and Disease.'' New York: Academic Press, pp 181–188.

Garvin JE (1960): A new method for the determination of taurine in tissues. Arch Biochem Biophys 9:219–225.

Gaull GE, Jensen RG, Rassin DK, Mallory MH (1982): Human milk as food. In Milunsky A, Friedman EA, Gluck L (eds): ''Advances in Perinatal Medicine.'' New York: Plenum Publishing, pp 47–117.

Gaull GE, Rassin DK, Raiha NCR, Heinonen K (1977): Milk protein quantity and quality in low-birth-weight infants. III. Effects of sulfur amino acids in plasma and urine. J Pediatr 90:348–355.

Geggel HS, Ament ME, Heckenlively JR, Martin DA, Martin DS, Kopple JD (1985): Nutritional requirements for taurine in patients receiving long-term parenteral nutrition. N Engl J Med 312:142–146.

Griffin WST, Woodward DJ, Chanda R (1977): Malnutrition-induced alterations of developing Purkinje cells. Exp Neurol 56:298–311.

Halsted JA, Smith JC and Irwin MJ (1974): A conspectus of research on zinc requirement of man. J Nutr 104:345–351.

Hambridge KM, Krebs NF, Jacobs MA, Favier A, Guyette L (1983): Zinc nutritional status during pregnancy: A longitudinal study. Am J Clin Nutr 37:429–442.

Hayes KC, Carey RE, Schmidt SY (1975): Retinal degeneration associated with taurine deficiency in the cat. Science 188:949–951.

Hayes KC, Sturman JA (1981): Taurine in metabolism. Annu Rev Nutr 1:401–425.

Hayes KC, Sturman JA (1982): Taurine Deficiency: A rationale for taurine depletion. In Huxtable RJ, Pasantes-Morales H (eds): ''Taurine in Nutrition and Neurology.'' New York: Plenum Press, pp 79–87.

Hill GM, Miller ER, Stowe HD (1983): Effect of dietary zinc levels on health and productivity of gilts and sows through two parities. J Anim Sci 57:114–122.

Hunt IF, Murphy NJ, Gómez J, Smith JC (1979): Dietary zinc intake of low-income pregnant women of Mexican descent. Am J Clin Nutr 32:1511–1518.

Hurley LS, Baly DL (1982): The effects of zinc deficiency during pregnancy. In Prasad AS (ed): ''Clinical, Biochemical and Nutritional Aspects of Trace Elements.'' New York: Alan R. Liss Inc., pp 145–159.

Huxtable RJ, Bressler R (1973): Effect of taurine on a muscle intracellular membrane. Biochim Biophys Acta 323:573–583.

Huxtable RJ, Laird HE, Lippincott SE (1979): The transport of taurine in the heart and the rapid depletion of tissue taurine content by guanidinoethyl sulfonate. J Pharmacol Exp Ther 211:465–471.

Huxtable RJ, Lippincott SE (1982a): Diet and biosynthesis as source of taurine in the mouse. J Nutr 112:1003–1010.

Huxtable RJ, Lippincott SE (1982b): Relative contribution of diet and biosynthesis to the taurine content of the adult rat. Drug Nutr Interact 1:153–168.

Huxtable RJ, Lippincott SE (1983): Relative contribution of the mother, the nurse and endogenous synthesis to the taurine content of the newborn and suckling rat. Ann Nutr Metab 27:107–116.

Jacobsen JG, Smith LH (1968): Biochemistry and physiology of taurine and taurine derivatives. Physiol Rev 48:424–511.

Jacobsen JG, Thomas LL, Smith LH (1964): Properties and distribution of mammalian L-cystein sulfinate carboxylases. Biochim Biophys Acta 85:103–108.

Jameson S (1976): Effects of zinc deficiency in human reproduction. Acta Med Scand Suppl 593:3–89.

King JC, Stein T, Doyle M (1981): Effect of vegetarianism on the zinc status of pregnant women. Am J Clin Nutr 34:1049–1055.

Kramer JH, Chovan JP, Schaffer SW (1981): Effect of taurine on calcium paradox and ischemic heart failure. Am J Physiol 60:20–40.

Krebs NF, Hambridge KM, Jacobs AM, Rasbach JO (1985): The effect of dietary zinc supplement during lactation on longitudinal changes in maternal zinc status and milk zinc concentrations. Am J Clin Nutr 41:560–570.

Lahdesmaki P (1986): Determination of taurine and other acidic amino acids in plants. Phytochemistry 25:2409–2411.

Lake N (1981): Depletion of retinal taurine by treatment with guanidinoethyl sulfonate. Life Sci 29:445–448.

Lake N (1982a): Depletion of taurine in the adult rat retina. Neurochem Res 7:1385–1390.

Lake N (1982b): Is taurine an essential amino acid? Retina 2:261–262.

Leuré-Dupreé AE, Bridges CD (1982): Changes in retinal morphology and vitamin A metabolism as a consequence of decreased zinc availability. Retina 2:294–302.

Marthur RL, Klethi J, Ledig M, Mandel P (1976): Cystein sulfinate decarboxylase in the visual pathway of adult chicken. Life Sci 18:75–80.

McConnell P, Berry H (1981): The effects of feeding after varying periods of neonatal undernutrition on the morphology of Purkinje cells in the cerebellum of the rat. J Comp Neurol 200:463–479.

Moser PB, Reynolds RD (1983): Dietary zinc intake and zinc concentrations of plasma, erythrocytes, and breast milk in antepartum and postpartum lactating and nonlactating women: A longitudinal study. Am J Clin Nutr 38:101–108.

Mutch PB, Hurley LS (1980): Mammary gland function and development: Effect of zinc deficiency in rat. Am J Physiol 238:E26–31.

Nakashima T, Takino T, Kuriyama K (1983): Therapeutic and prophylactic effects of taurine on experimental liver injury. In Kuriyama K, Huxtable RJ, Iwata H (eds): "Sulfur Amino Acids: Biochemical and Clinical Aspects." New York: Alan R. Liss, pp 449–459.

Noell WK, Walker US, Kang BS, Berman S (1966): Retinal damage by light in rats. Invest Ophthalmol Vis Sci 5:450–473.

O'Dell BL (1969): Effect of dietary components upon zinc availability: A review with original data. Am J Clin Nutr 22:1315–1330.

Osis D, Kramer L, Wiatrowski E (1972): Dietary zinc intake in man. Am J Clin Nutr 25:582–586.

Pasantes-Morales H (1986): Current concepts on the role of taurine in the retina. In Osborne NN, Chader J (eds): "Progress in Retinal Research." New York: Pergamon Press, pp 207–229.

Pasantes-Morales H, Ademe RM, Quesada O (1981): Protective effect of taurine on the light-induced disruption of isolated frog rod outer segments. J Neurosci Res 6:337–348.

Pasantes-Morales H, Cruz C (1984): Protective effect of taurine and zinc on peroxidation induced damage in photoreceptor outer segments. J Neurosci Res 11:303–311.

Pasantes-Morales H, Loriette C, Chatagner F (1977): Regional and subcellular distribution of taurine synthesizing enzymes in the rat central nervous system. Neurochem Res 2:671–680.

Pasantes-Morales H, Quesada O, Cárabez A, Huxtable R (1983): Effect of taurine transport antagonist, guanidinoethane sulfonate and alanine on the morphology of the rat retina. J Neurosci Res 9:135–144.

Pasantes-Morales H, Wright CE, Gaull GE (1984): Protective effect of taurine, zinc and tocopherol on retinal induced damage in human lymphoblastoid cells. J Nutr 114:2256–2261.

Physh JJ, Perkins RE, Back LS (1979): The effect of postnatal undernutrition on the development of the mouse Purkinje cell dendritic tree. Brain Res 163:165–170.

Quesada O, Huxtable RJ, Pasantes-Morales H (1984): Effect of guanidinoethane sulgonate on taurine uptake by rat retina. J Neurosci Res 11:179–186.

Rakic P, Sidman R (1973): Organization of cerebellar cortex secondary to deficit of granule cells in weaver mutant mice. J Comp Neurol 152:133–162.

Rapp LP, Wiegand RD, Anderson RE (1982): Ferrous ion mediated retinal degeneration: Role of rod outer segment peroxidation. In Clayton R, Heywood I, Reading H, Wright A (eds): "Biology of Normal and Genetically Abnormal Retinas." New York: Academic Press, pp 109–119.

Rassin DK, Sturman JA, Gaull GE (1978): Taurine and other free amino acids in milk of man and other mammals. Early Hum Dev 2:1–13.

Robin B, Nicolasi RJ, Hayes KC (1976): Dietary influence on bile acid conjugation in the cat. J Nutr 106:1241–1246.

Roe DA, Weston MO (1965): Potential significance of free taurine in the diet. Nature 205:287–288.

Salceda R, Pasantes-Morales H (1982): Uptake, release and binding of taurine in degenerated rat retinas. J Neurosci Res 8:631–642.

Sandstead HH, Wallwork JC, Halas ES, Tucker DH, Dvergesten CI, Strobel DA (1983): Zinc and central nervous function. In Sarkar B (ed): "Biological Aspects of Metals and Metal-Related Diseases." New York: Raven Press, pp 225–241.

Schmidt SY (1981): Taurine in retinas of taurine-deficient cats and RCS rats. In Baskin SI, Schaeffer SE (eds): "The Effect of Taurine in Excitable Tissues." New York: Spectrum Press, pp. 177–185.

Schmidt SY, Berson EL, Hayes KC (1976): Retinal degeneration in cats fed casein. I. Taurine deficiency. Invest Ophthalmol 15:47–52.

Skyes SM, Robinson GW, Waxler M, Kuwabara T (1981): Damage to the monkey retina by broad spectrum fluorescent light. Invest Ophthalmol Vis Sci 20:425–434.

Sotelo C (1975): Anatomical, physiological and biochemical studies of the cerebellum from mutant mice. II. Morphological study of cerebellar cortical neurons and circuits in the weaver mouse. Brain Res 94:19–44.

Spaeth DG, Schneider DL (1974): Taurine synthesis, concentration and bile-salt conjugation in rat, guinea pig and rabbit. Proc Soc Exp Biol Med 147:855–858.

Sturman JA, Hayes KC (1980): The biology of taurine in nutrition and development. In Draper HH (ed): "The Biology of Taurine in Nutrition and Development." New York: Plenum Publishing, pp 231–299.

Sturman JA, Moretz RC, French JH, Wisniewski HM (1985): Taurine deficiency in the developing cat: Persistence of the cerebellar external granule cell layer. J Neurosci Res 13:405–416.

Sturman JA, Rassin DK, Hayes KC, Gaull GE (1978): Taurine deficiency in the kitten: Exchange and turnover of ^{35}S-taurine in brain, retina and other tissues. J Nutr 108:1462–1476.

Sturman JA, Wen GY, Wisniewski HM, Neuringer MD (1984): Retinal degeneration in primates raised on a synthetic human infant formula. Int J Dev Neurosci 2:121–126.

Turnland JR, King JC, Wahbeh CJ, Ishkanian I, Tannous RI (1983): Zinc status and pregnancy outcome of pregnant Lebanese women. Nutr Res 3:309–315.

Underwood EJ (1977): Zinc. In Underwood EJ (ed): "Trace Elements in Human and Animal Nutrition." New York: Academic Press, pp 196–242.

Vuori E, Kuitunen P (1979): The concentration of copper and zinc in human milk. Acta Paediatr Scand 68:33–37.

West CD, Kemper TL (1976): The effect of low protein diet on the anatomical development of the rat brain. Brain Res 104:221–237.

Wiegand RD, Giusto NM, Rapp LM, Anderson RE (1983): Evidence of rod outer segment lipid peroxidation following constant illumination of the rat retina. Invest Ophthalmol Vis Sci 10:1433–1435.

Current Topics in Nutrition and Disease, Volume 16
Basic and Clinical Aspects of Nutrition and Brain Development,
pages 245–254
© 1987 Alan R. Liss, Inc.

Sulfur Amino Acids in Brain Development

J.A. Sturman
Department of Developmental Biochemistry, Institute for Basic Research
in Developmental Disabilities, Staten Island, New York 10314

Methionine is an essential amino acid for mammals, including man (Rose et al., 1955), and several of its metabolites have an important impact on development (Fig. 1). Cyst(e)ine is not essential for mature mammals, although it can spare up to 90% of the dietary requirement for methionine (Rose and Wixom, 1955). Biosynthesis of cyst(e)ine in developing tissues is limited or absent (Sturman et al., 1970; Gaull et al., 1972; Zlotkin and Anderson, 1982), however, which suggests that some dietary cyst(e)ine may be necessary for normal development. In this respect it is worth noting that human milk protein contains 50% more cyst(e)ine than methionine and thus is an excellent nutritional source (see Gaull et al., 1982). Cysteine is an especially important amino acid in proteins by virtue of its sulfhydryl group which is responsible for molecular configurations formed by a disulfide bond to another cysteine molecule in the same protein and by disulfide bonds to cysteine molecules in separate proteins and polypeptides. In utero, cysteine is obtained from the mother's circulation, as are other amino acids. It is unique in that the placenta restricts its access to the fetus whereas other amino acids are actively concentrated by the placenta resulting in 2- to 3-fold greater fetal plasma concentrations than maternal plasma concentrations (Gaull et al., 1973). These controls on the production and accumulation of cysteine in developing tissues may be necessary because of its toxicity to developing nervous tissues (Olney and Ho, 1970; Olney et al., 1972).

The immediate metabolic precursor of cysteine, cystathionine, is present in mature brain in high concentrations, especially in brains of primates and man. The concentration of cystathionine in developing brain is lower and increases throughout development, suggesting that its function, although presently unknown, may be primarily in mature brain (see Tallan et al., 1983).

The last metabolite of methionine metabolism, taurine, has been the subject of intense study during the last decade, with several international meetings and books being devoted to it. Major areas of interest are its role in

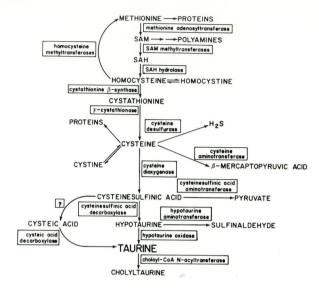

Fig. 1. Transsulfuration pathway of methionine metabolism.

such excitable tissues as brain, retina, and heart, and its possible importance as a nutrient, especially during development. Taurine is one of the most abundant free amino acids in mammalian tissues and is present in especially high concentrations in developing brain. The concentration of taurine in brain declines from birth to maturity, approximately by the time of weaning, as illustrated for rat brain (Fig. 2). A major advance in taurine research was the discovery that an inadequate dietary intake of taurine in cats resulted in taurine depletion and retinal degeneration (Hayes et al., 1975) (Fig. 3). Further studies revealed that the tapetum lucidum, a layer of cells behind the retina, also showed degenerative changes associated with taurine depletion (Wen et al., 1979) (Fig. 4). Study of the early stages of taurine depletion suggested that the initial mechanism involved disruption of the membrane surrounding the individual tapetal rods followed by loss of structure of the tapetal rods (Sturman et al., 1981) (Fig. 5).

The possibility of involvement of taurine with human infant nutrition and development was raised by the results from a feeding study with human preterm infants (Gaull et al., 1977). The concentration of taurine in plasma and urine of those infants fed synthetic formulas containing little or no taurine was reduced in comparison to similar infants fed pooled human milk. Taurine was unusual in this respect because most other amino acids were present in greater concentrations in plasma and urine of the infants fed the synthetic formulas than in those fed pooled human milk (Rassin et al., 1977a; Gaull et al., 1977). Similar findings were reported for term human infants fed

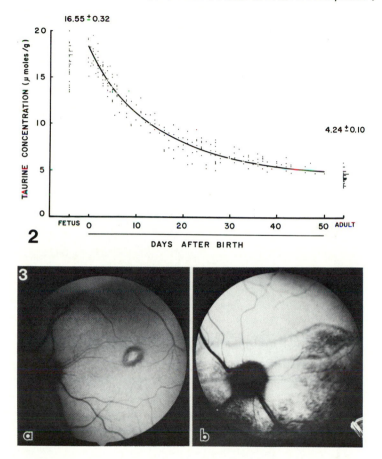

Fig. 2.   Concentration of taurine in rat brain as a function of age. Each point represents the value obtained from a separate animal, except for rat fetuses, in which several brains of fetuses from the same mother were pooled. The mean value ± S.E.M. for fetal and adult brains is given.

Fig. 3.   Fundus photographs (taken with a Kowa RC 2 fundus camera) of taurine-depleted adult cats. a) An early lesion; b) an advanced lesion.

synthetic formulas or pooled human milk (Rassin and Gaull, 1981; Jarvenpaa et al., 1982). Such infants showed no obvious signs of retinal abnormalities, although there was concern that subclinical effects might be present. Such a possibility was examined by raising infant rhesus monkeys on human infant formula alone or supplemented with taurine (Sturman et al., 1984). The concentration of taurine in plasma of those monkeys fed the formula alone was approximately half that of the monkeys fed the formula supplemented with taurine, resembling the results obtained with human infants fed

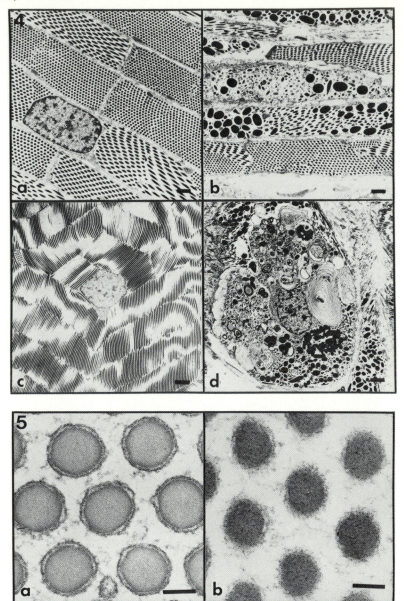

synthetic formulas or human milk, respectively. The monkeys showed no obvious signs of retinal abnormalities, but ultrastructural examination of the retinas when the monkeys were killed at 26 months after birth revealed degenerative changes in the cone photoreceptors of the monkeys fed the formula alone but not in those of the monkeys fed the formula supplemented with taurine (Fig. 6). This finding contributed to the decision of manufacturers of synthetic human infant formulas to add taurine to their products.

Our continuing research into the role of taurine in development has revealed that in kittens, at least, normal brain development requires normal taurine concentrations. Taurine-depleted female cats exhibit increased reproductive wastage and frequently resorb or abort their fetuses and have stillborn or low-birth-weight live kittens at term (Sturman et al., 1985). Severe hydrocephalus was observed in two aborted fetuses and in a surviving liveborn kitten, and anencephaly in one stillborn kitten (Fig. 7). The live kittens have a poor survival rate, grow at a lower than normal rate, and exhibit a number of neurologic abnormalities. These include an abnormal hind limb development, a peculiar gait, and radiologically obvious thoracic kyphosis (Fig. 8). Morphologic examination of the brains of such kittens revealed a persistence of cells in the cerebellar external granule cell layer at 8 weeks after birth, long after all cells should have migrated to the internal granule cell layer (Fig. 9). Moreover, numerous mitotic figures were present in the cells in the external granule cell layer indicating that cell division is still occurring, an event normally terminated by 3 weeks after birth in the kitten (Smith and Downs, 1978). Abnormal ontogeny was also evident in the visual cortex (Fig. 10) (Palackal et al., 1986). At birth, neuroblasts have failed to migrate and differentiate properly and have aggregated at the ventricular and pial zones. By weaning at 8 weeks after birth, only few pyramidal and non-pyramidal neurons are found, with heavily spined dendritic processes and poor arborization. More recently we have noted abnormal morphology of the spinal cord in such kittens in which the dorsal root nerves do not have the normal alignment, do not connect with the spinal

---

←Fig. 4. (Facing page) Electron micrographs of cross-sections of center of tapetum from (a) cat fed synthetic diet supplemented with taurine and (b) cat fed synthetic diet alone. Scale bars 1 μm. Electron micrographs of tangential sections of center of tapetum from (c) cat fed synthetic diet supplemented with taurine and (d) cat fed synthetic diet alone. Scale bars 2 μm. The tapetal cell in (d) is in an advanced state of degeneration and shows transformation to a phagosome, with remnants of tapetal rods, large electron-dense droplets, and whirls of membranes and myelin-like material.

Fig. 5. High magnification electron micrograph from ultrathin (gray interferance color) cross-sections of center of tapetum from (a) cat fed synthetic diet supplemented with taurine and (b) cat fed synthetic diet alone. Scale bars 0.1 μm.

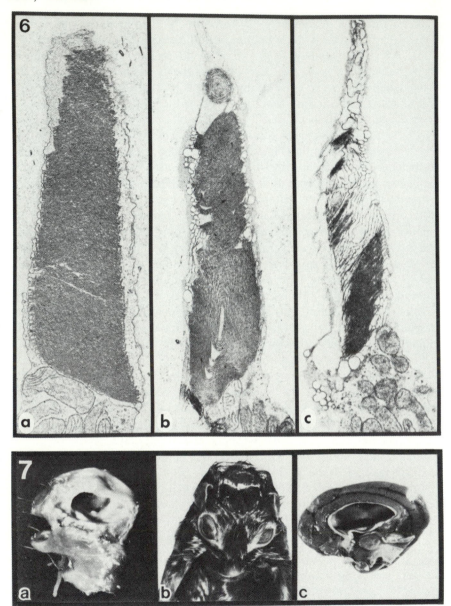

←Fig. 6. (Facing page) Electron micrographs of the outer segments of cone photoreceptors from (a) infant rhesus monkey raised on Nutramigen supplemented with taurine, (b) and (c) infant rhesus monkeys raised on Nutramigen alone. b) A cone with moderate disorientation and vesiculation of the disc membranes in the outer segment. c) A more severe degeneration. In both of these cones, the outer membrane is also disorganized, whereas the outer membrane of the cone from the taurine-supplemented monkey is intact. × 10,000.

Fig. 7. Abnormal offspring from taurine-depleted mothers. a) Fetus aborted preterm showing extreme hydrocephalus. b) Full term stillborn showing anencephaly. c) Brain from a 1-year-old kitten showing severe hydrocephalus.

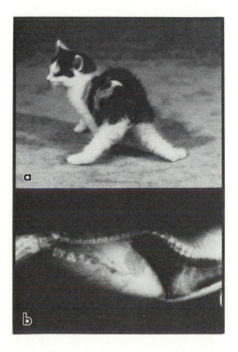

Fig. 8. (a) Photograph of 8-week-old kitten from a taurine-deficient mother illustrating the abnormal hind leg development. (b) X-ray of the same kitten illustrating thoracic kyphosis.

cord in the correct fashion, and have a greatly reduced proportion of white matter. These results may be important in understanding the human disease, Friedreich's ataxia, which shows many of the neurological signs and symptoms observed in taurine-deficient kittens and is associated with increased taurine excretion which may result in taurine deficiency (see Barbeau, 1984).

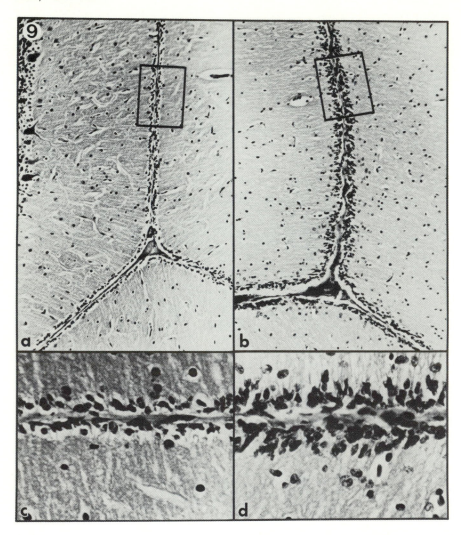

Fig. 9. Light micrographs of the external granule cell layer of midline sagittal sections of cerebellum (lobe VI) of 8-week-old kittens from taurine-supplemented (a,c) and taurine-depleted, (b,d) mothers. Note the increased thickness of the external granule cell layer of the taurine-deficient kittens as compared to the controls. a,b ×25; c,d, ×60.

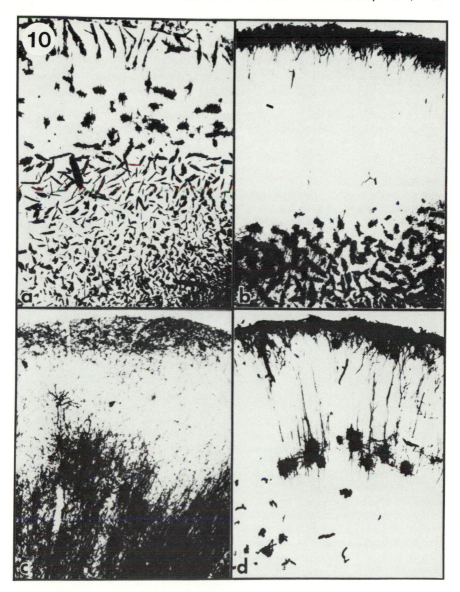

Fig. 10. Sections of kitten visual cortex stained by the rapid Golgi method. a) Newborn kitten from taurine-supplemented mother. b) Newborn kitten from taurine-deficient mother. c) 8-week-old kitten from taurine-supplemented mother. d) 8-week-old kitten from taurine-deficient mother. a,b ×40. c,d ×60.

REFERENCES

Barbeau A (1984): The Quebec cooperative study of Friedreich's ataxia: 1974–1984. 10 years of research. Can J Neurol Sci 11:646–660.

Gaull GE, Rassin DK, Raiha NCR, Heinonen K (1977): Milk protein quantity and quality in low-birth-weight infants. III. Effects on sulfur amino acids in plasma and urine. J Pediatr 90:348–355.

Gaull GE, Sturman JA, Raiha NCR (1972): Development of mammalian sulfur metabolism: Absence of cystathionase in human fetal tissues. Pediatr Res 6:538–547.

Gaull GE, von Berg W, Raiha NCR, Sturman JA (1973): Development of methyltransferase activity of human fetal tissues. Pediatr Res 7:527–533.

Hayes KC, Carey RE, Schmidt SY (1975): Retinal degeneration associated with taurine deficiency in the cat. Science 188:949–951.

Jarvenpaa A, Rassin DK, Raiha NCR, Gaull GE (1982): Milk protein quantity and quality in the term infant. II. Effects on acidic and neutral amino acids. Pediatrics 70:221–230.

Olney JW, Ho OL (1970): Brain damage in infant mice following oral intake of glutamate, aspartate or cysteine. Nature 227:609–610.

Olney JW, Ho OL, Rhee V, Schainker B (1972): Cysteine-induced brain damage in infant and fetal rodents. Brain Res 45:309–313.

Palackal T, Moretz RC, Sturman JA, Wisniewski HM (1986): Abnormal visual cortex development in the cat associated with dietary taurine deprivation. J Neurosci Res 15:223–239.

Rassin DK, Gaull GE (1981): Taurine: Significance in human nutrition. In Schaffer SW, Baskin SI, Kocsis JJ (eds): "The Effects of Taurine on Excitable Tissues." New York: Spectrum, pp 379–390.

Rassin DK, Gaull GE, Heinonen K, Raiha NCR (1977a): Milk protein quantity and quality in low-birth-weight infants. 2. Effects on selected aliphatic amino acids in plasma and urine. Pediatrics 59:407–522.

Rassin DK, Gaull GE, Raiha NCR, Heinonen K (1977b): Milk protein quantity and quality in low-birth-weight infants. 4. Effects on tyrosine and phenylalanine in plasma and urine. J Pediatr 90:356–360.

Rose WC, Coon MJ, Lockhart HB, Lambert GF (1955): The amino acid requirements of man. XI. The threonine and methionine requirements. J Biol Chem 215:101–110.

Rose WC, Wixom RL (1955): The amino acid requirements of man. XIII. The sparing effect of cystine on the methionine requirement. J Biol Chem 216:763–773.

Smith DE, Downs I (1978): Postnatal development of the granule cell in the kitten cerebellum. Am J Anat 151:527–538.

Sturman JA, Gaull GE, Raiha NCR (1970): Absence of cystathionase in human fetal liver: Is cystine essential? Science 169:74–76.

Sturman JA, Moretz RC, French JH, Wisniewski HM (1985): Postnatal taurine deficiency in the kitten results in a persistence of the cerebellar external granule cell layer: Correction by taurine feeding. J Neurosci Res 13:521–528.

Sturman JA, Wen GY, Wisniewski HM, Hayes KC (1981): Histochemical localization of zinc in the feline tapetum: Effect of taurine depletion. Histochemistry 72:341–350.

Sturman JA, Wen GY, Wisniewski HM, Neuringer MD (1984): Retinal degeneration in primates raised on a synthetic human infant formula. Int J Dev Neurosci 2:121–130.

Tallan HH, Rassin DK, Sturman JA, Gaull GE (1983): Methionine metabolism in brain. In Lajtha A (ed): "Handbook of Neurochemistry." Vol. 3, 2nd ed. New York: Plenum Publishing, pp 535–558.

Wen GY, Sturman JA, Wisniewski HM, Lidsky AA, Cornwell AC, Hayes KC (1979): Tapetum disorganization in taurine-depleted cats. Invest Ophthalmol Vis Sci 18:1201–1206.

Zlotkin HS, Anderson GH (1982): The development of cystathionase activity during the first year of life. Pediatr Res 16:65–68.

Current Topics in Nutrition and Disease, Volume 16
Basic and Clinical Aspects of Nutrition and Brain Development,
pages 255–267
© 1987 Alan R. Liss, Inc.

Brain Development and Neurotransmitter Receptors: Analysis Using Cerebral Cortical Neurons in Primary Culture

Kinya Kuriyama and Seitaro Ohkuma

Department of Pharmacology, Kyoto Prefectural University of Medicine,
Kawaramachi-Hirokoji, Kamikyo-Ku, Kyoto 602, Japan

INTRODUCTION

It has been well established that the development of the central nervous system (CNS) is accompanied not only by developmental changes in metabolism of various neurotransmitters but also changes in neurotransmitter receptors. For example, the ontogenic development of muscarnic cholinergic (Enna et al., 1976), GABA (Coyle and Enna, 1976), and β-adrenergic (Pittman et al., 1980) receptors in the brain have been well documented.

On the other hand, it is well known that the CNS consists of several different types of cells including neuronal, glial, and endothelial cells. Although neuronal cells play an important role in the transmission of neuronal signals to other neuronal cells and/or effector cells, the proportion of neurons occupying the brain mass is known to be approximately 40% (Pope, 1978), and 60 to 80% of protein in brain homogenates is attributed to glial cells (Hauser et al., 1980). In addition, it has been reported that more than 40% of protein in synaptosomal fractions originates from glial cells (Henn et al., 1976). Moreover, several investigators have detected benzodiazepine and β-adrenergic receptor binding sites in membrane fractions prepared from glial and endothelial cells (Bender and Hertz, 1984; Harden and McCarthy, 1982; Harik et al., 1981; Kobayashi et al., 1981; Tardy et al., 1981) dissociated from rodent brains. These facts clearly indicate that neuronal cell fractions well separated from non-neuronal cells are more suitable for studying the development of neurotransmitter receptors in the brain than other, frequently used cerebral preparations such as cerebral homogenates and subcellular fractions. In the present study, we have, therefore, investigated the developmental patterns of γ-aminobutyric acid (GABA) and β-adrenergic receptors as well as those of GABA and taurine metabolism using well-defined cerebral cortical neurons in primary culture.

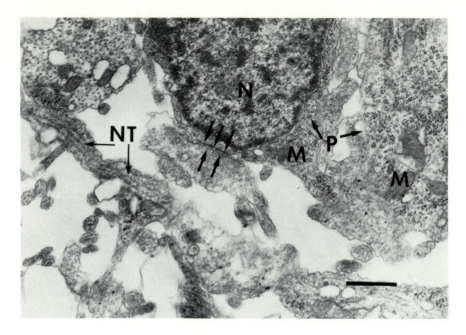

Fig. 1. Transmission electron micrograph of 14-day-old cultured neurons. Arrows indicate axosomatic synaptic contact with asymmetric membrane thickening and vesicle-filled boutons. N: nucleus, M: mitochondria, P: clustered polyribosome, NT: neural tubules. Bar, 0.5 μm.

MORPHOLOGIC CHARACTERISTICS OF PRIMARY CULTURE NEURONS

Dissociated cerebral cortical neurons were obtained from the neopallium of STD:ddy strain mouse fetuses by trypsin treatment (Ohkuma et al., 1986). Primary culture cerebral cortical neurons used in this study showed bipolar or pyramidal shapes with neuronal processes which formed fine networks and were aggregated during neuronal growth in vitro. Transmission electron microscopic studies revealed the formation of synaptic contacts which were completed 7 to 10 days after the inoculation (Fig. 1), although incomplete synapses with vesicle-filled boutons but no asymmetric membrane thickening were also observed in neurons cultured for 3 days. These morphologic investigations clearly indicate that cells cultured on polylysine-coated surfaces possess the morphologic characteristics specific for neurons.

In addition, more than 95% of the cells used in this study showed no immunoreactivity to anti-glial fibrillary acidic protein (GFAP), a specific marker for astroglial cells. This result indicates that the contamination of astroglial cells into the cultured neurons is negligible.

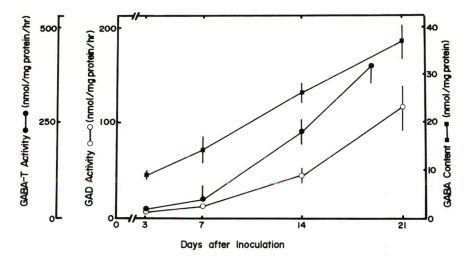

Fig. 2. Developmental pattern of γ-aminobutyric acid (GABA) content and activities of glutamic acid decarboxylase (GAD) and GABA-transaminase (GABA-T) in cerebral cortical neurons in primary culture. Each value represents the mean ± S.E.M. of three to eight separate experiments.

DEVELOPMENT OF GABA METABOLISM AND GABA RECEPTORS IN CULTURED NEURONS

GABA content was determined by HPLC (Ida and Kuriyama, 1983), and the activities of glutamic acid decarboxylase (GAD) (Kimura and Kuriyama, 1975) and GABA-transaminase (GABA-T) (Nishimura et al., 1981), enzymes involved in the metabolism of GABA, were assayed as previously described.

GABA content showed a linear increase during neuronal growth in vitro (Fig. 2). The progressive elevations of GAD and GABA-T activities were also observed with time in culture (Fig. 2). It is noteworthy that the developmental pattern of GABA content paralleled that of GAD activity. On the other hand, it was found that the magnitude of elevation of GABA-T activity was greater than those of GAD activity and GABA content, especially during the third week of primary culture (Fig. 2). The remarkable increase in GABA-T activity during this period may be, at least in part, due to the proliferation of glial cells, since the increase of astroglial cells possessing GABA-T (Hansson, 1984) in cultured neuronal cell preparations during the third week after seeding has been reported (Yu et al., 1984). These developmental patterns of GABA content and activities of GAD and GABA-T are essentially in agreement with those described previously (Yu et

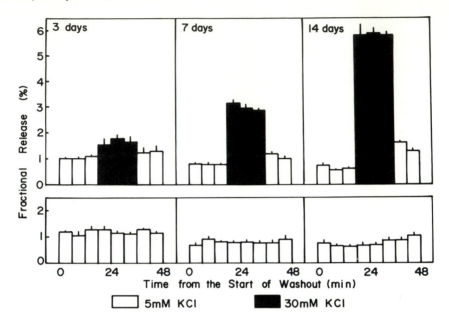

Fig. 3. Developmental pattern of high K⁺-evoked [³H]GABA release from cerebral cortical neurons in primary culture. Cells preloaded with [³H]GABA in the presence of 10^{-4} M aminooxyacetic acid (AOAA), a GABA-T inhibitor, were transferred successively to Krebs-Ringer bicarbonate buffer containing 10^{-4} M AOAA and 5 mM or 30 mM KCl at an interval of 6 min. The medium collected in each interval was then subjected to the measurement of the radioactivity released from cultured neurons. Each value represents the mean ± S.E.M. of three separate experiments.

al., 1984; Larsson et al., 1985). Furthermore, it can be said that primary cultured neurons used in this study definitely possess the biosynthesizing and degrading systems for GABA.

As described above, neuronal cells in primary culture exhibited the formation of synapses at 7 to 10 days after inoculation. Furthermore, it has been found that a progressive increase of the evoked release of preloaded [³H]GABA from these cells indeed occurs, as shown in Figure 3. These results indicate that presynaptic functions also develop during neuronal growth in vitro.

To investigate the development of postsynaptic membrane function of GABA-containing neurons, we investigated the developmental changes of GABA$_A$ receptors in the cells. [³H]Muscimol was used as a radiolabeled ligand for the assay of GABA$_A$ receptor binding. As shown in Table I, the number of GABA$_A$ receptor binding sites (Bmax value) with both high and low affinities showed a tendency to increase with time in culture, although the affinity of receptor to the ligand showed no significant changes. In

TABLE I. Developmental Changes of Kinetic Parameters for [³H]Muscimol and [³H]Flunitrazepam Binding to Particulate Fractions of Mouse Cerebral Cortical Neurons in Primary Culture[a]

| | [³H]Muscimol | | | | [³H]Flunitrazepam | |
| | High affinity | | Low affinity | | | |
	K_d (nM)	B_{max} (fmol/mg protein)	K_d (nM)	B_{max} (fmol/mg protein)	K_d (nM)	B_{max} (fmol/mg protein)
7 Days	76.3 ± 13.5	345 ± 53	497.9 ± 51.5	803 ± 29	1.27 ± 0.27	970 ± 91.7
14 Days	77.1 ± 10.4	525 ± 68	564.2 ± 71.9	1,290 ± 65	1.05 ± 0.01	1,240 ± 80.8

[a]Mean ± S.E.M. of four to six separate experiments.

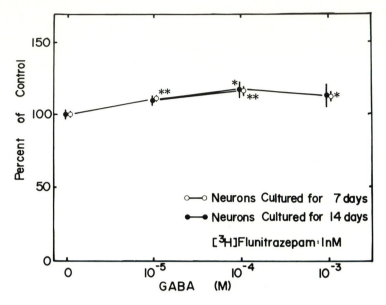

Fig. 4. Developmental pattern of the enhancement of [³H]flunitrazepam ([³H]FLN) binding by GABA in cerebral cortical neurons in primary culture. Each value is expressed as percentage of control and represents the mean ± S.E.M. of 4 separate experiments. The control value for [³H]FLN binding to particulate fractions obtained from neurons cultured for 7 and 14 days in the absence of GABA were 326.6 ± 7.8 and 411.7 ± 26.3 fmol/mg protein, respectively. *P < 0.05, **P < 0.02.

addition, [³H]muscimol binding was inhibited by bicuculline, a GABA$_A$ antagonist, in a dose-dependent manner. These developmental patterns of GABA$_A$ receptors have been found to be similar to those found in developing mammalian brain in vivo (Coyle and Enna, 1976; Enna et al., 1976).

It is well known that GABA$_A$ receptor forms a functional complex with benzodiazepine (BZP) receptor and Cl⁻ ionophore (Olsen, 1981). In this study, we also examined the developmental changes of BZP receptor using [³H]flunitrazepam ([³H]FLN) as a radiolabeled ligand. The developmental pattern of the binding of [³H]FLN, a ligand specific to the central type of BZP receptor, was essentially identical to that of [³H]muscimol binding. Namely, it was found that the Bmax value showed an increase without changing its affinity (Table I). Moreover, it is noteworthy that the enhancement of [³H]FLN binding by GABA has been observed not only in neurons cultured for 14 days but also in 7 day-old neurons in culture (Fig. 4). These results indicate that the functional coupling between GABA$_A$ receptor and BZP receptor is achieved at an early stage of neuronal development.

On the other hand, the binding of [³H]Ro 5-4864, a ligand binding

TABLE II. Developmental Changes of Kinetic Parameters for [³H]Dihydroalprenolol (DHA) Binding to Particulate Fractions Obtained From Cerebral Cortical Neurons in Primary Culture[a]

	[³H]DHA binding	
	Kd (nM)	B_{max} (fmol/mg protein)
7 Days	0.50 ± 0.06	32.55 ± 6.36
14 Days	0.54 ± 0.16	52.33 ± 7.11

[a]Mean ± S.E.M. of four separate experiments.

specifically to the peripheral type of BZP receptor, to the particulate fraction obtained from cultured neurons was not detected in the present study, as has been previously reported (Bender and Hertz, 1984; Syapin et al., 1985). These results strongly suggest that the BZP receptor detected in the neuronal cell membrane may be of the central type.

DEVELOPMENT OF A CYCLIC AMP GENERATING SYSTEM COUPLED WITH β-RECEPTORS IN CULTURED NEURONS

It is well established that the β-receptor is coupled with adenylate cyclase in various tissues including that of the CNS. Adenylate cyclase sensitive to neurotransmitters and hormones has been detected recently in both dissociated neurons (Breen et al., 1978; Chneiweiss et al., 1984, 1985) and astroglial cells (Ebersolt et al., 1981a, b; McCarthy and De Vellis, 1978; Van Calker et al., 1980). Therefore, we have investigated the development of the β-receptor/adenylate cyclase system in primary cultured neuronal cells.

The developmental pattern of the β-adrenergic receptor in these cells was examined using [³H]dihydroalprenolol ([³H]DHA) as a radiolabeled ligand. The number of [³H]DHA binding sites (Bmax) showed a progressive increase during neuronal growth in vitro, while the affinity of the receptor did not show any noticeable changes (Table II). The binding of [³H]DHA to the particulate fraction from cultured neurons was dose-dependently inhibited by propranolol and isoproterenol, β-receptor antagonist and agonist, respectively. Similar developmental changes in the β-receptor of the brain in vivo have been reported (Harden et al., 1977; Smith et al., 1980; Pittman et al., 1980).

The activity of adenylate cyclase coupled with β-receptor was also examined by a pulse-labeling procedure using [¹⁴C]adenine as previously described (Shimizu et al., 1969), and the [¹⁴C]cyclic AMP formed was determined by thin layer chromatograph (Keirns et al., 1974). Both basal and isoproterenol-stimulated adenylate cyclase activities showed a parallel elevation during neuronal growth in vitro (Fig. 5). The ratio of adenylate

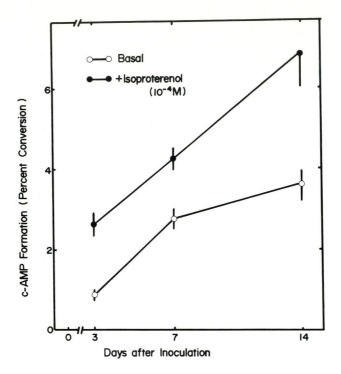

Fig. 5. Developmental pattern of basal and isoproterenol-stimulated cyclic AMP formations (% conversion) in cerebral cortical neurons in primary culture. The formation of [^{14}C]cyclic AMP was measured by the pulse labeling. Each value represents the mean ± S.E.M. of four to eight separate experiments.

cyclase activity found in 14-day-old neurons to that in neurons cultured for 7 days was approximately 2.0. This value was basically identical to the ratio found in the numbers of [^{3}H]DHA binding sites detected in neurons grown in vitro for 14 and 7 days. In addition, it was found that GppNHp-, NaF-, and forskolin-stimulated adenylate cyclase activities determined using [^{3}H]ATP as substrate also showed progressive increases during neuronal development in vitro (Fig. 6).

The above results clearly indicate that primary cultured neurons possess a cyclic AMP generating system coupled with β-adrenergic receptors. These results also strongly suggest that several subunits consisting of the cyclic AMP generating system such as adenylate cyclase and GTP binding protein may also develop in these neurons simultaneously with the development of the β-receptor.

Inspite of these findings, several investigators have suggested that β-receptors and catalytic sites in the brain develop independently in vivo

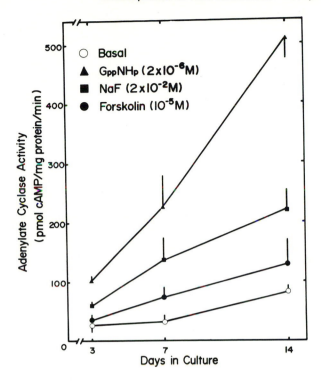

Fig. 6. Developmental pattern of basal, GppNHp-stimulated, NaF-stimulated, and forskolin-stimulated adenylate cyclase activities in particulate fractions obtained from primary cultured neurons. Each value represents the mean ± S.E.M. of five to six separate experiments.

(Harden and McCarthy, 1982). This discrepancy in the developmental pattern of adenylate cyclase coupled with β-adrenergic receptors found in primary cultured neurons and brain in vivo may be due to the presence of glial cells in the brain in vivo, since glial cells which possess a cyclic AMP generating system proliferate and mature during the third week after delivery (Pope, 1978).

DEVELOPMENT OF A TAURINE BIOSYNTHESIZING SYSTEM IN CULTURED NEURONS

Taurine is a highly concentrated amino acid in the CNS, but its exact functional role in the brain has not been elucidated (Kuriyama, 1980). The biochemical mechanisms underlying the well-known postmortem decline of taurine content have been recently clarified (Agrawal et al., 1966; Oja and Piha, 1966).

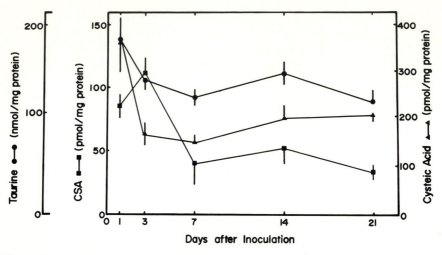

Fig 7.   Developmental pattern of taurine, cysteine sulfinic acid (CSA), and cysteic acid (CA) contents in mouse cerebral cortical neurons in primary culture. Each value represents the mean ± S.E.M. of three to eight separate experiments.

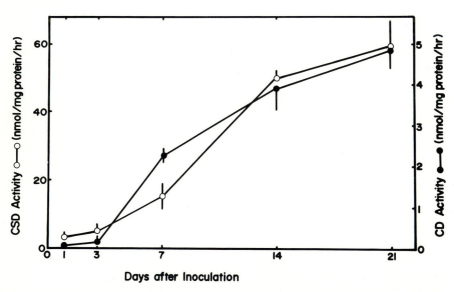

Fig. 8.   Developmental pattern of cysteine sulfinic acid decarboxylase (CSD) and cysteine dioxygenase (CD) activities in mouse cerebral cortical neurons in primary culture. Each value represents the mean ± S.E.M. of four to five separate experiments.

In neuron growth in vitro, the taurine content as well as cysteic acid (CA) and cysteine sulfinic acid (CSA) content, metabolic intermediates converted from cysteine, were found to be decreased, especially during the first week after inoculation, which corresponds to the perinatal stage in age-matched mice in vivo (Fig. 7). These results suggests that the developmental decline in taurine, CA, and CSA contents found in brain grown in vivo may be attributed to the decline in neuronal cells, although possible participation of non-neuronal cells, such as glial cells, may be involved.

In contrast to the developmental decline of taurine and its metabolic intermediates, the activities of enzymes such as cysteine sulfinic acid decarboxylase and cysteine dioxygenase, both of which are involved in taurine biosynthesis from cysteine, showed a progressive elevation during neuronal development in vitro (Fig. 8). These changes in activities were essentially similar to those found in developing brain in vivo (Agrawal et al., 1971; Misra and Olney, 1966). These results suggest that the developmental elevation in taurine biosynthesizing systems observed in brain in vivo may also be attributed, at least in part, to the developmental changes in neuronal cells.

CONCLUSIONS

In the present study, we have demonstrated that primary cultured neurons that developed synaptic contacts possess not only GABA-metabolizing systems but also $GABA_A$ receptors functionally coupled with BZP receptors. The content of GABA and the activities of GAD and GABA-T in these cells also show a progressive increase with time of incubation. Furthermore, $GABA_A$ and BZP receptors in these neurons showed a progressive increase in the number of binding sites without changing Km values. Similar developmental patterns of β-adrenergic receptors were also found in developing neurons in vitro. These β-adrenergic receptors were also found to be coupled with adenylate cyclase, which exhibited increased activity in parallel with that in β-adrenergic receptor binding sites. On the other hand, these primary cultured neurons have been shown to possess metabolic developmental patterns of neuroactive compounds such as GABA, taurine, and cyclic AMP, similar to those found in developing brain in vivo.

Since these primary cultured neurons exhibit progressive development not only of receptor binding capacity but also functional coupling of receptors with intracellular effector systems, it has been concluded that these cells are useful experimental tools for analyzing the developmental characteristics of various neurotransmitter receptors in the brain. These cells may also be useful for investigating the effects of various modulating factors of the CNS, such as nutritional deficiencies, and the application of centrally acting drugs on the metabolic development and function of cerebral neurons.

ACKNOWLEDGMENTS

This work was supported in part by research grants (No. 59480120 and 61219020, 1986) from the Ministry of Education and Culture, Japan.

REFERENCES

Agrawal HC, Davis JM, Himwich WA (1966): Postnatal changes in free amino acid pool of rat brain. J Neurochem 13:607–615.

Agrawal HC, Davison AN, Kaczmarek LK (1971): Subcellular distribution of taurine and cysteine sulfinate decarboxylase in developing rat brain. Biochem J 122:759–763.

Bender AS, Hertz L (1984): Flunitrazepam binding to intact and homogenized astrocytes and neurons in primary culture. J Neurochem 43:1319–1327.

Breen GAM, McGinnis JF, De Vellis J (1978): Modulation of the hydrocortisone induction of glycerol phosphate dehydrogenase by N^6, $O^{2'}$-dibutyryl cyclic AMP, norepinephrine and isobutylmethylxanthine in rat brain cell cultures. J Biol Chem 253:2554–2562.

Chneiweiss H, Prochiantz A, Glowinski J, Premont J (1984): Biogenic amine-sensitive adenylate cyclases in primary culture of neuronal and glial cells from mesencephalon. Brain Res 302:363–370.

Chneiweiss H, Glowinski J, Premont J (1985): Modulation by monoamines of somatostatin-sensitive adenylate cyclase on neuronal and glial cells from the mouse brain in primary cultures. J Neurochem 44:1825–1831.

Coyle JT, Enna SJ (1976): Neurochemical aspects of the ontogenesis of GABAergic neurons in the rat brain. Brain Res 111:119–133.

Ebersolt C, Perez M, Bockaert J (1981a): α_1 and α_2 adrenergic receptors in mouse brain astrocytes from primary cultures. J Neurosci Res 6:643–652.

Ebersolt C, Perez M, Vassent G, Bockaert J (1981b): Characteristics of the β_1 and β_2 adrenergic-sensitive adenylate cyclases in glial cell primary cultures and their comparison with α_2-adrenergic sensitive adenylate cyclase of meningeal cells. Brain Res 213:151–161.

Enna SJ, Yamamura HI, Snyder SH (1976): Development of muscarinic cholinergic and GABA receptor bindings in chick embryo brain. Brain Res 101:177–183.

Hansson E (1984): Enzyme activities of monoamine oxidase, catechol-O-methyltransferase and γ-aminobutyric acid transaminase in primary astroglial cultures and adult rat brain from different brain regions. Neurochem Res 9:45–57.

Harden TK, McCarthy KD (1982): Identification of the beta adrenergic receptor subtype on astroglia purified from rat brain. J Pharmacol Exp Ther 222:600–605.

Harden TK, Wolfe BB, Sporn JR, Perkins JP, Molinoff PB (1977): Ontogeny of β-adrenergic receptors in rat cerebral cortex. Brain Res 125:99–108.

Harik SI, Sharma VK, Wetherbee JR, Warren RH, Banerjee SP (1981): Adrenergic and cholinergic receptors of cerebral microvessels. J Cerebral Blood Flow Metab 1:329–338.

Hauser K, Balcar VJ, Bernasconi R (1980): Development of GABA neurons in dissociated cell culture of rat cerebral cortex. Brain Res Bull 5(Suppl 2):37–41.

Henn FA, Anderson DJ, Rustad DG (1976): Glial contamination of synaptosomal fractions. Brain Res 101:341–344.

Ida S, Kuriyama K (1983): Simultaneous determination of cysteine sulfinic acid and cysteic acid in rat brain by high-performance liquid chromatography. Anal Biochem 130:95–101.

Keirns JJ, Wheeler MA, Bitensky MW (1974): Isolation of cyclic AMP and cyclic GMP by thin-layer chromatography. Application to assay of adenylate cyclase, guanylate cyclase and cyclic nucleotide phosphodiesterase. Anal Biochem 61:336–348.

Kimura H, Kuriyama K (1975): A new microassay method for L-glutamic acid decarboxylase activity. Jpn J Pharmacol 25:189–195.

Kobayashi H, Memo M, Spano PF, Trabucci M (1981): Identification of β-adrenergic receptor binding sites in rat brain microvessels, using [^{125}I]iodohydroxybenzylpindolol. J Neurochem 36:1383–1388.

Kuriyama K (1980): Taurine as a neuromodulator. Fed Proc 39:2680–2684.

Larsson OM, Drejer J, Kvamme E, Svenneby G, Hertz L, Schousboe A (1985): Ontogenic development of glutamate and GABA metabolizing enzymes in cultured cerebral cortex interneurons and in cerebral cortex in vivo. Int J Dev Neurosci 3:177–185.

McCarthy KD, De Vellis J (1978): Alpha-adrenergic receptor modulation of beta-adrenergic, adenosine and prostaglandin E increased adenosine 3':5'-cyclic monophosphate levels in primary cultures of glia. J Cyclic Nucleotide Res 4:15–26.

Misra CH, Olney JW (1975): Cysteine oxidase in brain. Brain Res 97:117–126.

Nishimura C, Ida S, Kuriyama K (1981): Alteration of GABA system in frog retina following short light and dark adaptation—a quantitative comparison with retinal taurine. Brain Res 219:433–438.

Oja SS, Piha RS (1966): Changes in the concentration of free amino acids in the rat brain during postnatal development. Life Sci 5:865–870.

Ohkuma S, Tomono S, Tanaka Y, Kuriyama K, Mukainaka T (1986): Development of taurine biosynthesizing system in cerebral cortical neurons in primary culture. Int J Dev Neurosci 4:383–395.

Olsen RW (1981): GABA-benzodiazepine-barbiturate receptor interactions. J Neurochem 37:1–13.

Pittman RN, Minneman KP, Molinoff PB (1980): Ontogeny of β$_1$ and β$_2$-receptors in rat cerebellum and cerebral cortex. Brain Res 188:357–368.

Pope A (1978): Neuroglia: Quantitative aspects. In Schoffeniels E, Frank G, Hertz L, Tower DB (eds): "Dynamic Properties of Glial Cells." Oxford: Pergamon Press, pp 13–20.

Shimizu H, Daly JW, Creveling CR (1969): A radioisotopic method for measuring the formation of adenosine 3', 5'-cyclic monophosphate in incubated slices in brain. J Neurochem 16:1609–1619.

Smith RM, Patel AJ, Kingsbury AE, Hunt A, Balázs R (1980): Effects of thyroid state on brain development: β-Adrenergic receptors and 5'-nucleotidase activity. Brain Res 198:375–387.

Syapin PJ, Cole R, De Vellis J, Noble EP (1985): Benzodiazepine binding characteristics of embryonic rat brain neurons grown in culture. J Neurochem 45:1797–1801.

Tardy M, Costa MF, Rolland B, Fages C, Gonnard P (1981): Benzodiazepine receptors on primary cultures of mouse astrocytes. J Neurochem 36:1587–1589.

Van Calker D, Müller M, Hamprecht B (1980): Regulation by secretin, vasoactive intestinal peptide, and somatostatin of cyclic AMP accumulation in cultured brain cells. Proc Natl Acad Sci USA 77:6907–6911.

Yu ACH, Hertz E, Hertz L (1984): Alterations in uptake and release rates for GABA, glutamate, and glutamine during biochemical maturation of highly purified cultures of cerebral cortical neurons, a GABAergic preparation. J Neurochem 42:951–960.

SECTION IV: CORRELATIONS OF BRAIN DEVELOPMENT AND MALNUTRITION

Current Topics in Nutrition and Disease, Volume 16
Basic and Clinical Aspects of Nutrition and Brain Development,
pages 271–285
© 1987 Alan R. Liss, Inc.

Subtle Defects in the Regulation of the Free Amino Acid Balance in Friedreich Ataxia: A Relative Deficiency of Histidine Combined With a Mild But Chronic Hyperammonemia?

N. M. van Gelder, M. Roy, F. Bélanger, S. Paris, and A. Barbeau

Clinical Research Institute of Montréal, Department of Neurobiology, Montréal, Québec H2W 1R7, Canada

INTRODUCTION

Previous amino acid studies on Friedreich ataxia patients suggested but did not definitely establish defects in tissue retention and/or excretion mechanisms for certain amino acids. Determinations by Lemieux et al. (1976, 1978) of amino acid profiles in CSF and plasma as well as of renal clearance rates, particularly with respect to taurine, raised the possibility of abnormalities for this amino acid. Further investigations pointed to disturbances of valine and glycine (hippuric acid) metabolism (Barbeau, 1982; Barbeau et al., 1982; Bertraud et al., 1982).

In an attempt to more clearly define these data, a study was undertaken with Friedreich ataxia patients to examine plasma amino acid concentrations over a 5-hr period following a single oral dose of a particular amino acid. A special effort was made to select control subjects who closely matched the patients in terms of age and sex; they also were paired in time with the patients on or near the same day. As will be reported here, using this protocol, no major differences were observed between healthy individuals and ataxia patients, even though many of these patients are no longer ambulatory and have serious cardiac disease. Not only was it surprising that the generally sedentary condition of the patients was not reflected by altered plasma amino acid profiles when compared to healthy, active, and relatively young (average age 28 years) subjects, but over the period of 1 year these profiles varied markedly in the same subject, and especially in the ataxia patient. This, despite the fact that in the control as well as in the patient groups the trial conditions were standardized as much as possible—the same personnel took samples, fasting for 18 hr, processing of blood to yield plasma, etc. Variability in amino acid analysis of duplicate blood samples did not exceed 7% and thus could not explain such fluctuations.

From these and previous data (van Gelder, 1981), it is becoming increasingly evident that for each individual, and even a family or species, the plasma amino acid profile is quite characteristic and is difficult to perturb. It also suggests that such profiles are determined by a combination of factors, including most importantly, the genetic influences which establish a typical plasma amino acid pattern by balancing absorption in the alimentary tract, renal excretion rates, and cellular metabolism (Visek, 1984). When an individual is presented with an (abnormal) amino acid load, the resulting plasma increases are predictably transient and more determined by the physiochemical properties of the amino acid than by temporal fluctuations in dietary habits or even large and chronic changes in the health status not specifically associated with a genetic defect in the metabolism of an amino acid. This led us to re-examine previous amino acid data from Friedreich ataxia studies, choosing as an "internal standard" an essential amino acid (valine) which reflects, on the one hand, these genetic directives but which, on the other hand, may possibly mirror long-term variations in dietary habits. Alterations in digestive absorption and/or renal handling as a consequence of disease, as well as amino acid assimilation into proteins, should also influence the free level of this amino acid.

Valine is an essential amino acid with a ubiquitous distribution in most diets and protein structures, while this branched chain amino acid is also ketogenic (Barbeau et al., 1982). The plasma levels of this amino acid will, therefore, provide some indication of the in vivo energy balance, in addition to protein metabolism and the other parameters cited. As will be seen, when the concentrations of the other amino acids are expressed relative to the valine concentration (taken as 1), very consistent amino acid patterns emerge, reflecting the relative abundance of free amino acids in specific tissue types and highlighting the metabolic difference between a healthy individual and one suffering from a serious genetic neurological degenerative disease.

METHODS
Protocol

A total of 23 healthy control subjects, 12 males (28 ± 7 years) and 11 females (28 ± 7 years), were compared with 16 Friedreich ataxia patients (9 males, 26 ± 4 years and 7 females, 26 ± 7 years). The subjects were requested to start fasting at 20:00 hours on the evening before the test. The following morning, subjects took a single oral dose of an amino acid, and four blood samples were subsequently drawn by venipuncture over a 5-hr period. Aside from non-sugared tea, the subjects did not receive any sustenance, and they remained reposed. As much as possible, for each patient a matching control individual was either tested the same day, a closely preceding day, or within a few days thereafter.

On a number of occasions, the same patient or control subject volunteered to participate in more than one amino acid loading trial. For that reason, several baseline fasting values for plasma amino acid concentrations were obtained from the same individual over a period of 8–12 months. In each such instance, the final values for amino acid concentrations assigned to a single individual represent the average of all these amino acid determinations; in the data presentations (Figs. 1–3 and Table I), N refers to the number of subjects and not to the number of blood samples.

Patients

The diagnosis of Friedreich ataxia in the 16 patients who volunteered for this study was based on strict criteria established by Geoffroy et al. (1976). Only one of the 16 was still ambulatory at the time of the trials; the remaining 15 patients had been confined to a wheelchair for 0.5–16 yr (mean = 6 yr). In ten patients for whom such data were available, varyious degrees of cardiomyopathy were present. Two patients demonstrated, respectively, a slight and a very elevated total bilirubin value, but bilirubin abnormalities in Friedreich ataxia have been reported to be a probable occurrence (Barbeau et al., 1976). Similarly, even though in only one patient clinically defined diabetes mellitus was diagnosed, some disturbance of insulin metabolism may be present in most Friedreich ataxia patients, whether or not they exhibit clinical or chemical signs of this type of diabetes (Shapcott et al., 1976). Finally, none of the patients in this group had any clinical or biochemical evidence for possible impaired digestive, hepatic, or renal function.

Blood Processing

Each venous blood sample (10 ml) was taken with a syringe already containing EDTA and stored on ice for the duration of the 5-hr blood sampling period. Following the last sampling, they were all centrifuged at 1,000g for 15 min, and the serum was then subjected for 20 min to centrifugation at 20,000g to remove platelets. Water was added, 1 or 2 ml, to 1 ml plasma and placed in a boiling water bath for 20 min to coagulate soluble proteins. After cooling to 4°C, the volume was adjusted to 10 times the original plasma volume with water. Following homogenization and centrifugation for 60 min at 30,000g, the deproteinized plasma was passed through a 0.22-μ millipore filter, 10 times concentrated (v/v) amino acid buffer was added, and the solutions were stored at −20°C until analysis.

Amino Acid Analysis

A ninhydrin, postcolumn derivitization technique was employed, using HPLC pumps and a two-buffer system consisting of lithium hydroxide

(0.2 N) and lithium citrate buffer (0.15N). At a constant temperature of 43.5°C, total elution time up to GABA was 60 min. The sensitivity of the system now allows detection of 50 pmoles of an amino acid (see below), and reproducibility of duplicate standard samples was ± 7%. The standard used for plasma amino acid analysis was a commercially available "physiological fluid" 2.5-μmole amino acid mixture, modified to contain a 5 to 1 ratio of glutamine to glutamate and a 2 to 1 ratio of glycine to alanine.

At the time of this study, the low glutamic acid concentrations relative to glutamine in the plasma samples and an inefficient column heater did not allow for an accurate estimate of the glutamate values (15–20% duplicate variability), even though the peaks were well separated. Although values represent roughly 4–7 μmole/100 ml plasma, they have not been reported in Table I; similarly and for the same reason phosphoserine and phosphoethanolamine values are also omitted. (Improvements in the analysis method have now eliminated these deficiencies, but they came too late for this report.)

TABLE I. Free Amino Acids in Serum μmole/100 ml Plasma of Control and Friedreich Ataxia Subjects

| | Male | | Female | | Percentage normal fluctuations[b] |
	Control (12)[a]	F.A. (9)	Control (11)	F.A. (7)	
TAU	5.04	4.58	5.09	4.95	15
THR	9.21	7.71	9.32	10.06	30
SER	8.90	7.88	8.99	9.76	15
GLY	23.10	20.83	23.18	21.19	31
ALA	34.36	37.21	34.02	39.14	24
VAL	22.49	23.52	22.31	19.19	17
GLN	51.65	49.29	51.80	51.47	13

[a]Values in parentheses = number of subjects. To obtain concentrations relative to valine (Tables II and III), divide all values by valine concentration.
[b]S.D./mean.

RESULTS

With respect to possible differences between Friedreich ataxia patients and comparable control subjects, baseline plasma amino acid concentrations in the two groups were very similar (Table I); the values obtained are comparable to those reported by Lemieux et al. (1976), whose study covered a larger population. Nevertheless, despite this lack of statistical divergence, it was noteworthy that repeated blood sampling from several patients, 2–4 times over a period of 1 year, showed a wider fluctuation in amino acid

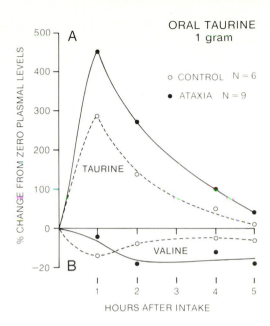

Fig. 1.   Taurine and valine changes in plasma following a 1-g oral dose of taurine. Note scale change from A to B (bottom). These and curves in Figures 2 and 3 have been fitted by eye estimation. At highest divergences between control and ataxia values, significance of Student's t test was 0.05 or better. Other plasma amino acids measured did not change significantly from their levels before the trial began (zero plasma levels). N = number of subjects.

values than those seen in control subjects (not shown). This wider variation in the ataxia group may be due to long-term influences of variability in the diet, as patients feel better or worse during the year, or it may indeed reflect a greater instability in the metabolic regulation of amino acid patterns, inherent to the disease process. The latter possibility is supported by the results obtained when patients or control subjects were subjected to selective amino acid loading. Ataxia patients appeared to respond to these amino acid loads in a manner which, while in general similar to control subjects, did reveal differences.

Following ingestion of 1 g taurine under fasting conditions, seven out of nine patients exhibited peak plasma taurine concentrations higher than the most elevated concentrations measured in control subjects (Fig. 1). This must reflect enhanced digestive absorption in patients since urinary excretion increases dramatically following a taurine load and, apparently, in proportion to the rise in plasma concentrations (Filla et al., 1979). In addition, the depression in plasma valine levels seen in both groups tended to be more accentuated in the patients. For both groups, taurine concentrations returned

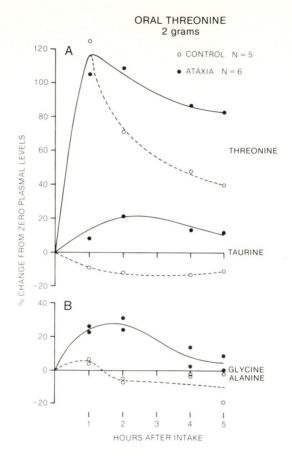

Fig. 2.   Oral threonine administration to Friedreich ataxia patients results in a slower plasma clearance of the amino acid, an increase of taurine in all six patients rather than a slight fall in plasma levels as seen in five control subjects, and a more pronounced and persistent rise in plasma glycine and alanine. N = number of subjects.

to base values by 5 hr, whereas valine levels remained below the initial concentrations, especially in the patients.

In contrast to the 300–400% increase of taurine, twice the amount of threonine did not elevate plasma levels by much more than double the initial concentrations (Fig. 2). Peak levels in patients and control subjects were identical, but in the patients these high levels seemed to persist much longer. Also, in all ataxic individuals, taurine, glycine, and alanine concentrations increased 20–30% in the first hour; taurine levels stayed elevated during the entire 5-hr period, but glycine and alanine had returned to normal by that time even though threonine concentrations had still not diminished much. In

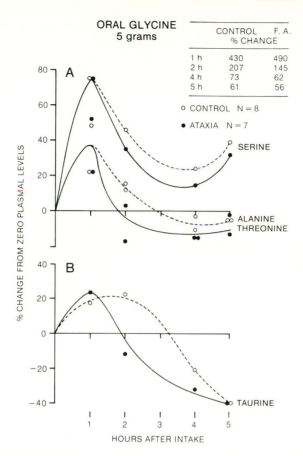

ORAL GLYCINE 5 grams	CONTROL % CHANGE	F. A.
1 h	430	490
2 h	207	145
4 h	73	62
5 h	61	56

○ CONTROL N = 8

● ATAXIA N = 7

Fig. 3. A 5-g glycine load in Friedreich ataxia patients (table, top right) causes plasma increases of serine, alanine, threonine, and taurine which are almost identical to those seen in control subjects. Only the 2-hr percentage change of taurine (B) differs significantly (P = 0.04) from control subjects. However, for all amino acids mentioned, patients demonstrate a very consistent accelerated decrease from peak plasma levels following a rise in glycine, even though urinary excretion of these amino acids appears either diminished (glycine) or unchanged (see Table II and Lemieux et al., 1976). These data and opposite changes for some of these same amino acids when plasma threonine is high (Fig. 2) indicate that plasma clearance rates are under metabolic control and do not simply reflect urinary excretion patterns. N = number of subjects.

control subjects, taurine, glycine, and alanine tended to decrease rather than increase following threonine loading, and these changes were less pronounced. In both control and ataxia patients, glutamine rose to 60% above resting concentrations during the first 2 hr and then decreased to normal within 5 hr.

In order to obtain an elevation of plasma concentrations in the same range as that obtained following 1 g of taurine ingestion, 3–5 g of glycine needed to be administered. The concentration changes for the patients and control subjects were practically identical (see table insert, Fig. 3), as were those for serine, which also increased significantly in response to the glycine load (Fig. 3). Conversely, the oral intake of 1 g serine (not shown) did not force a change in plasma glycine levels; on the other hand, serine levels never rose by more than 40%. Glycine loading also caused initial increases in alanine, threonine, and taurine, but with the persistence of the high glycine concentrations, the levels of these amino acids tended to become depressed (Fig. 3). This depression consistently occurred earlier in patients than in control subjects.

These data indicate that changes in the plasma concentration of one amino acid influence those of others and, moreover, that patients respond somewhat differently than control subjects to such changes. The question thus arises as to the significance of previously reported differences between healthy subjects and Friedreich ataxia patients, with respect to palsma amino acids or the free amino acids in other tissues. For reasons stated in the Introduction, valine was selected to serve as an internal "reference" amino acid, against which the levels of other free amino acids can be expressed in terms of their relative abundance.

When the data obtained by Lemieux et al. (1976, 1978) is expressed in this manner, it is seen that for CSF, plasma, and urine, a characteristic amino acid pattern emerges, for each of the body fluids (Table II). In additon, if more than a 30% change from the norm is considered to exceed a chance fluctuation (see Table 1), one observes that patients and control subjects exhibit remarkably similar plasma amino acid profiles relative to valine concentrations. The two exceptions are ornithine and histidine which decreased by approximately 50% in the ataxia patients. A comparable decrease of histidine excretion in urine is observed, but ornithine excretion proportionaly to valine remained unchanged. At the same time, two products required to maintain adequate body reserves of histidine, carnosine (histidine-beta-alanine) and beta-alanine, are increased in urine of ataxic individuals. These data indicate that, relative to the other free amino acids, histidine availability for tissue needs may be severely limited in Friedreich ataxia. The excretion of glutamic acid and its metabolities, and of glycine, are also selectively decreased by 30–50%.

In CSF (Table II), the doubling of the valine concentration on first examination explains the relative decrease of many of the other amino acids. Yet, this decrease appears more selective for certain amino acids than for others. For example, threonine, together with serine and glycine are more decreased than alanine (van Gelder and Drujan, 1980), and so are isoleucine

TABLE II. Free Amino Acid Abundance in CSF, Plasma, and Urine Relative to Valine (= 1) in Control and Friedreich Ataxia Subjects

	CSF		Plasma		Urine	
	Control (7)	F.A (14)	Control (37)	F.A. (38)	Control (24)	F.A. (19)
THR	1.50	0.94 ↓	0.59	0.55	5.11	4.97
SER	2.26	0.94 ↓	0.63	0.56	7.67	8.46
GLY	0.66	0.32 ↓	1.22	0.91	70.49	38.32
ALA	1.58	1.30	1.56	1.55	10.45	9.75
MET	0.17	0.08 ↓	0.09	0.08	0.27	0.44
ILE	0.46	0.37	0.31	0.29	0.57	0.65
LEU	1.09	0.83	0.60	0.52	1.48	1.12
TYR	0.73	0.62	0.26	0.23	3.10	3.22
PHE	0.77	0.54 ↓	0.28	0.21	1.78	1.40
TAU	0.96	0.51 ↓	0.23	0.21	27.53	29.24
GLU	5.76	3.95 ↓	0.84	0.67	4.90	3.63
GLN	22.60	8.95 ↓	2.49	2.59	11.70	7.50 ↓
ASP	0.28	0.19 ↓	0.09	0.05	4.54	2.92 ↓
ORN	0.46	0.43	0.44	0.22 ↓	4.98	4.67
LYS	1.87	1.63	0.82	0.71	3.18	2.30
HIS	0.89	0.80	0.43	0.28 ↓	27.33	16.84 ↓
ARG	1.77	1.36	0.33	0.26	n.d.	0.16
(H)CAR	0.25	0.22			1.86	2.58 ↑
BALA			n.d.	Trace	0.48	2.06 ↑
BAIB			n.d.	n.d.	2.68	3.22
VAL	9.3	17.5	19.27	20.87	1.72	3.13
	μmole/1,000 ml[a]		μmole/100 ml[b]		μmole/min/1.73 m[2c]	

[a]Data from Lemieux et al., 1978.
[b]Data from Lemieux et al., 1976.
[c]Data from Lemieux et al., 1976.

and phenylalanine when compared, respectively, with leucine and tyrosine. The basic amino acids remain constant with reference to valine, while glutamine and other products of the glutamic acid cycle, combined with taurine (van Gelder, 1982), do not follow the rise in valine. These amino acids thus demonstrate a more pronounced decrease relative to valine and several other amino acids than might be anticipated if the phenomenon were due to generalized tissue destruction or breakdown of the CFS-blood barriers in ataxia patients. The observation rather suggests a specific disturbance of metabolic events within the CNS which in part determine CSF amino acid composition.

In order to establish whether changes in the CSF of ataxia patients are in fact a reflection of some type of (degenerating) CNS changes, the amino acid data of Huxtable et al. (1979) was also re-expressed relative to valine (Table III; 35% plus change considered beyond chance). As can be observed, cerebellar hemispheres (CH) of Friedreich ataxia patients show a very pronounced overabundance of taurine and glutamine in their tissue. Moreover, with the exception of the inferior olivary nucleus (ION), this relative taurine increase also exists in other structures of cerebellar-brainstem regions. Furthermore, instead of an elevated glutamine level and no change in glutamic and aspartic acids, as is found in the dorsal root ganglion (DRG) in addition to the cerebellar hemispheres, the anterior and posterior cerebellar vermis (ACV, PCV), the inferior olivary nucleus as well as the dentate nucleus (DN) all exhibit decreases in glutamic acid and its metabolites, including GABA. The relative loss of the inhibitory amino acid is especially marked in the olivary and dentate nuclei, where glutamic acid decreases are also the most severe. In this connection, it should be stated that an increase of glutamine or a decrease of glutamic acid in the CNS may represent equivalent reflections of the same metabolic process, namely enhanced glutamic acid turnover or release. The observed changes depend on glial configuration and abundance in a particular brain region (van Gelder et al., 1983). The decrease of glutamic acid in combination with taurine and glutamine accumulation in certain CNS regions would seem compatible with the decrease of these same amino acids in CSF (Table II).

Both nuclei and the vermis exhibit a consistent 30–40% relative loss of two essential amino acids threonine and phenylalanine, with isoleucine demonstrating a similar trend (compare CSF, Table II); in the dorsal root ganglion the two amino acids are increased. In general, the ganglion, which undergoes severe involution because of a retrograde degeneration of the peripheral sensory nervous system, shows changes of neutral and essential amino acids which are opposite (increases) to those seen in the cerebellar-brainstem structures. The cerebellar hemispheres seem least affected; except for the pronounced relative increase in taurine and glutamine, most other amino acids are observed to remain in normal balance.

Finally, the internal consistency of the data when expressing amino acid levels relative to valine appear validated by the fact that the patients' absolute valine values compared to the control group can be lower (PCV, CH), similar ACV, DRG, plasma), or higher (ION, DN, CSF, urine). The observed changes in the total amino acid profile appear quite different in the various neural tissues or body fluids and not always in the same direction. It probably signifies that in tissues and body fluids a continuous readjustment of the free amino acid balance occurs, relative to each other, as the level of one or of several amino acids becomes altered. This might be expected when a number of amino acids are co-transported inward or outward together, are required in

TABLE III. Free Amino Acid Abundance in Cerebellar and Brainstem Structures Relative to Valine (= 1) in Control and Friedreich Ataxia Subjects

	PCV[a]		ACV		ION		DN		DRG		CH	
	Control (4)	F.A. (2)	Control (4)	F.A. (2)	Control (3)	F.A. (1)	Control (3)	F.A. (2)	Control (1)	F.A. (1)	Control (4)	F.A. (2)
THR	1.26	0.88 ↓[b]	1.41	0.98 ↓	1.15	0.73 ↓	1.18	0.83 →[c]	0.83	1.16 ◆	1.25	1.26
SER	1.61	1.22	1.72	1.38	1.39	1.49	1.67	1.41	1.02	0.97	1.55	1.68
GLY	2.86	2.21	2.94	2.22	3.11	2.18	2.80	2.24	1.45	2.37 ↑	2.61	3.08
ALA	3.10	2.17	3.36	2.38	3.39	1.92 ↓	2.67	2.42	2.43	3.59 ↑	2.81	3.29
MET	0.53	0.50	0.62	0.63	0.67	0.67	0.50	0.58	0.35	0.51 ↑	0.52	0.63
ILE	0.61	0.53 ◆	0.71	0.25 ↓	0.70	0.47 ↓	0.64	0.45 ◆	0.59	0.70	0.63	0.55
LEU	1.36	1.02	1.59	0.82 ↓	1.29	1.06	1.23	1.05	0.83	1.11	1.33	1.13
TYR	0.68	0.60	0.78	0.75	0.80	0.55	0.70	0.56	0.54	0.97 ↑	0.65	0.97 ↑
PHE	0.81	0.55 ↓	0.91	0.70	0.90	0.42 ↓	0.79	0.46 ↓	0.57	0.89 ↑	0.79	0.84
TAU	2.55	4.10 ↑	2.77	4.27 ↑	1.75	1.98	2.05	3.36 ↑	1.27	1.70 ↑	2.95	9.95 ↑
GLU	16.25	7.84 ↓	13.29	6.87 ↓	9.22	2.61 ↓	10.23	3.96 ↓	2.95	2.62	13.52	11.63
GLN	8.26	8.84	6.19	9.33 ↑	9.87	2.64 ↓	9.38	8.91	0.57	3.43 ↑	7.17	13.11 ↑
ASP	2.27	1.59 ↓	2.48	1.67 ↓	1.22	0.78 ↓	1.85	0.89 ↓	1.02	0.83	2.09	1.97
GABA	2.58	1.64 ↓	2.67	1.62 ↓	1.89	0.54 ↓	4.81	1.46 ↓	n.d.	0.19	1.88	1.92
VAL	0.77	0.58	0.58	0.60	0.54	1.54	0.66	1.04	0.37	0.37	0.75	0.38

(μmole/g wet weight)

[a]PCV, ACV = posterior and anterior cerebellar vermis; ION = inferior olivary nucleus; DN = dentate nucleus; DRG = dorsal root ganglion; CH = cerebellar hemispheres. Data from Huxtable et al., 1979. To obtain absolute concentrations, multiply valine content × relative values (μmole/g wet weight).

[b]Thin arrows = ± 35% difference from control values.

[c]Heavy arrows = ± 30%.

adequate amounts and in precise proportions for protein assimilation, and, for some, represent precursor-product relationships (Smith, 1980).

In practical terms, the comparative amino acid pattern is obtained independent of sample dilution (errors) or whether or not the unit of reference (mg protein, volume) is equivalently valid for different samples. Each amino acid determination generates a defined profile which is distinctive for a tissue type, while at the same time reflecting the metabolic condition at time of sampling.

DISCUSSION

Friedreich ataxia patients respond to a particular amino acid loads by either enhanced absorption or retention of certain amino acids (taurine, threonine, Fig. 2), or the normal response to such amino acid loading appears exaggerated (valine, glycine, alanine, taurine). The differences are subtle but appear real and consistent. In addition, no major deviations in resting plasma amino acid levels were observed in this study, indicating that the patients may be having difficulty maintaining a balanced pattern of free amino acids when they are stressed nutritionally. One obvious reason would be the altered dynamics of muscle activity in the patients, which in healthy individuals is interposed as a metabolic buffer between free amino acids in plasma and their excretion.

Both Visek (1984) and Smith (1980) have emphasized that a comparative amino acid profile rather than absolute values of individual amino acids, may be more significant in terms of determining the tissue needs for amino acids. Such profiles take into account the many interacting metabolic, dietary, genetic, and health factors which eventually establish a tissue-specific free amino pattern. When such comparative profiles are generated from a data base provided by Lemieux et al. (1976, 1978) and Huxtable et al. (1979), using valine as a reference amino acid for reasons outlined in the introduction, internally consistent amino acid abnormalities appear to emerge in Friedreich ataxia patients.

No doubt, this manner of expressing free amino acid data may initially meet with some reluctance, given the accepted practice of presenting such data per unit weight or unit volume. However, considering the enormous variations in tissue composition and water content in different matabolic and disease states, and that volume regulation represents an ongoing, dynamic process, these units of reference are more a convention than an accurate basis for comparison. Moreover, the metabolism of the amino acids is interdependent through many uncontrollable factors such as individual variations of hormonal fluctuations, dietary habits, appetites, alimentary efficiency, health status, and physical activity, to mention only the most obvious. It is perhaps most remarkable that normal fluctuations of average values are not larger than those reported here and in the literature. Only the mature brain seems to escape somewhat from this problem for the obvious reason that its internal free amino acid content is tightly controlled by endogenous metabolism and is far more independent from nutritional factors or environmental conditions.

On the other hand, despite these many natural variables, each individual of a species nevertheless maintains itself in overall metabolic amino acid balance as a consequence of its genetic and evolutionary endowment. The end result is such that in each organ tissue a specific and typical pattern of free amino acids is regulated despite varying conditions. In the adult, as long as this amino acid profile and the relative balance of a free amino acid against the others remains preserved, an absolute decrease of amino acid availability will be less damaging than will be a disequilibrium in the amino acid profile. Increased metabolic (e.g., muscle) catabolism can for a long time compensate for undernutrition (in the adult), but a specific relative deficiency of one amino acid may neither provide the trigger for such generalized catabolism nor be sufficient to maintain an adequate supply of an essential amino acid (Smith, 1980). The observed deviations from the norm in Friedreich ataxia patients may in fact illustrate this point.

Ataxia patients exhibit an overall plasma amino acid spectrum which very closely resembles that of healthy subjects (Bergström et al., 1974). The only exception appears to be ornithine and histidine, which, relative to the other amino acids, are decreased by approximately 50%. This fall in histidine seems matched by decreased histidine excretion in the urine. Ornithine is of course an essential constituent of the liver urea cycle and ammonia detoxification. Histidine has recently been upgraded to represent a "semi" essential amino acid (Lunde et al., 1986; Visek, 1984), especially in the young (Snyderman et al., 1963). A sufficient dietary supply of this amino acid appears needed to maintain a positive nitrogen balance, and its endogenous synthesis entails incorporation of ammonia. Thus, the lowered plasma ornithine (Table II) may reflect increased ammonia levels as a consequence of reduced histidine availability or synthesis relative to other plasma amino acids. Histidine deficiency moreover induces a slower rate of plasma amino acid assimilation (Visek, 1984), as some of the data from the loading tests indeed suggest (Figs. 1–3). One important body reserve of histidine is carnosine in muscle (Visek, 1984), which, however, is also excreted at a higher rate by ataxia subjects, together with its precursor beta-alanine (Table II).

In addition to the relatively large decrease in glycine excretion, these patients also exhibit a diminished urinary output of products related to the glutamine/glutamate cycle which, in the kidney, represents another major control mechanism for ammonia regulation. Quite interestingly, experimental hyperammonemia in animals produces in certain CNS regions an increase in glutamine or a fall in glutamic acid and its products, as can be observed here in the patients (Table III); taurine values increase (Giguère and Butterworth, 1984; Hamberger and Nyström, 1984).

Hence, without overstating the case in view of the very circumstantial evidence, one working hypothesis may be that Friedreich ataxia patients suffer from a chronic insufficiency of histidine relative to other essential amino acids, and perhaps an equally persistent but not so obvious hyperammonemia. Whether the relative loss in the CNS of two essential amino acids—threonine and phenylalanine (possibly isoleucine)—combined with their decreased appearance in the CSF, can be connected to such a metabolic imbalance is certainly not clear. Glial edema and damage might be one explanation.

SUMMARY

The data presented here suggest once again (Barbeau, 1982) that a possible defect exists in the regulatory mechanisms controlling a balanced free amino acid pattern in Friedreich ataxia patients. Potentially, the defect may involve a persistent histidine deficiency which could also be a cause for mild but chronic hyperammonemia. Whether this contributes directly to the course of the disease or whether it is a consequence of the general degenerative process in these patients remains entirely undetermined.

ACKNOWLEDGMENTS

This study was supported by funds provided by the Quebec Cooperative Study of Friedreich's Ataxia. A generous private donation by D. Bloom to N.v.G. is also gratefully acknowledged.

EPILOGUE

It has been largely through the personal and persistent efforts and dedication of Dr. A. Barbeau and Mr. Claude Saint-Jean that in 1975 l'Association Canadienne de l'Ataxie de Friedreich was founded. Today, the program has partially or totally funded studies leading to more than 150 published papers, involving 250 investigators (Barbeau, 1984). A valuable data bank has been created in this manner, which investigators can use to guide their future studies. André Barbeau died on March 9, 1986, too early to see realized his conviction that the cause and the cure for this disease will be found eventually. His colleagues and collaborators intend to continue their efforts to find the scientific information needed to successfully treat this neurological disorder.

One day, the conviction of Dr. André Barbeau will become a reality to serve as a lasting monument to this remarkable neurobiologist.

REFERENCES

Barbeau A (1982): Friedreich's Disease 1982: Etiologic hypotheses. A personal analysis. Can J Neurol Sci 9:243–263.

Barbeau A (1984): The Quebec Cooperative Study of Friedreich's Ataxia: 1974–1984: 10 Years of Research. Can J Neurol Sci 11:646–660.

Barbeau A, Breton G, Lemieux B, Butterworth RF (1976): Bilirubin metabolism–preliminary investigation. Can J Neurol Sci 3:365–372.

Barbeau A, Bertrand M, Bouchard R, Gauthier GL, Bouchard JP (1982): Effect of valine load test on plasma alpha-keto acids in Friedreich Ataxia. Can J Neurol Sci 9:239–242.

Bergström J, Fürst P, Norée LO, Vinnars E (1974): Intracellular free amino acid concentration in human muscle tissue. J Appl Physiol 36:693–697.

Bertrand MJ, Bouchard R, Gauthier GL, Bouchard JP, Barbeau A (1982): Quantitative metabolic profiling of alpha-keto acids in Friedreich's Ataxia. Can J Neurol Sci 9:231–234.

Filla A, Butterworth RF, Barbeau A (1979): Pilot studies on membranes and some transport mechanisms in Friedreich's Ataxia. Can J Neurol Sci 6:285–289.

Geoffroy G, Barbeau A, Breton G, Lemieux B, Aubé M, Léger C, Bouchard JP (1976): Clinical description and roentgenologic evaluation of patients with Friedreich's Ataxia. Can J Neurol Sci 3:279–286.

Giguère JF, Butterworth RF (1984): Amino acid changes in regions of the CNS in relation to function in experimental portal-systemic encephalopathy. Neurochem Res 9:1309–1321.

Hamberger A, Nyström B (1984): Extra- and intracellular amino acids in the hippocampus during development of hepatic encephalopathy. Neurochem Res 9:1181–1192.

Huxtable R, Azari J, Reisine T, Johnson P, Yamamura H, Barbeau A (1979): Regional distribution of amino acids in Friedreich's Ataxia brains. Can J Neurol Sci 6:255–258.

Lemieux B, Barbeau A, Beroniade V, Shapcott D, Breton G, Geoffroy G, Melançon S (1976): Amino acid metabolism in Friedreich's Ataxia. Can J Neurol Sci 3:373–378.

Lemieux B, Giguerre R, Barbeau A, Melançon S, Shapcott D (1978): Taurine in cerebrospinal fluid in Friedreich's Ataxia. Can J Neurol Sci 5:125–129.

Lunde HA, Gjessing LR, Sjaastad O (1986): Homocarnosinosis: Influence of dietary restriction of histidine. Neurochem Res 11:825–838.

Shapcott D, Melançon S, Butterworth RF, Khoury K, Collu R, Breton G, Geoffroy G, Lemieux B, Barbeau A (1976): Glucose and insulin metabolism in Friedreich's Ataxia. Can J Neurol Sci 3:361–364.

Smith RH (1980): Comparative amino acid requirements. Proc Nutr Soc 39:71–78.

Snyderman SE, Boyer A, Roitman E, Holt LE, Prose PH (1963): The histidine requirements of the infant. Pediatrics 31:786–801.

van Gelder NM (1981): The role of taurine and glutamic acid in the epileptic process: A genetic predisposition. Rev Pure Appl Pharmacol Sci 2:293–316.

van Gelder NM (1982): Changed taurine-glutamic acid content and altered nervous tissue cytoarchitecture. Adv Expt Med Biol 139:239–256.

van Gelder NM, Drujan BD (1980): Alterations in the compartmentalised metabolism of glutamic acid with changed cerebral conditions. Brain Res 200:443–455.

van Gelder NM, Siatitsas I, Ménini C, Gloor P (1983): Feline generalized penicillin epilepsy: Changes of glutamic acid and taurine parallel the progressive increase in exertability of the cortex. Epilepsia 24:200–213.

Visek WJ (1984): An update of concepts of essential amino acids. Annu Rev Nutr 4:137–155.

Current Topics in Nutrition and Disease, Volume 16
Basic and Clinical Aspects of Nutrition and Brain Development,
pages 287–304
© 1987 Alan R. Liss, Inc.

Thiamin Malnutrition and Brain Development

Roger F. Butterworth

Laboratory of Neurochemistry, André-Viallet Clinical Research Centre, Hôpital Saint-Luc, University of Montreal, Montreal, Quebec H2X 3J4, Canada

INTRODUCTION

Thiamin, vitamin B_1, is a water-soluble vitamin found in high concentrations in brewer's yeast, wheatgerm, and spinach. Lesser amounts are found in pork muscle, whole grains, dried peas, and beans. The thiamin content of various foodstuffs is shown in Table I.

Thiamin levels may vary with the growing season; synthesis of the vitamin is stimulated by light and thiamin content of oats, wheat, and peas is found to increase with maturation (Thiessen, 1978). Dry storage of cereal grains or freezing of fish and vegetables does not lead to appreciable loss of thiamin. However, milling of grain removes as much as 85% of the vitamin, and prolonged cooking also leads to substantial thiamin loss.

The normal daily thiamin requirement by man is of the order of 1.0–1.5 mg. However, thiamin requirements may increase in childhood. In addition, physical exercise as well as genetic factors may play a role in determining thiamin requirements. Thiamin needs in pregnancy and lactation are substantially greater than normal, and it is generally recommended that daily allowances for thiamin be increased by 0.5 mg during pregnancy and lactation (Rassin, 1984). Mature human milk contains approximately 21 μg thiamin per 100 kcal, and thiamin content of infant formulas is generally in excess of these concentrations (Rassin, 1984). Infectious disease may aggravate thiamin malnutrition. For example, prisoners in the Far East during World War II who ate thiamin-deficient diets but showed no overt symptoms, rapidly developed beri beri following an outbreak of infectious diarrhea (Marks, 1975).

Measurement of Thiamin Status

Classic criteria for the measurement of thiamin status include assessment of dietary intake and urinary thiamin excretion. Levels of urinary thiamin below 30 μg/g creatinine are generally associated with a high risk for development of thiamin deficiency (Sauberlich et al., 1974). However, the

TABLE I. Thiamin Content of Various Foodstuffs

	Food	Thiamin content (μg/100 g)
Excellent source of thiamin	Brewer's yeast	2,000–10,000
	Wheat germ	2,000
	Spinach	1,600
Moderately good source of thiamin	Fresh pork	800
	Dried beans, peas	700
	Whole grain cereal	400
	Eggs	100–200
Poor source of thiamin	Unfortified white bread	50
	Cow's milk	40
	Milled rice	20–40
	Jams, jellies	0
	Alcoholic beverages	0

technique currently most widely used to assess thiamin status is by measurement of the activity of a thiamin-dependent enzyme, transketolase, in hemolysates of red blood cells. This method, originally described by Brin et al. in 1960, has undergone many modifications (Dreyfus, 1962; Massod et al., 1971). According to this method, transketolase is measured in the absence of and in the presence of excess added thiamin pyrophosphate (TPP), the enzyme cofactor. The incremental increase of transketolase resulting from TPP addition is found to be inversely related to the degree of thiamin deficiency. This so-called "TPP-effect" is generally found to be less than 15% in normal subjects, i.e. addition of excess TPP to the incubation medium leads to increased transketolase activity of 15% or less. Typical results taken from healthy laboratory personnel in the author's research department are shown in Figure 1.

In one recent study, 19 male volunteer medical students participated in a double-blind assessment of the effects of partial thiamin deficiency for a period of 4 to 5 weeks. The ten thiamin-deficient subjects were correctly identified by low urinary thiamin excretion and by elevated TPP-Effect parameters, and a linear relationship was found to exist between the TPP-Effect and log (urinary thiamin excretion) for each subject (Wood et al., 1980).

Thiamin Status in Different World Populations

A joint WHO-FAO report in 1967 suggested that thiamin deficiency was still an important problem in certain countries including The Philippines, Vietnam, Burma, and Thailand (WHO Technical Report #302, Rome, 1967). Although a more recent study suggested a drastic reduction in the

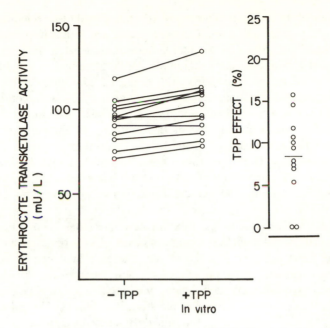

Fig. 1.   Erythrocyte transketolase activities and percentage TPP-Effect in healthy volunteers.

incidence of beri beri (Burgess and Burgess, 1976), subclinical thiamin deficiency, as evaluated by measurement of erythrocyte transketolase, may still represent a problem of considerable importance in certain world populations (Brin, 1974). For example, a study carried out on Ghanaian children aged from 6 months to 6 years revealed evidence of severe thiamin deficiency in 34% of those studied (Neumann et al., 1979). Subclinical thiamin deficiency, defined as erythrocyte transketolase TPP-Effect greater than 15%, was reported in 36% of malnourished children in a study from Jamaica (Hailemariam et al., 1985), and similar evidence of thiamin deficiency was found in 21% of a large population of individuals of mainly Melanesian extraction in Australia (Duffy et al., 1981). Another study revealed evidence of thiamin deficiency in children from an area of northeastern Thailand (Sornmani et al., 1981). It has been suggested that thiamin deficiency in these populations may not only be due to inadequate or inappropraite diets. There is evidence to suggest that methods of food preparation together with the presence of thiamin-degrading enzymes (thiaminases) may also be involved. For example, in the Ghanaian study, it was suggested that the widely practiced method of making of soups and stews involving prolonged heating of ingredients as well as the increasing tendency to refining of grains may have been an important contributory factor in the development of thiamin deficiency in this population (Neumann et al., 1979). Heat-stable antithiamin factors have been found in pumpkin leaves, merit betal, and cow pea, vegetables commonly eaten in certain areas of Ghana and Thailand (Nakornchai et al., 1975; Neumann et al., 1979). Some species of fish, such as carp and tuna, contain appreciable levels of thiaminases, and thiamin deficiency may therefore occur in countries where such fish is eaten raw. In addition, certain bacteria of both the *Bacillus* and *Clostridium* genera are capable of the synthesis of thiaminases, and these bacteria have been isolated from fecal material in a group of Japanese patients suffering from hypothiaminosis (Evans, 1975). A similarly high incidence of thiaminase activity of probable bacterial origin was reported in fecal material from thiamin-deficient patients in the Australian study (Duffy et al., 1981).

It is generally assumed that thiamin deficiency has been eradicated from most industrialized societies. Certainly cases of beri beri are rarely encountered in these communities. However, there is evidence to suggest that significant segments of the population of such countries may be at risk for the development of thiamin deficiency, as revealed by biochemical testing. Separate studies in the United States by Dibble et al. (1965) and Morse et al. (1965) provided evidence of thiamin deficiency in significant numbers of schoolchildren in New York state and Vermont, respectively. A subsequent study published in 1969 suggested that as much as 25% of the general population of the United States may show biochemical evidence of thiamin deficiency (Davis et al., 1969). Such findings led Brin in 1974 to suggest that thiamin malnutrition in the U.S. was increasing. He went on to propose that this phenomenon might be due to decreased consumption of enriched bread in favor of refined carbohydrates in candy and snack foods. Such foods are not only poor sources of thiamin, but high carbodydrate input is associated with an increased requirement for dietary thiamin (Marks, 1975). A survey by Nutrition Canada (#H58-36, 1973) published in 1973, provided data suggesting that up to 20% of the Canadian population was at risk for development of thiamin deficiency.

Thiamin Requirements in Pregnancy and Lactation

In pregnancy, maternal nutrients are ingested, processed by the placenta, and provided to the fetus. As the fetus develops and biochemical maturation takes place, nutritional requirements change to respond to changing fetal demands. Nutritional deficits in the mother result in an increased incidence of low birth-weight infants, and it is generally recommended that pregnant and lactating mothers receive dietary supplements (Rassin, 1984). It is currently recommended that thiamin supplements of 0.5 mg per day be provided during pregnancy and lactation (Munro, 1980). In a U.S. study published in 1975, vitamin profiles in 174 mothers and their newborns at parturition were investigated. A considerable percentage of mothers had been receiving suboptimal levels of thiamin (Baker et al., 1975). Evidence of thiamin deficiency was also reported during the 1970's in pregnant women in Malaysia (Chong and Ho, 1970) and in central Europe (Heller et al., 1974). Thiamin malnutrition still remains a problem in some parts of Asia where it has been repeatedly shown that babies suckling from thiamin-deficient mothers have developed clinical signs of beri beri (Kywe-Thein et al., 1968; Pongparich et al., 1974). Beri beri frequently occurs in infants breast-fed by mothers who themselves have no clinical symptoms of thiamin deficiency but who secrete milk with a low thiamin content (Davidson et al., 1975). Milk synthesis is a complex metabolic process, known to be influenced by nutritional factors. Studies in rat pups suckling from dams receiving a thiamin-deficient diet revealed evidence of memory deficits (Bell and Stewart, 1979) and significant growth retardation (Trostler and Sklan, 1977). Analysis of milk composition from thiamin-deficient rats revealed that the percentage transfer of thiamin was significantly reduced. Lactose content of the milk was decreased, whereas fatty acid levels were increased, and it was suggested that such changes in milk composition resulting from thiamin deficiency may have clinical significance (Trostler and Sklan, 1977).

In 1968, Lemoine and associates reported a high incidence of intrauterine growth retardation (IUGR), psychomotor abnormalities, and congenital defects in children born to alcoholic mothers. Ulleland reported an incidence in excess of 80% of IUGR in offspring of alcoholic mothers (Ulleland, 1972). Since then, numerous other studies have confirmed these findings, and the syndrome is now generally referred to as the ''fetal alcohol syndrome'' (Jones and Smith, 1973). Chronic alcoholism results in severe thiamin deficiency, and even when a normal diet is ingested, chronic alcohol abuse may lead to thiamin deficiency due to alcohol-induced reduction of thiamin absorption or decreased synthesis of the cofactor form of thiamin, thiamin pyrophosphate (TPP) (Leevy, 1982). Thiamin deprivation in the pregnant rat results in IUGR in the offspring, and it has been suggested that thiamin deficiency in addition to a direct toxic effect of alcohol may be the cause of the fetal alcohol syndrome (Roecklin et al., 1985). Further studies are clearly required to evaluate this hypothesis.

THIAMIN DEFICIENCY AND CNS FUNCTION

Neurological Disorders Associated With Thiamin Deficiency in Man

The classic form of thiamin malnutrition in man is beri beri. Three forms of the disease are known, namely wet beri beri, characterized by edema, high output cardiac failure, and elevated blood pyruvate levels; dry beri beri, a polyneuropathy; and the infantile form. Thiamin deficiency in infants, infantile beri beri, is characterized by failure to gain weight, vomiting, and constipation, all of which respond promptly to thiamin administration to either the nursing mother or the infant. Infantile beri beri usually presents in the first year of life and is particularly dangerous in the first few months postnatally when it generally is of sudden onset and runs a fulminating course with acute cardiovascular symptoms and subsequent death, often within hours. The central nervous system is frequently involved as evidenced by nystagmus and convulsions (Sturman and Rivlin, 1975). In industrialized nations, the major disease associated with thiamin deficiency is Wernicke's encephalopathy or the Wernicke-Korsakoff syndrome which is characterized by ophthalmoplegia, ataxia, and loss of memory. Although most commonly associated with chronic alcoholism, the disease is also encountered in cases of hyperemesis gravidarum, gastrointestinal carcinoma, and anorexia nervosa. Infants born to alcoholic mothers are prone to develop the fetal alcohol syndrome and, as discussed in the previous section, an etiological role for thiamin deficiency in this disorder has been suggested.

There is also evidence to support the contention that a disorder of thiamin neurochemistry may play a role in the etiology of the Sudden Infant Death syndrome (SIDS). Sudden unexpected deaths have been described in apparently thriving infants of thiamin-deficient mothers (Read, 1978), and a sleep apnea, a symptom frequently encountered in "near-miss" SIDS cases, has been described in Leigh disease, a genetic disease of infants associated with an inherited abnormality of a thiamin-requiring enzyme (Sorbi and Blass, 1982; Butterworth 1982). However, direct studies of transketolase activities of erythrocyte hemolysates from cases of SIDS did not reveal any evidence of thiamin deficiency (Peterson et al., 1981).

Pharmacologic doses of thiamin have occasionally been found to be efficacious in the treatment of certain neurological diseases of children associated with inherited defects of thiamin-dependent enzymes (Butterworth, 1985). Such diseases are generally referred to as thiamin-responsive genetic disorders.

Neuropathology of Thiamin Deficiency

Chronic thiamin deficiency results in selective destruction of certain cells of the central nervous system, with sparing of neighboring ones. Such selective vulnerability is characteristic of many metabolic encephalopathies. The relationship of thiamin deficiency to specific brain lesions in man is derived mainly from cases of Wernicke encephalopathy of a nutritional etiology, such as that reported in association with chronic gastritis or gastric carcinoma (Campbell and Biggart, 1939) as well as that encountered in prisoners of war (de Wardner and Lennox, 1947) and in infantile beri beri

(Davis and Wolf, 1958). Lesions are consistently found in mammillary bodies, thalamus, hypothalamus, and pons in such cases. Feeding of thiamin deficient diets to laboratory rats results in neuropathologic damage limited to pontine structures. In particular, lateral vestibular nucleus is found to be lesioned (Tellez and Terry 1968; Collins and Converse, 1970). When the central thiamin antagonist, pyrithiamin, is used to induce thiamin deficiency in the rat, more extensive lesions are observed, and structures such as mammillary bodies, thalamus, hypothalamus, and cerebellum, in addition to pons, are affected by this treatment (Troncoso et al., 1981). Thus the pattern of neuropathologic damage observed in the rat following pyrithiamin treatment resembles that encountered in Wernicke encephalopathy in man (Butterworth, 1986) and treatment of rats with pyrithiamin is currently the most widely used experimental approach for studies of pathogenetic mechanisms involved in this disease.

Horita et al. (1983) evaluated the neuropathologic consequences of daily pyrithiamin administration to the offspring of rats from thiamin-deficient mothers. Starting around 22 days of age, acute pathologic changes were apparent in vestibular nuclei, mammillary bodies, and thalamus of these animals.

Neurochemistry of Thiamin Deficiency

Thiamin content of brain. Thiamin deprivation results in decreased tissue thiamin stores. Dreyfus (1961) studied the effects of thiamin deficiency on the quantitative histochemical distribution of thiamin in the central nervous system. Stores of total (free plus phosphorylated) thiamin were found to be depleted at a uniform rate, and animals became symptomatic when thiamin levels in brain fell below 20% of normal levels. No correlation was found between total thiamin concentration in any particular brain region and that region's susceptibility to thiamin deprivation. This finding was later confirmed by Rindi and coworkers (1980). Thiamin content and thiamin turnover rate of different brain regions of the rat are shown in Table II.

Thus, it can be observed that thiamin turnover rates are significantly greater in vulnerable brain regions (cerebellum, pons, medulla) than in less vulnerable, rostrally situated brain structures. In an earlier study, Pincus and Grove (1970) demonstrated that chronic thiamin deprivation in the rat led to greatest loss of TPP in pons.

Thiamin-dependent enzymes. TPP serves as cofactor in three enzymatic reactions involved in cerebral carbohydrate metabolism. These enzyme systems are the pryruvate dehydrogenase complex (PDHC, EC 1.2.4.1), α-ketoglutarate dehydrogenase (αKGDH, EC 1.2.4.2), and transketolase (EC 2.2.1.1). The position of these enzymes in glucose metabolism is shown schematically in Figure 2.

TABLE II. Thiamin Content and Turnover Rates of Different Rat CNS Regions[a]

	Thiamin content (µg/g)	Thiamin turnover rate (µg/g/hr)
Cerebellum	4.38 ± 0.07	0.551
Medulla	3.32 ± 0.16	0.543
Pons	3.27 ± 0.11	0.454
Spinal cord	2.07 ± 0.10	0.389
Hypothalamus	2.86 ± 0.12	0.357
Midbrain	3.10 ± 0.11	0.294
Striatum	3.32 ± 0.16	0.268
Cerebral cortex	2.62 ± 0.15	0.159

[a]Data from Rindi et al., 1980. Values are means of at least 25 samples ± S.E.

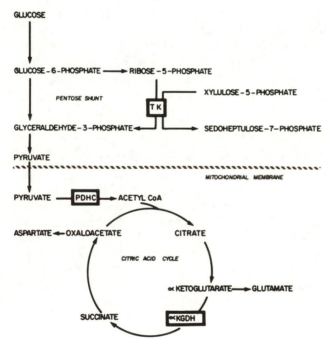

Fig. 2. Thiamin-dependent enzymes involved in cerebral glucose metabolism (from Butterworth, 1986, with permission).

Measurement of PDHC in homogenates of whole brain from symptomatic thiamin-deprived rats revealed no significant alterations (Heinrich et al., 1973). However, when PDHC activity was measured in dissected vulnerable brain stem structures, decreases of the order of 20–30% were consistently recorded (Dreyfus and Hauser, 1965; McCandless and Schenker, 1968; Pincus and Wells, 1972; Butterworth et al., 1985). Reductions of αKGDH of

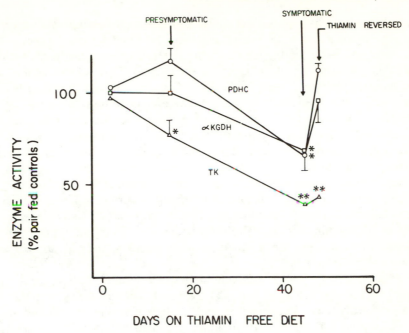

Fig. 3. Effect of progressive thiamin deprivation and supplementation on activities of thiamin-dependent enzymes in lateral vestibular nucleus of the rat. Significantly different from pair-fed control values indicated by *P < 0.05, **P < 0.01 by analysis of variance.

a similar magnitude are also found in brain stem structures of thiamin-deprived rats (Butterworth et al., 1986). Studies of cerebral glucose utilization in thiamin deprivation have repeatedly demonstrated that onset of neurological symptoms of thiamin deficiency is associated with reduced glucose utilization of a comparable magnitude to the reductions of PDHC and αKGDH (Robertson et al., 1975; Sharp et al., 1982; Hakim and Pappius, 1983). Such decreased enzyme activities probably result from selective loss of TPP from brain stem structures during thiamin deprivation (Pincus and Grove, 1970). Reversal of neurological symptoms of thiamin deficiency following administration of the vitamin to symptomatic thiamin-deprived rats leads to prompt reversal of the abnormalities of PDHC and αKGDH (Butterworth et al., 1985, 1986). The effect of thiamin deprivation and subsequent thiamin refeeding on enzyme activities in lateral vestibular nucleus is shown in Figure 3.

Transketolase activities in the brain of thiamin-deprived rats have consistently been found to be severely decreased with vulnerable brain stem structures being affected earlier and more severely than other brain regions (McCandless and Schenker, 1968; Pincus and Wells, 1972; Giguère and Butterworth, 1987). In contrast to PDHC and αKGDH, defective transketolase activities are not fully normalized following incubation of tissue homogenates with excess TPP in vitro (Pincus and Grove, 1972; Giguère and Butterworth, 1987) or after reversal of encephalopathy following thiamin administration to symptomatic animals (Fig. 3) (McCandless and Schenker, 1968; Pincus and Wells, 1972; Giguère and Butterworth, 1987). It has been suggested that the early reduction of transketolase in lateral vestibular nucleus of thiamin-deprived rats may relate to the early glial cell changes observed in this brain structure (Collins, 1967; Butterworth, 1986). The irreversibility of the transketolase deficit following thiamin administration to symptomatic thiamin-deprived rats appears to apply also to extracerebral tissues. Diminished activities of transketolase in erythrocytes from thiamin-deficient rats are not readily reversed following thiamin supplementation (Butterworth et al., 1985), and transketolase defects in the blood of thiamin-deficient alcoholic patients were found to be slow to normalize following daily thiamin administration for up to 10 days (Waldenlind et al., 1981).

In a study of the effect of thiamin deficiency on brain development, Geel and Dreyfus (1974) fed a thiamin-deficient diet to pregnant rats from the 14th day of pregnancy. The brain weight of the offspring was found to be decreased, and neurological symptoms appeared by 25 days of age. The normal developmental increase in brain transketolase activity was found to occur between 5 and 18 days of age. During this same time interval, transketolase activities of the thiamin-deficient group declined significantly and by 25 days of age were depressed to less than 30% of control values (Fig. 4). Similar results were subsequently reported by Trostler et al. (1977).

In contrast to the developing young, thiamin-deficient mothers remained asymptomatic, and brain transketolase activity declined only slightly (to 80% of control values) after 5 weeks on the thiamin-deficient diet. It was concluded from these studies that immature animals are much more susceptible to dietary thiamin deficiency than are adults (Dreyfus, 1974). There are no reports in the literature of the effect of maternal thiamin deficiency on the development of adult patterns of PDHC and αKGDH. However, pyruvate levels were found to be significantly increased in the brain of rat pups born to mothers fed a thiamin-deficient diet during pregnancy and lactation (Trostler et al., 1977), and increased pyruvate content of brain was described in pyrithiamine-treated newborn rats (McCandless et al., 1976).

Brain lipids. Since chronic thiamin deprivation results in loss of myelin in the CNS (Dreyfus, 1974; Collins, 1974), several studies have been performed to evaluate the effect of maternal thiamin deficiency on myelination in the developing brain. The period of myelination, which is most rapid between 10 and 20 days post partum in the rat, is considered to be a particularly vulnerable period in brain development (Davison and Dobbing,

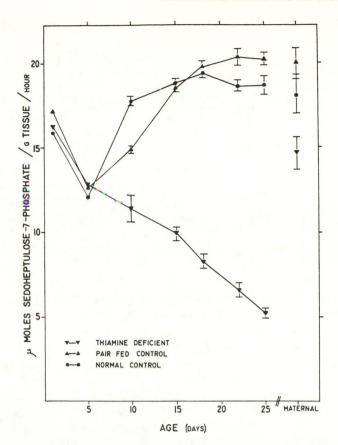

Fig. 4. Whole brain transketolase of thiamin-deficient and control rats during development. Points are means ± S.E. for 8–25 animals (from Geel and Dreyfus, 1974, with permission).

1966). Accordingly, Geel and Dreyfus (1975) examined brain lipid composition of 25-day-old offspring of rats exposed to thiamin deprivation from the 14th day of gestation. No changes in brain lipids of either whole brain or dissected cerebellum or brain stem were observed that were distinct from the effects of undernutrition. A subsequent study of Trostler et al. (1977) described alterations of phosopholipids and cerebrosides in the brain of rat pups from mothers fed a low thiamin diet during pregnancy and lactation. Rehabilitation with thiamin led to normalization of phospholipid changes, but cerebrosides were still found to be lower than normal even after 23 days of thiamin supplementation. It was suggested that such alterations may suggest damage to the myelin sheath. The authors proposed that the differences between their findings and those of Geel and Dreyfus (1975) may

TABLE III. Effect of Chronic Thiamin Deprivation on Cerebral Amino Acids in Rats

	Amino acid concentration (μmol/g)[a]			
	Cerebellum		Brain stem	
	Pair-fed controls	Thiamin-deficient	Pair-fed controls	Thiamin-deficient
Glutamate	10.47 ± 0.16	7.57 ± 0.20[**]	5.40 ± 0.13	3.98 ± 0.25[**]
Aspartate	3.12 ± 0.28	2.11 ± 0.18[*]	5.22 ± 0.17	3.42 ± 0.27[**]
GABA	2.48 ± 0.19	1.84 ± 0.14[*]	2.12 ± 0.14	1.72 ± 0.33
Glutamine	5.96 ± 0.14	5.14 ± 0.28[*]	3.47 ± 0.22	3.45 ± 0.26
Glycine	1.09 ± 0.08	0.75 ± 0.06[*]	3.75 ± 0.08	2.99 ± 0.20[*]
Taurine	5.31 ± 0.48	3.88 ± 0.24[*]	0.89 ± 0.14	0.98 ± 0.15

[a]Means ± S.E. of results obtained from seven rats per treatment group (data from Hamel et al., 1979). Significant differences between thiamin-deficient and pair-fed groups by Student T test.
[*]$P < 0.05$.
[**]$P < 0.01$.

have resulted from differing severities of thiamin deficiency in the two studies (Trostler et al., 1977; Trostler and Sklan, 1978). In another study, the thiamin antagonist, pyrithiamin, was administered to newborn rats during the critical period for myelinogenesis (McCandless et al., 1976). Myelination, measured both morphologically and biochemically proceeded at normal rates. The authors went on to suggest that alternative metabolic pathways may operate in developing rat brain enabling it to circumvent certain metabolic changes induced by thiamin deficiency. The question of the effect of maternal thiamin deficiencies on lipid composition of brain was recently re-evaluated by Reddy and Ramakrishnan (1982). Mothers were fed a thiamin-deficient diet from day 14 of gestation through lactation. Significant deficits of galactolipids, phospholipids, and plasmalogens were observed in the brains of pups from both thiamin-deficient and pair-fed control mothers. It was again concluded that thiamin deficiency and undernutrition affect cerebral lipid concentration but, of the two, thiamin deficiency appeared to have a more severe effect on white matter lipids.

Neurotransmitter function. There is a substantial body of evidence to suggest that the encephalopathy resulting from thiamin deficiency may result from impairment of neurotransmitter function. Abnormalities of several neurotransmitter systems in the CNS have been recorded, and their role in the pathogenesis of thiamin deficiency encephalopathy has been discussed (see review articles by Butterworth, 1982, and Witt, 1985). For example, acetylcholine synthesis is markedly decreased in the brain of rats fed a thiamin-deficient diet (Vorhees et al., 1977) or administered pyrithiamine (Vorhees et al., 1978; Barclay et al., 1981). Administration of arecoline, a muscarinic agonist, was found to reverse the neurological symptoms associated with pyrithiamin treatment, and it was suggested that pyrithiamine treatment, therefore, resulted in a central muscarinic cholinergic lesion in the CNS. Decreased synthesis of acetylcholine is most likely a consequence of diminished availability of acetyl CoA resulting from decreased activity of thiamin-dependent enzymes (Gibson et al., 1984).

Chronic thiamin deprivation in the rat leads to decreased concentrations of γ-aminobutyric acid (GABA) in cerebellum and brain stem (Table III). (Hamel et al., 1979), and it has been suggested that these changes may result from loss of Purkinje cell function following thiamin deprivation in these animals (Butterworth, 1982). Further evidence for a disorder of central GABA function is provided by a report that presymptomatic thiamin-deprived rats were found to be more susceptible to the development of seizures induced by the GABA antagonist, picrotoxin, than were pair-fed control animals (Butterworth, 1982).

Glutamate and aspartate meet many of the anatomical, physiological, and neurochemical criteria for neurotransmitter status in the mammalian CNS and, following thiamin deprivation, levels of both amino acids were found to be significantly decreased in brain stem and cerebellum (Table III). Synthesis of glutamate from ^{14}C-glucose by brain was reportedly decreased following thiamin deprivation (Takahashi, 1981), and conversion of intraventricularly injected ^{14}C-α-ketoglutarate into glutamate was found to be significantly reduced in the brain of symptomatic thiamin-deprived rats (Gubler et al., 1974).

Other reports have demonstrated defective serotoninergic function following thiamin deprivation. Feeding of a thiamin-deficient diet to adult rats resulted in decreased serotonin uptake by cerebellar synaptosomes (Plaitakis et al., 1978), and autoradiographic studies revealed a selective loss of indoleamine axons in these animals (Chan-Palay et al., 1977). It was suggested that these results may reflect a loss of serotoninergic cerebellar mossy fibers in thiamin deficiency.

No studies to date have addressed the issue of the effects of thiamin deficiency on neurotransmitter function in developing brain.

SUMMARY

Thiamin deficiency remains a potentially important health care problem in many world communities. Although the classic thiamin deficiency disorder beri beri is practically non-existent in industrialized countries and its prevalence in previously high risk rice-consuming countries of the Far East is nowadays very low, there is evidence to suggest that thiamin status in substantial numbers of individuals from both developed and underdeveloped nations may be marginal. Pregnant and lactating mothers have increased thiamin requirements and find themselves among those at high risk for development of thiamin deficiency. Appropriate supplementation of diets during pregnancy and lactation is therefore recommended. Studies with experimental animals suggest that consumption of a thiamin-inadequate diet during pregnancy leads to IUGR and altered neurochemical parameters in the CNS of the offspring.

Chronic alcoholism is associated with severe thiamin deficiency. The deficiency state results from inadequate dietary intake as well as from direct effects of alcohol on thiamin absorption and utilization. Thiamin-deficient alcoholic patients develop Wernicke encephalopathy (Wernicke-Korsakoff syndrome). Although some neurological symptoms of Wernicke encephalopathy, such as ophthalmoplegia, respond rapidly to thiamin treatment, others, such as ataxia, respond only partially. Infants born to alcoholic mothers have a high incidence of IUGR and congenital abnormalities (the fetal alcohol syndrome), and thiamin deficiency may play an important etiologic role in the development of this syndrome.

Chronic thiamin deprivation results in selective neuropathological lesions to certain brain structures with sparing of neighboring ones. Particularly vulnerable brain structures, such as pons, have a relatively high thiamin turnover rate. In addition, thiamin deprivation leads to selective depletion of TPP in pons. TPP is the cofactor for three important enzymes involved in glucose utilization. Activities of all three enzyme systems (pyruvate dehydrogenase complex, α-ketoglutarate dehydrogenase, and transketolase) are decreased following thiamin deprivation, with greatest changes being observed in affected brain stem structures. Maternal thiamin deficiency results in decreased transketolase in the brains of offspring. Defects of these cerebral thiamin-dependent enzymes may be responsible for the decreased synthesis of glucose-derived neurotransmitters (acetylcholine, GABA, glutamate) consistently observed in the brain in thiamin deficiency. Maternal thiamin deficiency does not appear to result in decreased myelination in developing brain.

ACKNOWLEDGMENTS

Studies from the author's laboratory were funded by grants from The Medical Research Council of Canada, Fonds de la recherche en santé du Québec, and La Foundation de l'Hôpital Saint-Luc. The author wishes to thank Françoise Trotier and Diane Malette for their assistance with the preparation of the manuscript.

REFERENCES

Baker H, Frank O, Thompson AD, Langer A, Munves ED, De Angelis B, Kaminetzsky A (1975): Vitamin profile of 174 mothers and newborn at parturition. Am J Clin Nutr 28:59–65.

Barclay LL, Gibson GE, Blass JP (1981): Impairment of behaviour and acetyl choline metabolism in thiamine deficiency. J Pharmacol Exp Ther 217:537–543.

Bell JM, Stewart CN (1979): Effects of fetal and early postnatal thiamin deficiency on avoidance learning in rats. J Nutr 109:1577–1583.

Brin M (1974); Recent information on thiamine nutritional status in selected countries. In Gubler CJ, Fujiwara M, Dreyfus PM (eds): "Thiamine." New York: John Wiley and Sons, pp 143–151.

Burgess HJL, Burgess AP (1976): Malnutrition in the Western Pacific. WHO Chron 30:64–77.

Butterworth RF (1982): Neurotransmitter function in thiamine-deficiency encephalopathy. Neurochem Int 4:449–464.

Butterworth RF (1985): Pyruvate dehydrogenase deficiency disorders. In McCandless DW (ed): "Cerebral Energy Metabolism and Metabolic Encephalopathy." New York: Plenum Publishing, pp 121–141.

Butterworth RF (1986): Cerebral thiamine-dependent enzyme changes in experimental Wernicke's encephalopathy. Metab Brain Dis 1:165–175.

Butterworth RF, Giguère JF, Besnard AM (1985): Activities of thiamine-dependent enzymes in two experimental models of thiamine-deficiency encephalopathy. 1. The pyruvate dehydrogenase complex. Neurochem Res 10:1417–1428.

Butterworth RF, Giguère JF, Besnard AM (1986): Activities of thiamine-dependent enzymes in two experimental models of thiamine-deficiency encephalopathy. 2. α-Ketoglutarate dehydrogenase. Neurochem Res 11:567–577.

Campbell ACP, Biggart JH (1939): Wernicke's encephalopathy (polioencephalitis hemorrhagica superior): Its alcoholic and non-alcoholic incidence. J Pathol Bacteriol 48:245–262.

Chan-Palay V, Plaitakis A, Nicklas WJ, Berl S (1977): Autoradiographic demonstration of loss of labeled indoleamine axons of the cerebellum in chronic diet-induced thiamine deficiency. Brain Res 138:380–384.

Chong YH, Ho GS (1970): Erythrocyte transketolase activity. Am J Clin Nutr 23:261–266.

Collins GH (1967) Glial cell changes in the brainstem of thiamine deficient rats. Am J Pathol 50:791–802.

Collins GH (1974): The morphology of myelin degeneration in thiamine deficiency. In Gubler CJ, Fujiwara M, Dreyfus PM (eds): "Thiamine," New York: John Wiley and Sons, pp 261–269.

Collins GH, Converse WK (1970): Cerebellar degeneration in thiamine deficient rats. Am J Pathol 50:219–233.

Davidson S, Passmore R, Brock JP, Truswell AS (1975): "Human Nutrition and Dietetics." 6th Ed. Edinburgh: Churchill Livingstone, pp 338–339.

Davis RA, Wolf A (1958): Infantile beri beri associated with Wernicke's encephalopathy. Pediatrics 21:409–420.

Davis TRA, Gershoff SN, Gamble DF (1969): J Nutr Ed Suppl 1:39.

Davison AN, Dobbing J (1966): Br Med Bull 22:40–44.

de Wardner HE, Lennox B (1947): Cerebral beri beri (Wernicke's encephalopathy). Lancet 252:11–17.

Dibble MV, Brin M, McMullen E, Peel A, Chen N (1965): Some preliminary biochemical findings in junior high school children in Syracuse and Orondaga County, New York. Am J Clin Nutr 17:218–239.

Dreyfus PM (1961); The quantitative biochemical distribution of thiamine in deficient rat brain. J Neurochem 8:139–146.

Dreyfus PM (1962): Clinical application of blood transketolase determinations. N Engl J Med 267:596–xxx.

Dreyfus PM (1974): Thiamine-deficiency encephalopathy: Thoughts on its pathogenesis. In Gubler CJ, Fujiwara M, Dreyfus PM (eds): "Thiamine." New York: John Wiley and Sons, pp 229–239.

Dreyfus PM, Hauser G (1965); The effects of thiamine deficiency on the pyruvate decarboxylase system of the central nervous system. Biochim Biophys Acta 104:78–84.

Duffy P, Morris H, Neilson G (1981): Thiamin status of a Melanesian population. Am J Clin Nutr 34:1584–1592.

Evans WC (1975): Thiaminases and their effects on animals. Vitamins Hormones 33:467–470.

Geel SE, Dreyfus PM (1974): Thiamine deficiency encephalopathy in the developing rat. Brain Res 76:435–445.

Geel SE, Dreyfus PM (1975): Brain lipid composition of immature thiamine-deficient and undernourished rats. J Neurochem 24:353–360.

Giguère JF, Butterworth RF (1987): Activities of thiamine-dependent enzymes in two experimental models of thiamine-deficiency encephalopathy. 3. Transketolase. Neurochem Res 12, in press.

Gubler CJ, Adams BL, Hammond B, Yuan EC, Guo SM, Bennon M (1974): Effect of thiamine deprivation and thiamine antagonists on the level of γ-aminobutyric acid and on 2-oxoglutarate metabolism in rat brain. J Neurochem 22:831–836.

Hailemariam B, Landman JP, Jackson AA (1985): Thiamin status in normal and malnourished children in Jamaica. Br J Nutr 53:477–483.

Hakim AM, Pappius HM (1983): Sequence of metabolic, clinical and histological events in experimental thiamine deficiency. Ann Neurol 13:365–375.

Hamel E, Butterworth RF, Barbeau A (1979): Effect of thiamine deficiency on levels of putative amino acid transmitters in affected regions of the rat brain. J Neurochem 33:575–577.

Heinrich CP, Stadler H, Weiser H (1973): The effect of thiamine deficiency on the acetyl CoA and acetylcholine levels in rat brain. J Neurochem 21:1273–1281.

Heller S, Salkeld RM, Korner WF (1974): Vitamin B_1 status in pregnancy. Am J Clin Nutr 27:1221–1224.

Horita N, Okuno A, Izumiyama Y (1983); Neuropathologic changes in suckling and weanling rats with pyrithiamine-induced thiamine deficiency. Acta Neuropathol (Berl) 61:27–35.

Jones KL, Smith DW (1973); Recognition of the fetal alcohol syndrome in early infancy. Lancet 2:999–1001.

Kywe-Thein, Thane-Toe, Tin-Tin-Oo, Khin-Khin-Tway (1968): A study of infantile beri beri in Rangoon, Union of Burma. J Life Sci 1:62–72.

Leevy CM (1982); Thiamin deficiency and alcoholism. Ann NY Acad Sci 378:316–326.

Marks J (1975): "A Guide to the Vitamins: Their Role in Health and Disease." Baltimore: University Park Press, pp 14–21.

Massod MF, McGuire SL, Werner KR (1971): Analysis of blood transketolase activity. Am J Clin Pathol 55:465–470.

McCandless DW, Malone MJ, Szoke M (1976): Pyrithiamine-induced thiamine deficiency: Effects on rat myelination. Int J Vit Nutr Res 46:24–32.

McCandless DW, Schenker S (1968): Encephalopathy of thiamine deficiency: Studies of intracerebral mechanisms. J Clin Invest 47:2268–2280.

Morse EH, Merrow SB Clarke RF (1965): Some biochemical findings in Burlington (Vt) junior high school children. Am J Clin Nutr 17:211–214.

Munro HN (1980): The Ninth edition of recommended dietary allowances. In Scarpa IS, Kiefer HC, Garmon G (eds): "Sourcebook of Food and Nutrition." Chicago: Marquis Academic Media, pp 82–85.

Nakornchai S, Sriphojanart S, Termtenand O, Vimokesant S, Dhannamita S, Sakorn S (1975): A comparative study of antithiamin activity in vegetables from different parts of Thailand. J Med Assoc 58:81–90.

Neumann CG, Swendseid ME, Jacob M, Stiehm ER, Dirige OV (1979): Biochemical evidence of thiamin deficiency in young Ghanaian children . Am J Clin Nutr 32:99–104.

Peterson DR, Labbe RF, van Belle G, Chinn NM (1981): Erythrocyte transketolase activity and sudden infant death. Am J Clin Nutr 34:65–67.

Pincus JH, Grove I (1970): Distribution of thiamine phosphate esters in normal and thiamine-deficient brain. Exp Neurol 28:477–483.

Pincus JH, Wells K (1972): Regional distributuion of thiamine-dependent enzymes in normal and thiamine-deficient brain. Exp Neurol 37:495–501.

Plaitakis A, Nicklas WJ, Berl S (1978): thiamine deficiency: Selective impairment of the cerebellar serotonergic system. Neurology 28:691–698.

Pongparich B, Spikrikkrich N, Dhanamitta S, Valyasevi A (1974); Biochemical detection of thiamine deficiency in infants and children in Thailand. Am J Clin Nutr 27:1399–1408.

Rassin DK (1984): Nutritional requirements for the fetus and the neonate. In Ogra PL (ed): "Neonatal Infections: Nutritional and Immunologic Interactions." New York: Grune and Stratton, pp 205–227.

Read DJC (1978): The aetiology of the Suddent Infant Death syndrome: current ideas on breathing and sleep and possible links to deranged thiamine neurochemistry. Aust NZ Med 8:322–336.

Reddy TS, Ramakrishnan CV (1982); Effects of maternal thiamine deficiency on the lipid composition of rat whole brain, gray matter and white matter. Neurochem Int 4:495–499.

Rindi G, Patrini C, Comincioli V, Reggiani C (1980): Thiamine content and turnover rates of some rat nervous regions using labeled thiamine as a tracer. Brain Res 181:369–380.

Robertson DM, Manz HJ, Haas RA, Meyers N (1975): Glucose uptake in the brainstem of thiamine-deficient rats. Am J Pathol 79:107–118.

Roecklin B, Levin SW, Comly M, Mukherjee AB (1985): Intrauterine growth retardation induced by thiamine deficiency and pyrithiamine during pregnancy in the rat. Am J Obstet Gynecol 151:455–460.

Sauberlich HE, Dowdy RP, Skala JH (1974); "Laboratory Tests for the Assessment of Nutritional Status." Cleveland, Ohio: CRC Press, pp 24–26.

Sharp FR, Bolger E, Evans K (1982): Thiamine deficiency limits glucose utilization and glial proliferation in brain lesions of symptomatic rats. J Cerebr Blood Flow Metab 2:203–207.

Sorbi S, Blass JP (1982); Abnormal activation of pyruvate dehydrogenase in Leigh disease fibroblasts. Neurology 32:555–558.

Sornmani S, Schelp FP, Vivatanasesth P, Pongpaew P, Sritabutra P, Supawan V, Vudhivai N, Egormaiphol S, Harinasuta C (1981): An investigation of the health and nutritional status of the population in the Nam Pong Water Resource Development Project, Northeast Thailand. Ann Trop Med Parasitol 75:335–346.

Sturman JA, Rivlin RS (1975): Pathogenesis of brain dysfunction in deficiency of thiamine, riboflavin, pantothenic acid, or vitamin B_6. In Gaull GE (ed): "Biology of Brain Dysfunction," Vol. 3. New York: Plenum Publishing, pp 425–475.

Takahashi H (1981); The effect of thiamine deficiency on glucose metabolism in rat cerebral cortex. Nippon Ika Daig Zasshi (Japan) 48:643–656; also published in Chem Abs 96:33744f (1982).

Tellez I, Terry RD (1968): Fine structure of the early changes in the vestibular nuclei of the thiamine deficient rat. Am J Pathol 52:77–94.

Thiessen I (1978): The role of thiamine in research with animals and in humans. J Orthomol Psychiatr 7:107–113.

Troncoso SC, Johnston MV, Hess KM, Griffin JW, Price DL (1981): Model of Wernicke's encephalopathy. Arch Neurol 38:350–354.

Trostler N, Guggenheim K, Havivi E, Sklan D (1977): Effect of thiamine deficiency in pregnant and lactating rats on the brain of their offspring. Nutr Metab 21:294–304.

Trostler N, Sklan D (1977): Milk composition and thiamine transfer in thiamine deficient rats. Am J Clin Nutr 30:681–685.

Trostler N, Sklan D (1978): Lipogenesis in the brain of thiamine-deficient rat pups. J Nutr Sci Vitaminol 24:105–111.

Ulleland C (1972): The offspring of alcoholic mothers. Ann NY Acad Sci 197:167–169.

Vorhees CV, Schmidt DE, Barrett RJ (1978): Effects of pyrithiamine and oxythiamine on acetylcholine levels and utilization in rat brain. Brain Res Bull 3:493–496.

Vorhhes CV, Schmidt DE, Barrett RJ, Schenker S (1977): Effects of thiamin deficiency on acetylcholine levels and utilization in vivo in rat brain. J Nutr 107:1092–1908.

Waldenlind L, Borg S, Vikander B (1981); Effect of peroral thiamine treatment on thiamine contents and transketolase activity of red blood cells in alcoholic patients. Acta Med Scand 209:209–212.

Witt ED (1985): Neuroanatomical consequences of thiamine deficiency: A comparative analysis. Alcohol Alcoholism 20:201–221.

Wood B, Gijsbers A, Goode A, Davis S, Mulholland J, Breen K (1980): A study of partial thiamin restriction in human volunteers. Am J Clin Nutr 33:848–861.

Current Topics in Nutrition and Disease, Volume 16
Basic and Clinical Aspects of Nutrition and Brain Development,
pages 305–313
© *1987 Alan R. Liss, Inc.*

Interactions Between Nutritional States and Some Brain Biogenic Amines

A.V. Juorio

Psychiatric Research Division, University of Saskatchewan, Saskatoon, Saskatchewan S7N OWO, Canada

INTRODUCTION

Trace amines is a general term that refers to biogenic amines that are present in neural tissues in concentrations ranging from 0.1 to 100 ng g^{-1} (Boulton, 1976a). The *p*- and *m*-isomers of tyramine, β-phenylethylamine, and tryptamine are present in the mammalian brain. Their concentrations in comparison with that of dopamine or 5-hydroxytryptamine are quite small but show an uneven regional distribution. The highest concentration of β-phenylethylamine, *p*-tyramine, *m*-tyramine, and tryptamine are present in the caudate nucleus followed by the hypothalamus and brain stem (Table I). A portion of cerebral β-phenylethylamine, *p*-tyramine, and tryptamine were found associated with a subcellular particulate fraction (Boulton and Baker, 1975). Notwithstanding their small concentrations, the turnover rate of the trace amines is quite rapid, as is suggested by the higher endogenous concentrations of their respective acid metabolites (Table I) and the rate of accumulation of the trace amines observed after monoamine oxidase inhibition (Philips and Boulton, 1979). The synthesis rate calculated for β-phenylethylamine and tryptamine is similar to that exhibited by the classic transmitters (Durden and Philips, 1980; Juorio and Durden, 1984).

β-Phenylethylamine and tryptamine are formed by decarboxylation of phenylalanine or tryptophan, respectively (Lovenberg et al., 1962; Saavedra and Axelrod, 1973; Saavedra, 1974; Juorio and Durden, 1984). The case for *p*- and *m*-tyramine is somewhat more complex because *p*-tyrosine decarboxylation is very slow (Fellman et al., 1976), and attempts to demonstrate the presence of endogenous *m*-tyrosine have been so far unsuccessful (Durden et al., unpublished). Recent experiments, however, have shown that the parenteral administration of L-phenylalanine or *p*-tyrosine increase the mouse striatal concentration of *p*-tyramine, an effect that is enhanced by monoamine oxidase inhibition and reduced by administration of aromatic-L-amino acid decarboxylase inhibitors (Juorio

TABLE I. Regional Distribution of β-Phenylethylamine (PE), Phenylacetic Acid (PAA), *p*-Tyramine (*p*-TA), *p*-Hydroxyphenylacetic Acid (*p*-HPAA), *m*-Tyramine (*m*-TA), *m*-Hydroxyphenylacetic Acid (*m*-HPAA), Tryptamine (T), and Indoleacetic Acid (IAA) in Rat Brain (ng g^{-1})

	PE	PAA	*p*-TA	p-HPAA	*m*-TA	*m*-HPAA	T	IAA
Whole brain	1.8[a]	31.8[c]	2.0[d]	10.6[e]	0.3[f]	2.3[e]	0.5[g]	11.6[h]
Hypothalamus	2.1[b]	60.1[c]	1.2[b]	4.5[e]	0.2[b]	1.2[e]	0.9[g]	23.7[h]
Striatum	4.2[b]	64.6[c]	11.1[b]	28.3[e]	3.0[b]	5.3[e]	2.9[g]	63.6[h]
Brain stem	1.6[b]	33.1[c]	0.4[b]	8.6[e]	0.1[b]	1.8[e]	0.2[g]	11.7[h]
Cerebellum	2.1[b]	31.3[c]	0.1[b]	8.1[e]	0.01[b]	1.2[e]	0.3[g]	10.1[h]
Rest	1.4[b]	27.6[c]	0.5[b]	5.3[e]	0.2[b]	1.7[e]	0.3[g]	—

[a]Durden et al., 1973.
[b]Philips unpublished, cited by Boulton, 1976b.
[c]Durden and Boulton, 1982.
[d]Philips et al., 1974a.
[e]Durden and Boulton, 1981.
[f]Philips et al., 1975.
[g]Philips et al., 1974b.
[h]Warsh et al., 1977.

and Boulton, 1982; Juorio, 1983). The parenteral administration of L-phenylalanine or *m*-tyrosine also increased the striatal *m*-tyramine concentration and was further enhanced by monoamine oxidase inhibition (Juorio and Boulton, 1982). These experiments show that after in vivo administration, *m*-tyrosine is a better substrate for decarboxylation than *p*-tyrosine. Quite surprisingly, the administration of various aromatic-L-amino acid decarboxylase inhibitors, at low or moderate doses, all increased striatal *m*-tyramine concentrations (Juorio and Boulton, 1982; Juorio, 1983). Only when the doses were markedly increased was a substantial reduction in striatal *m*-tyramine achieved. This finding suggests that the brain concentrations of β-phenylethylamine, *p*-tyramine, *m*-tyramine, and tryptamine depend on the availability of the respective precursor amino acids and could be altered by conditions such as diabetes or protein undernutrition that affect the concentrations of these amino acids.

EFFECTS OF INSULIN AND DIABETES

It has been known for some time that insulin administration increases the brain concentration of tryptophan and *p*-tyrosine (Fernstrom and Wurtman, 1971; Tagliamonte et al., 1975; DeMontis et al., 1978) (Table II), while the opposite effect is observed in diabetic rats (Fernando et al., 1976; Crandall

TABLE II. Effect of Streptozotocin-Induced (65 mg kg^{-1}, 14 d) Diabetes and Insulin (2 IU kg^{-1}, 2 h) Administration on Rat Striatal Concentration of *p*-Tyrosine, *p*-Tyramine (*p*-TA), *m*-Tyramine (*m*-TA) Dopamine (DA), 3,4-Dihydroxyphenylacetic Acid (DOPAC), Homovanillic Acid (HVA), Tryptophan, 5-Hydroxytryptamine (5-HT), 5-Hydroxyindole Acetic Acid (5-HIAA), and Blood Glucose

	Diabetes			Insulin		
	Concentration	Controls	% of Controls	Concentration	Controls	% of Controls
p-Tyrosine[a]	6.5 μg g^{-1}*	12.2	53	13.4 μg g^{-1}*	10.2	131
p-TA[a]	9.1 ng g^{-1}*	14.0	65	17.5 ng g^{-1}*	12.2	143
m-TA[a]	5.3 ng g^{-1}*	2.4	220	3.0 ng g^{-1}*	4.8	63
DA[a]	14.0 μg g^{-1}	13.4	104	11.3 μg g^{-1}	12.3	92
DOPAC[a]	1.2 μg g^{-1}*	1.5	80	2.4 μg g^{-1}*	1.8	133
HVA[a]	0.6 μg g^{-1}*	0.7	86	1.2 μg g^{-1}*	0.7	171
Tryptophan[b]	2.7 μg g^{-1}*	5.5	49	7.5 μg g^{-1}*	6.5	115
5-HT[b]	0.6 μg g^{-1}*	0.7	86	0.7 μg g^{-1}	0.6	117
5-HIAA[b]	0.6 μg g^{-1}*	0.8	75	1.0 μg g^{-1}*	0.8	125
Blood glucose[a]	12.4 mM L^{-1}*	3.8	368	0.8 mM L^{-1}*	3.9	21

*Significantly different from controls.
[a]Kwok and Juorio, 1986.
[b]Kwok and Juorio, 1987.

and Fernstrom, 1983) (Table II). In addition, diabetic rats show a decrease in dopamine and 5-hydroxytryptamine metabolism (Trulson and Himmel, 1983; MacKenzie and Trulson, 1978; Saller, 1984; Kwok et al., 1985; Kwok and Juorio, 1986, 1987), while the concentration of striatal *p*-tyramine decreases and that of *m*-tyramine increases (Kwok and Juorio, 1986a) (Table II). These reciprocal changes in *p*- and *m*-tyramine were observed after insulin administration (Kwok and Juorio, 1986) at a time when the metabolism of dopamine and 5-hydroxytryptamine was markedly increased (Table II). Such changes could be explained by the lower affinity of aromatic-L-amino acid decarboxylase toward *p*-tyrosine than towards *m*-tyrosine, so that the limiting factor in the synthesis of *p*-tyramine would be the availability of *p*-tyrosine while for that of *m*-tyramine would be the activity of aromatic-L-amino acid decarboxylase. Similar reciprocal changes in brain *p*- and *m*-tyramine have been observed following the administration of dopamine receptor blocking agents (chlorpromazine, spiroperidol, etc.) which reduced availability of *p*-tyrosine as opposed to dopamine receptor agonists that increased it (Juorio, 1977, 1979).

The reduction in brain tryptophan observed in diabetic rats (Table II) occurred concomitantly with a decrease in the rate of accumulation of striatal tryptamine (Table III), but no changes were detected following insulin

TABLE III. Effect of Streptozotocin (65 mg kg^{-1}, 14 d) and Insulin (2 IU kg^{-1}, 2 h) on Pargyline-Induced Accumulation of Tryptamine in the Rat Striatum[a]

	Tryptamine (ng g^{-1})	% of Controls
Controls	93.4	—
Diabetes	64.0*	69
Controls	92.1	—
Insulin	94.4	103

*Values are significantly lower than controls.
[a]Data from Kwok and Juorio, 1987.

administration. Some prelininary experiments have also shown that the concentration of rat striatal β-phenylethylamine is not significantly changed by streptozotocin-induced diabetes (Kwok and Juorio, in preparation).

EFFECT OF PROTEIN UNDERNUTRITION

Lasting effects of early undernuturition on the behavior of rats (Frankova and Barnes, 1968) prompted several investigators to study the effects of early undernutrition on neurotransmitter metabolism (see review by Wiggins et al., 1984). With respect to the effect of early undernutrition on brain dopamine levels, there is agreement that it produces either a reduction (Shoemaker and Wurtman, 1971; Ramanamurthy, 1977) or no change (Sobotka et al., 1974), while the activity of tyrosine hydroxylase tends to increase (Shoemaker and Wurtman, 1971; Marichich et al., 1979). In a series of experiments in our laboratory, preweaning undernutrition was induced by rearing normal rat pups with mothers kept since the birth of the litter on a 5% (low) protein diet or an 18% (control) diet. The pups were killed 3 weeks after birth (Bhave et al., 1987a). The undernourished pups showed no significant changes in their concentrations of dopamine, 3, 4-dihydroxyphenylacetic acid or homovanillic acid in either the striatum or the olfactory tubercles (Table IV). The determination of dopamine turnover either by the rate of accumulation of dopamine or the rate of decline of 3,4-dihydroxyphenylacetic acid or homovanillic acid was carried out in both control and undernourished pups following monoamine oxidase inhibition (Table IV). Analysis of the data by two-way analysis of variance and by searching for main effects showed that rats subjected to preweaning undernutrition showed a moderate reduction in striatal dopamine turnover, while the reduction in the olfactory tubercles was more marked (Table IV).

The endogenous concentrations of p-tyramine in the striatum of pups subjected to preweaning undernutrition showed a significant reduction (to 72% of controls), whereas m-tyramine levels were significantly increased (to

TABLE IV. Effects of Preweaning Undernutrition on Dopamine (DA) Turnover in the Rat Striatum and Olfactory Tubercles[a]

	Control (nmol g^{-1} h^{-1})	Experimental (nmol g^{-1} h^{-1})	% of Controls
Striatum			
DA	8.0	6.1	76
DOPAC	7.9	4.2	53
HVA	6.4	4.9	77
Olfactory tubercles			
DA	5.9	4.5	76
DOPAC	4.9	4.1	84
HVA	3.1	1.5	48

[a]The turnover rates of DA were determined from the increase in or decrease of ln [DOPAC] or ln [HVA] from the regression coefficient at 0, 30, and 60 min after pargyline administration (200 mg kg^{-1}) and the DOPAC or HVA intercept. When compared using two-way analysis of variance for main effects, the turnover in the striatum was reduced slightly ($P = 0.065$) and in the olfactory tubercles reduced significantly ($P = 0.032$). Data from Bhave et al., 1987a.

TABLE V. Effects of Early Undernutrition on *p*-TA and *m*-TA Concentrations in the Rat Striatum[a]

	Age (wk)	Control (ng g^{-1})	Experimental (ng g^{-1})	% of Controls
Preweaning undernutrition				
p-TA	3	5.0	3.6*	72
m-TA	3	0.9	1.7*	189
Postweaning protein deficiency				
p-TA	9	11.7	7.6*	65
m-TA	9	2.9	5.7*	197

*Values significantly different from controls.
[a]The results are from Bhave et al., 1987a.

189% of controls) (Table V). Other experiments with rat pups reared by normally fed mothers and kept after weaning on a low protein (5%) diet to an age of 9 weeks (postweaning undernutrition) showed a reduction in the concentration of striatal *p*-tyramine (to 65% of controls), while *m*-tyramine was significantly increased (to 197% of controls). An explanation of these findings could be similar to that of diabetic rats (Table II) or attributable to the fact that after antipsychotic drug treatment (Juorio, 1977, 1979) there is a reduction in the availability of *p*-tyrosine with a consequent reduction in *p*-tyramine and increase in *m*-tyramine. Since protein malnutrition also markedly reduces plasma insulin concentration (Anthony and Faloona, 1974), it may be that the changes induced by preweaning undernutrition on brain dopamine, *p*-tyramine, and *m*-tyramine are a consequence of the

TABLE VI. Effect of Preweaning Undernutrition on 5-Hydroxytryptamine (5-HT) Turnover in Rat Brain Regions[a]

	Compound	Control (nmol g^{-1} h^{-1})	Experimental (nmol g^{-1} h^{-1})	% of Controls
Striatum	5-HT	1.2	0.8	67
	5-HIAA	1.6	0.6	38
Olfactory tubercles	5-HT	2.2	1.6	72
	5-HIAA	2.2	0.8	36
Hypothalamus	5-HT	3.6	2.2	61
	5-HIAA	4.9	2.3	47
Hippocampus	5-HT	2.7	0.8	30
	5-HIAA	1.5	0.8	53
Pons medulla	5-HT	4.8	4.0	83
	5-HIAA	2.8	3.1	111
All regions	5-HT and 5-HIAA	2.8	1.7	60

[a]The turnover rates of 5-HT were determined from the increase of 5-HT or decrease of 1n [5-HIAA] from the regression coefficient at 0, 30, and 60 min after pargyline administration (200 mg kg^{-1}) and the 5-HIAA intercept. When compared using two-way analysis of variance for main effects, 5-HT turnover decreased; as measured by 5-HT accumulation, $F = 12.4$, $p < 0.025$; or by 5-HIAA decrease, $F = 5.8$, $P < 0.084$; and when 5-HT and 5-HIAA data were combined, $F = 12.24$, $P < 0.005$. Data are from Bhave et al., 1987b.

changes in precursor amino acid availability induced by insulin reduction. In addition, it has been known that high-protein-containing diets protect against streptozotocin-induced diabetes (Eizirik and Migliorini, 1985). This finding suggests that the levels of biogenic trace amines would be affected by changes in dietary protein concentration.

The effects of early undernutrition on brain 5-hydroxytryptamine concentrations have been observed to produce no change (Hernandez, 1973; Dickerson and Pao, 1975), a decrease (Sereni et al., 1966; Ramanamurthy, 1977), or an increase (Sobotka et al., 1974; Stern et al., 1975). The differences in the results of these studies could be due to differences in the mode of induction of undernutrition and the degree of severity achieved. The experiments of Bhave et al., (1987b) show the effect of preweaning undernutrition on 3-week-old rat pups. (Bhave et al., 1987b). The determination of 5-hydroxytryptamine turnover either by the rate of accumulation of 5-hydroxytryptamine or the rate of decline of 5-hydroxyindole acetic acid were carried out in both control and undernourished pups after monoamine oxidase inhibition (Table VI). Analysis of the data by two-way analysis of variance and by searching for main effects showed that rats subjected to preweaning undernutrition had an overall reduction (60% of controls) in brain 5-hydroxytryptamine turnover (Table VI). The effects of preweaning undernutrition on brain tryptamine remain to be determined; the observed 5-hydroxytryptamine turnover reductions, however, suggest that the tryptamine concentrations could also be reduced.

CONCLUSIONS

The changes in trace brain amines induced by experimental diabetes or insulin administration in rats can be explained as a result of decreases in the availability of some of their precursor amino acids and their differential affinity for aromatic-L-amino acid decarboxylase. Similar explanations can be extended to the changes induced by preweaning undernutrition, especially in view of the reduction in plasma insulin levels produced by both experimental diabetes and protein undernutrition.

ACKNOWLEDGMENTS

I thank Dr. A.A. Boulton for helpful discussions and Saskatchewan Health for continuing financial support.

REFERENCES

Anthony LE, Faloona GR (1974): Plasma insulin and glucagon levels in protein-malnourished rats. Metabolism 23:303–306.

Bhave SV, Telang SD, Durden DA, Juorio AV (1987a): Effects of nutritional stress on tyramine concentration and dopamine turnover. Neurochem Res, in press.

Bhave SV, Telang SD, Durden DA, Juorio AV (1986b): Effects of nutritional stress on the regional metabolism of 5-hydroxytryptamine in rat brain, submitted for publication.

Boulton AA (1976a): In Usdin E, Sandler M (eds): "Trace Amines and the Brain." New York: Marcel Dekker, pp 21–39.

Boulton AA (1976b): Identification, distribution, metabolism and function of *meta-* and *para*-tyramine, phenylethylamine and tryptamine in brain. Adv Biochem Psychopharmacol 15:57–67.

Boulton AA, Baker GB (1975): The subcellular distribution of β-phenylethylamine, *p*-tyramine and tryptamine in rat brain. J Neurochem 25:477–481.

Crandall EA, Fernstrom JD (1983): Effects of experimental diabetes on the levels of aromatic and branched-chain aminoacids in rat blood and brain. Diabetes 32:222–230.

DeMontis MG, Olianas MD, Haber B, Tagliamonte A (1978): Increase in large neutral aminoacid transport into brain by insulin. J Neurochem 30:121–124.

Dickerson JWT, Pao SK (1975): Effect of pre- and post-natal maternal protein deficiency on free amino acids and amines of rat brain. Biol Neonate 25:114–124.

Durden DA, Boulton AA (1981): Identification and distribution of m- and *p*-hydroxyphenylacetic acid in the brain of the rat. J Neurochem 36:129–135.

Durden DA, Boulton AA (1982): Identification and distribution of phenylacetic acid in the brain of the rat. J Neurochem 38:1532–1536.

Durden DA, Philips SR (1980): Kinetic measurement of the turnover rates of phenylethylamine and tryptamine in vivo in the rat brain. J Neurochem 34:1725–1732.

Durden DA, Philips SR, Boulton AA (1973): Identification and distribution of β-phenylethylamine in the rat. Can J Biochem 51:995–1002.

Eizirik DL, Migliorini RH (1985): Protection against streptozotocin diabetes by high protein diets: Effect of a vegetable protein source (soya). Nutr Rep Int 32:41–47.

Fellman JH, Roth ES, Fujita TS (1976): Decarboxylation to tyramine is no major route of tyrosine metabolism in mammals. Arch Biochem Biophys 174:562–567.

Fernando JCR, Knott PJ, Curzon G (1976): The relevance of both plasma free tryptophan and insulin to rat brain tryptophan concentration. J Neurochem 27:343–345.

Fernstrom JD, Wurtman RJ (1971): Brain serotonin content: Increase following ingestion of carboyhdrate diet. Science 174:1023–1025.

Frankova S, Barnes RH (1968): Influence of malnutrition in early life on exploratory behavior of rats. J Nutr 96:477–484.

Hernandez RJ (1973): Developmental pattern of the serotonin synthesizing enzyme in the brain of post-natally nalmourished rats. Experientia 29:1487–1488.

Juorio AV (1977): Effect of chlorpromazine and other antipsychotic drugs on mouse striatal tyramines. Life Sci 20:1663–1668.

Juorio AV (1979): Drug-induced changes in the formation, storage and metabolism of tyramine in the mouse. Br J Pharmacol 66:377–384.

Juorio AV (1983): The effects of some decarboxylase inhibitors on mouse striatal tyramines. Neuropharmacology 22:71–73.

Juorio AV, Boulton AA (1982): The effects of some precursor amino acids and enzyme inhibitors on mouse striatal concentration of tyramines and homovanillic acid. J Neurochem 39:859–863.

Juorio AV, Durden DA (1984): The distribution and turnover of tryptamine in the brain and spinal cord. Neurochem Res 9:1281–1291.

Kwok RPS, Juorio AV (1986): The concentration of striatal tyramine and dopamine metabolism in diabetic rats and the effect of insulin administration. Neuroendocrinology, 590–596.

Kwok RPS, Juorio AV (1987): The facilitating effect of insulin on brain 5-hydroxytryptamine metabolism Neuroendocrinology 45:267–273.

Kwok RPS, Walls EK, Juorio AV (1985): The concentration of dopamine, 5-hydroxytryptamine and some of their metabolites in the brain of genetically diabetic rats. Neurochem Res 10:611–616.

Lovenberg W, Weissbach H, Udenfriend S (1962): Aromatic-L-aminoacid decarboxylase. J Biol Chem 237:89–93.

MacKenzie RG, Trulson ME (1978): Effects of insulin and streptozotocin-induced diabetes on brain tryptophan and serotonin metabolism in rats. J Neurochem 30:205–211.

Marichich ES, Molina VA, Orsingher OA (1979): Persistent changes in central catecholaminergic system after recovery of perinatally undernourished rats. J Nutr 109:1045–1050.

Philips SR, Boulton AA (1979): The effects of monoamine oxidase inhibitors on some arylalkylamines in rat striatum. J Neurochem 33:159–167.

Philips SR, Davis BA, Durden DA, Boulton AA (1975): Identification and distribution of *m*-tyramine in the rat. Can J Biochem 53:65–69.

Philips SR, Durden DA, Boulton AA (1974a): Identification and distribution of *p*-tyramine in the rat. Can J Biochem 52:366–373.

Philips SR, Durden DA, Boulton AA (1974b): Identification and distribution of tryptamine in the rat. Can J Biochem 52:447–451.

Ramanamurthy PSV (1977): Maternal and early post-natal malnutrition and transmitter amines in rat brain. J Neurochem 28:253–254.

Saavedra JM (1974): Enzymatic isotopic assay for and in the presence of β-phenylethylamine in rat brain. J Neurochem 22:211–216.

Saavedra JM, Axelrod J (1973): Effect of drugs on the tryptamine content of rat tissues. J Pharmacol Exp Ther 185:523–529.

Saller CF (1984): Dopaminergic activity is reduced in diabetic rats. Neurosci Lett 49:301–306.

Sereni F, Principi N, Perletti L, Sereni LP (1966): Undernutrition and the developing rat brain. 1. Influence on acetylcholinesterase and succinic acid dehydrogenase activities and on norepinephrine and 5-OH-tryptamine tissue concentrations. Biol Neonate 10:254–265.

Shoemaker WJ, Wurtman RJ (1971): Perinatal undernutrition: Accumulation of catecholamines in rat brain. Science 171:1017–1019.

Sobotka TJ, Cook MP, Brodie RE (1974): Neonatal malnutrition: Neurochemical, hormonal and behavioural manifestations. Brain Res 65:443–457.

Stern WC, Miller M, Forbes WB, Morgane PJ, Resnick O (1975): Ontogeny of the levels of biogenic amines in various parts of the brain and in peripheral tissues in normal and protein malnourished rats. Exp Neurol 49:314–326.

Tagliamonte A, DeMontis MG, Olianas M, Onali PL, Gessa GL (1975): Possible role of insulin in the transport of tyrosine and tryptophan from blood to brain. Pharmacol Res Commun 7:493–499.

Trulson ME, Himmel CD (1983): Decreased brain dopamine synthesis rate and increased [^{3}H]-spiroperidol binding in streptozotocin-diabetic rats. J Neurochem 40:1456–1459.

Warsh JJ, Chan PW, Godse DD, Coscina DV, Stancer HC (1977): Gas-chromatography-mass fragmentography determination of indole-3-acetic acid in rat brain. J Neurochem 29:955–958.

Wiggins RC, Fuller G, Enna SJ (1984): Undernturition and the development of brain neurotransmitter systems. Life Sci 35:2085–2094.

SECTION V: CLINICAL CORRELATIONS OF BRAIN DEVELOPMENT AND MALNUTRITION

Current Topics in Nutrition and Disease, Volume 16
Basic and Clinical Aspects of Nutrition and Brain Development,
pages 317–321
© 1987 Alan R. Liss, Inc.

Perspective: The Development of Studies of Nutrition, the Brain, and Mental Performance— A Brief Retrospect

Mervyn Susser

Gertrude H. Sergievsky Center, Columbia University, New York, New York 10032

In the early 1900s, interest in the possible effects of nutritional deprivation on the brain dissipated. Experimentalists had attempted and failed to produce detectable effects by withholding nutrients (Davison and Dobbing, 1966). In the late 1960s, however, interest revived. A new generation of researchers addressed the problem. Experimentalists like McCance and Widdowson (1974), by paying scrupulous attention to dietary content and especially to the timing of nutritional insults in relation to sensitive developmental periods, demonstrated profound effects on growth; in pigs protein deficiencies early in gestation produced irreversible stunting. Underlying this work was the guiding concept of critical periods of development, during which adverse exposures might wreak irreversible change (Stockard, 1921). Davison and Dobbing (1966) pointed out that previous research had ignored the variation among species in the rate of development of the brain. Sensitive or vulnerable periods could be expected to coincide with times of maximum growth, and these differed among species. For example, the maximum rate of brain growth in pigs, as in human beings, was attained prenatally and persisted into the early postnatal months (Fig. 1). In rats, maximum growth was attained only in the postnatal period. In this view, if persisting effects were to be detected, nturitional deprivation would need to center on the vulnerable periods of maximum brain growth for each species. The results of Winick and his colleagues offered corroboration (Winick and Noble, 1966). In rats, the normal proliferation and subsequent enlargement of brain cells was impeded by severe and early protein deficiency, but was not always reversible. Depletion of brain cells proved irrecoverable only when the nutritional deficiency coincided with the period of maximum brain growth. In other experiments with pigs, monkeys, and rodents, early and severe nutritional deprivation—especially protein deprivation—seemed also to affect behavior and learning (Barnes et al., 1968).

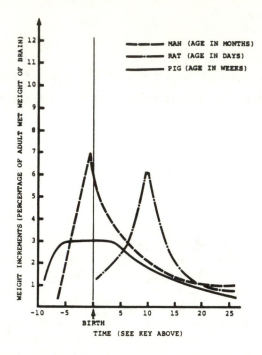

Fig. 1. Brain growth spurt in relation to conception and birth, compared in rat, pig, and man. (Adapted from Davison and Dobbing, 1966.)

The extent of malnutrition in children of the Third World came to be appreciated slowly. Kwashiorkor had been recognized as a manifestation of protein malnutrition by Cicely Williams (Williams, 1933) in Nigeria in 1933. The widespread nature of kwashiorkor and its analogues was not fully grasped before the 1950s (Brock and Autret). Clinicians began to observe and report the apathy, misery, and depressed functional performance of the affected children. By the mid 1960s, a number of followup studies of severe early malnutrition indicated that depressed mental performance persisted into later childhood (Scrinshaw and Gordon, 1968).

In view of the scale of Third World nutritional deprivation—often half the children in a community might be stunted and carry the stigmata of malnutrition—the potential effects on depressed mental performance were straggering. Indeed, many investigators at once declared themselves staggered. Their alarm outran the evidence. A close examination showed the human studies conducted up to that time to be poorly controlled or otherwise flawed (Stein and Kassab, 1970). More definitive studies were needed.

The studies that followed the recognition of this need provide the substance of our review (Stein and Susser, following chapter). (When overlap is unavoidable, it is mitigated by a perspective here that is historical; in the review it is developmental.) In its simplest form, the hypothesis was that at the time of maximum brain growth, prenatal nutritional deprivation (especially of protein) would produce an irreversible depletion of brain cells; a consequent postnatal deficit in mental performance would follow. Several large-scale studies in human beings were undertaken which were based more or less directly on the same hypothesis.

In our own studies of a well-defined situation of acute starvation in a developed country, namely the Dutch famine of 1944/1945, we found no support for the idea that prenatal nutrition during the period of the brain growth spurt had depressed the cognitive performance in young adults 20 years later (Stein et al., 1975). One alternative explanation was that passably good previous nutrition in the mothers protected their pregnancies in the prenatal period. These women had no overt signs of malnutrion and, during their growth period in the Netherlands before World War II, levels of nutrition were high. Perhaps then prenatal nutritional deprivation might affect subsequent development only in chronically malnourished mothers? This hypothesis would require testing in overtly malnourished mothers such as are found in less developed countries.

Another strong alternative was that, because the prenatal period covered only about 10% of the period of maximum brain growth during which the brain was sensitive to insults (Dobbing and Sands, 1973), the severe prenatal nutritional deprivation would still leave sufficient reserve in the brain to protect subsequent function. This hypothesis would require a test of the combined and independent effects of prenatal and postnatal malnutrition, again a likely situation only in less developed countries.

In two studies in less developed countries, both these alternative hypotheses could be simultaneously tested and eliminated. These studies of prenatal and postnatal nutritional supplementation in malnourished women, one a quasi-experiment in Guatemala (Habicht et al., 1974), and the other a controlled trial in Bogota (Mora et al., 1979), failed to support the contention that in malnourished women better *prenatal* nutrition alone could improve postnatal cognitive performance. In addition, prenatal nutrition had no demonstrable effect on cognition over and above that of postnatal nutrition (Waber et al., 1981; Freeman et al., 1980). (In controlled trials of high protein prenatal supplementation in New York as well as Bogota, however, effects on visual habituation occurred (Waber et al., 1981; Rush et al., 1980). Some studies, but not all, have suggested a link between habituation in infancy and later measured IQ).

Remaining alternative explanations were that the apparent variation in cognitive function with nutritional conditions was owed either to postnatal nutritional deprivation or to the social deprivation that invariably accompanies such malnutrition. The results of the intervention studies in Guatemala and Bogota both gave some support to the idea of a positive effect of *postnatal* nutrition on cognitive perofrmance (Waber et al., 1981a; Freeman et al., 1980). But here also a limiting negative emerged. In the Bogota study, the detectable effects on cognition were those of contemporaneous nutrition. This finding pointed to a pathway leading from nutrition to cognition through some current state of motivation, behavior, or health state.

Intensive longitudinal observation studies over many years in a Mexican village can be taken as supporting this result (Cravioto and Delicardie, 1975). The poor mental performance observed in malnourished children was largely accounted for by the mothers' access to external stimulation in the form of listening to the radio. Followup case-control studies of severe early malnutrition in Jamaica can also be taken to support the result. Differences between cases and control subjects were found mainly in the less stimulating environment and, when differences were found, the degree of social stimulation accounted for a good part of the differences (Hertzig et al., 1972; Richardson, 1976). In this study, the contribution of the current state of nutrition of the children is not known.

A study of postnatal intervention in Cali, Columbia, provided both good nutrition and social stimulation (McKay et al., 1978). In these children, well fed at the time of the last testing, there was marked cognitive improvement. In one group given nutritional supplementation alone, however, no effect cold be attributed to the intervention. For the present, then, one may conclude that the greatest postnatal influence on cognitive performance comes from social stimulation, or it is immediate and behaviorial.

The path of scientific development is never ending. It may be banal to say that our conclusions are always subject to revision, reversion, and subversion. Still, the moral that follows needs more than lip service. To arrive at a conclusion should not be to foreclose further study.

REFERENCES

Barnes RH, Moore AU, Reid IM, Pond WG (1968): Effect of food deprivation on behavioral patterns. In Scrimshaw NS, Gordon J (eds): "Malnutrition, learning and behavior." Cambridge, Mass.: MIT Press, pp 203–217.

Brock JF, Autret M (1952): "Kwashiorkor in Africa." Geneva: World Health Organization.

Cravioto J, DeLicardie ER (1975): Environmental and nutritional deprivation in children with learning disabilities. In Cruickshank WM, Hallahan DP (eds): "Perceptual and Learning Disabilities in Children." Vol. 2, "Research and Theory." Syracuse, N.Y.: Syracuse University Press, pp 3–102.

Davison AN, Dobbing J (1966): Myelination as a vulnerable period in brain development. Br Med Bull 22:40–44.

Dobbing J, Sands J (1973): Quantitative growth and development of the human brain. Arch Dis Child 48:757–767.

Freeman HE, Klein RE, Townsend JW, Lechtig A (1980): Nutrition and cognitive development among rural Guatemalan children. Am J Public Health 70:1277–1285.

Habicht JB, Yarbrough C, Lechtig A, Klein RE (1974): Relation of maternal supplementary feeding during pregnancy to birthweight and other sociobiological factors. In Winick M (ed): "Proceedings of the Symposium on Nutrition and Fetal Development." New York: John Wiley and Sons, pp 127–146.

Hertzig ME, Birch HG, Richardson SA, Tizad J (1972): Intellectual levels of school children severely malnourished in the first two years of life. Pediatrics 49:814–824.

McCance RA, Widdowson EM (1974): Review lecture. Determinants of growth and form. Proc Soc Lond (Biol) 185:1–17.

McKay H, Sinisterra L, McKay A, Gomez H, Lioreda P (1978): Improving cognitive ability in chronically deprived children. Science 200:270–278.

Mora JO, de Paredes B, Wagner M, deNavarro L, Suescun J, Christiansen N, Herrera MG (1979): Nutritional supplementation and the outcome of pregnancy. Am J Clin Nutr 32:455–462.

Richardson SA (1976): The relation of severe malnutrition in infancy to the intelligence of school children with differing life histories. Pediatr Res 10:57–61.

Rush D, Stein Z, Susser M (1980): Diet in pregnancy: A randomized controlled trial of prenatal nutritional supplementation. Birth Defects 16:3.

Scrimshaw NS, Gordon J (eds) (1968): "Malnutrition, Learning and Behavior." Cambridge, Mass.: MIT Press.

Stein Z, Susser M, Saenger G, Marolla FM (1975): "Famine and Human Development: Studies of the Dutch Winter 1944–5." New York: Oxford University Press.

Stein ZA, Kassab H (1970): Nutrition. In Wortis (ed): "Mental Retardation," Vol. 2. New York: Grune and Stratton, pp 92–116.

Stockard CR (1921): Developmental rate and structural expression: An experimental study of twins, "double monsters," and single deformities and the interaction among embryonic organs during their origin and development. Am J Anat 28:115–277.

Waber DP, Vuori-Christiansen L, Ortiz N, Clement JR, Christiansen N, Mora JO, Reed RB, Herrera G (1981): Nutritional supplementation, maternal education, and cognitive development of infants at risk of malnutrition. Am J Clin Nutr 34:807–813.

Williams CD (1933): A nutritional disease of childhood associated with a maize diet. Arch Dis Child 8:423–433.

Winick M, Noble A (1966): Cellular response in rats during malnutrition at various ages. J Nutr 89:300–306.

Current Topics in Nutrition and Disease, Volume 16
Basic and Clinical Aspects of Nutrition and Brain Development,
pages 323–338
© 1987 Alan R. Liss, Inc.

Early Nutrition, Fetal Growth, and Mental Function: Observations in Our Species

Zena Stein and Mervyn Susser

Gertrude H. Sergievsky Center, Columbia University and New York
Psychiatric Institute, New York, New York 10032

INTRODUCTION

This paper reviews the effects of early adverse nutritional experiences in human beings, with particular attention to the prenatal period. The outcome of interest is development, especially neurological and mental development. The scheme we present is based on the idea that in successive phases of development, the organism is sensitive to different types and degrees of insult, and that the timing of the insult therefore governs the types and degrees of effect.

The infant enters a particular psychosocial milieu from the moment of birth, and both physical and mental growth reflect this milieu. Hence it is difficult, and often misleading, to study the influence of early nutrition as if it were an isolated phenomenon. In practice, the opportunities to execute refined experiments that control the effects of milieu are rare. In the review that follows, we discuss a few planned experiments (none of them perfect), a closely documented "natural experiment," and several observational studies from which useful if not conclusive inferences may be drawn.

The development of the human infant, from zygote to formed fetus to infant, may be divided into four fairly distinct phases of varying susceptibility to stimuli that might affect development. Following the crucial initiating event of fertilization, the newly formed zygote divides into the many-celled blastocyst, travels down the Fallopian tube, and on the sixth day begins attaching to the uterus. Over the succeeding 5 weeks of embryonic development, virtually all the specialized organs of the human being emerge. Thus, by the end of the sixth week, at 42 days after fertilization, a formed fetus is present, with head, a human-looking face, a beating heart, limbs, and early separation of the phalanges. At a mode of 280 days, the infant is thrust into the world. It now encounters a varied and continually expanding social and physical environment, through developmental sequences marked by

Periconceptional

2 wks before fertilization till implanted (24 days LMP)

Embryonic

First trimester (organogenesis) (3–12 wks LMP)

Fetal

2nd trimester (neuronal hyperplasia);

3rd trimester (neuronal hypertrophy: glial hyperplasia)

Postnatal

Up to 2 yrs (rapid brain growth: myelination, arborization, synapses)

Fig. 1.   Timing of exposure.

1. Iodine deficiency disorders
2. (Uncontrolled) insulin-dependent diabetes
3. Hyperphenylalaninemia (HPA)
Each based on inference from prophylactic treatment **ineffective** after the periconceptional period.

Fig. 2.   Periconceptional: maternal.

staged behaviors like smiling, sitting, walking, and talking. The radical transformation from zygote to toddler, during which the main growth of the brain takes place, is completed over the short period of 2 years. It is not surprising that in this formative period, vulnerabilities and requirements for nutrients will also change radically. The successive steps of development are outlined in Figure 1.

PERICONCEPTIONAL EXPOSURE

In our reading of the literature, three disorders of nutrition can affect very early embryonic development. Each presents a specific problem of maternal metabolism, namely, iodine deficiency, insulin deficiency, and hyperphenylalaninemia (Fig. 2). The exposures are classed as periconceptional by negative inference: in each case, prophylactic treatment of the mother given after the first missed period has not proved effective.

Iodine Deficiency

Iodine deficiency in the mother before conception is associated with cretinism in the offspring, which may be either a myxoedematous type, a neurological type, or a mixed type (Hetzel and Hay, 1979). Cretinism of any form is endemic where iodine deficiency is prevalent, and throughout the world hundreds of millions reside in such areas. The child of myxoedematous type is small, dull or moderately retarded, often deaf, and with delayed development; the child of neurological type tends to be severely retarded, with spasticity and sometimes hemiparesis. Prophylactic randomized controlled trials show that iodized oil administered to the mother before conception prevents the condition. With the neurological type, treatment after birth, and even soon after pregnancy is far less effective (if effective at all) than prophylaxis before conception. The exact limits of usefulness of treatment begun late remain somewhat obscure. With the myxoedematous type, in which hypothyroidism is usually present, treatment of thyroid deficiency from a young age seems to lead to some intellectual improvement.

Diabetes

Uncontrolled insulin-dependent diabetes in the mother affects growth and produces an excess of congenital anomalies. Recent literature suggests that the main teratogenic phase is confined to a period before pregnancy, is established and recognized (Miller et al., 1981). In the weeks before the first missed period, high blood sugar levels (as indicated by retrospective interpretation of the glycosylate test) appear to be associated with an increased risk for congenital malformations of specific type, and also for mental retardation. Later during the fetal phase, blood sugar levels influence the growth and survival of the fetus, but seem not to affect the risk of malformations and mental retardation. A recent prospective study conducted by the National Institute of Child Health and Development (NICHD), in which diabetic pregnancies have been carefully monitored for blood sugar levels, should soon shed light on the role of the control of diabetes in the periconceptional period in teratogenesis.

Phenylketonuria

Phenylketonuria in a pregnant women exposes her offspring in utero to hyperphenylalaninemia. Prenatally, these offspring usually experience growth retardation; postnatally, mental retardation is a regular outcome, often together with microcephaly and congenital heart defects (Lenke and Levy, 1980). The dietary control of phenylalanine levels during pregnancy has not been shown to prevent these disorders. The hope that control before conception may do so is held out by a number of case reports. A collaborative controlled trial, undertaken by NICHD, aims to test the benefits of a phenylalanine-free maternal diet begun before a pregnancy is undertaken.

A	B
• Preterm births	• Lower social classes (UK; New England)
• Stillbirths and first week deaths	• Great depression (New England)
• CNS disorders (including NTD)	• Mutivite and iron, prepregnancy supplements
• Obesity	(Smithells et al.)

Fig. 3A.   Embryonic: acute nutritional deficiency. First trimester starvation: Dutch Famine.
Fig. 3B.   Embryonic: chronic nutritional deficiency. Neural tube defects.

EMBRYONIC PHASE

Nutritional deficiencies that seem to act in the embryonic phase have been sometimes acute, sometimes chronic. Acute starvation in the mother is exemplified by studies of the effects of exposure to the Dutch famine of 1944/5. Several adverse outcomes appeared in relation to exposure to the famine solely in the first trimester of pregnancy (Fig. 3A). Both length of gestation and organogenesis were affected. At birth, there was an excess of premature infants of very low birthweight and also an excess of stillbirths; an excess of first-week deaths also occurred (Stein et al., 1975a). Among survivors into young adulthood who were exposed in the embryonic phase, there was also an excess of obesity (Ravelli et al., 1976), a result since replicated experimentally in rats (Jones and Friedman, 1982).

Chronic dietary deficiency in the mother, extending from the woman's childhood and through the whole of pregnancy, has for some years been proposed as a cause of spina bifida and anencephaly. The hypothesis has seemed plausible in the light of the known social, geographic, and temporal variation of these neural tube defects (Fig. 3B). In Britain and in the United States, this disorder of organogenesis has been more common among the poorer classes, and in the United States prevalence reached a peak during the Great Depression of the 1930s (Edwards, 1958; Yen and MacMahon, 1968). Towards the end of World War II in Germany (Eichmann and Gesenius, 1952), as well as in the Netherlands (Stein et al., 1975a; Stein and Susser 1976), severe food shortage was associated with a rise in incidence of neural tube defects. Ethnic variation is quite marked; frequency is high in Celts, low in Japanese, Chinese, and Africans. The fact that among ethnic groups in the same locale differences persist—as with the Irish who migrated to New England compared with other New Englanders—indicates that some groups are more susceptible than others to the same environmental insults (Elwood, 1972). This susceptibility could be genetic or, perhaps less likely, cultural in origin.

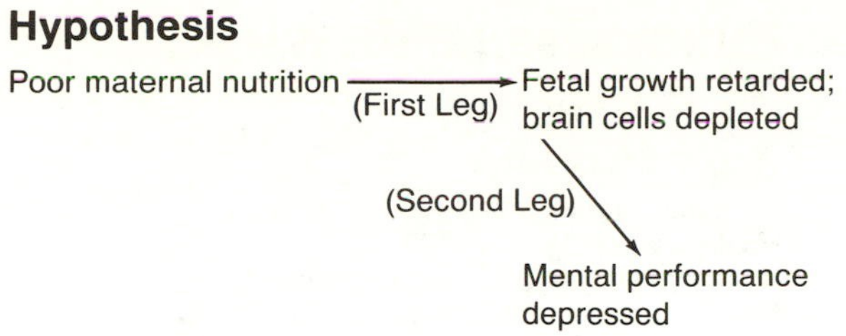

Hypothesis

Poor maternal nutrition ─────────▶ Fetal growth retarded;
(First Leg) brain cells depleted

(Second Leg)

Mental performance
depressed

Fig. 4.   Fetal stage.

More direct evidence has added plausibility to the dietary hypothesis. Dietary supplements of "multivite and iron," given to women with an affected child in anticipation of their next pregnancy, seem to have reduced the risk of recurrence. Non-randomized controls—women who were not given the special supplement before their pregnancies—had significantly higher frequencies of neural tube defects (Smithells et al., 1980). Parenthetically, one must note potential problems with the comparability of these controls (Laurence et al., 1980). Some subsequent reports support the hypothesis. Whether this presumed protection is conferred before conception, or during the periconception phase, or in the embryonic phase before the neuropore closes at the 28th day of gestation, must remain uncertain until the causal relationship is truly established (Mulinaire et al., 1981). The condition is discussed here because the effect is on organogenesis, and hence acts on development during the embryonic phase, even if it might arise earlier.

FETAL PHASE

In the fetal phase, evidence of developmental vulnerability is related chiefly to global nutrients and especially to calories in the diet. This contrasts with the periconception phase, in which the evidence pointed to metabolic imbalance, and with the embryonic phase, in which it pointed to specific micronutrients.

Again, a distinction is drawn between the effects of acute starvation of the mother and those of chronic malnutrition persisting from her childhood and through her pregnancy. The effects need to be analyzed in sequence: a first leg of a presumed causal chain involves prenatal exposure and effects seen at birth; a second leg is conditional on the state of the infant at birth, and involves effects on postnatal development (Fig. 4). In general, at birth the effects observed pertain only to indices of physical growth and survival. One must wait for development to unfold in order to observe function and performance. The following discussion will deal in turn with each leg of the

Nutrition and Birth Weight
(First Leg)

Acute Starvation

3rd trimester (Smith; Stein et al.; Antonov)
Maximum 3–400g
Asymmetrical: hierarchy bwt/length/head circ.
Mortality up to 3 mos. consistent with bwt (Stein et al.)

Prenatal Supplementation

North American: 40–50g
    New York (Rush, Stein, Susser)
    Montreal (Rush)

Latin American: 70–80g
    Bogota (Mora et al.)
    Guatemala (Habicht et al.)

Other
    Taiwan? (Heriot et al.)

Chronic Malnutrition

Low social class
Poverty   } Ecological
Third World

Fig. 5. Evidence from fetal stage.

sequence, that is, first, size at birth, and then subsequent development. The evidence for each leg stems from observational studies (both of acute starvation and of chronic malnutrition) and from experiments in which maternal diets were supplemented (Fig. 5).

Size at Birth

The strongest and most substantial effects of nutrition on birth weight were demonstrated during periods of acute starvation in World War II, especially during the 900 days of the Leningrad siege (Antonov, 1947), and in the aftermath of the Dutch famine (Smith, 1947). We further investigated the experience of the Dutch famine. With exposure in the third trimester of pregnancy, we found a maximum effect on birth weight of 300–400 grams or about 9–10% (Stein et al., 1975a). All dimensions of fetal growth including head circumference were affected, although not to the same degree. Effects occurred in a hierarchy, with maternal weight the most sensitive, followed by placental weight and birth weight, and then by length and head circumference (Stein and Susser, 1975). The Dutch famine study is unique also in demonstrating an effect of prenatal nutrition on infant mortality. Besides first trimester effects (possibly embryonic in origin) on stillbirths and first-week deaths, fetal phase exposure in the third trimester had a marked effect on the death rate up to 3 months of age (Stein et al., 1975b). Increased mortality in the same exposed cohorts continued through infancy and beyond, but could not be attributed unequivocally to the famine.

With regard to chronic malnutrition, all over the world low birth weight is associated with poor maternal nutrition. The greater part of the phenomenon of low birth weight occurring under conditions of deprivation is accounted for by a slower rate of growth in utero. Shortened gestation, while also more frequent in adverse nutritional conditions, does not account for the greater part of the lowered birth weight observed in surviving live births. Under these conditions, typically, size at birth is diminished in all dimensions, so that the infant is symmetrically small, with head, length, and weight affected proportionately. A current hypothesis is that—with chronic maternal malnutrition persisting from before conception—growth begins to slow down quite early, probably before mid-trimester, and continues slowly until delivery (Villar and Belizan, 1982). This growth pattern contrasts with that of most low birth weight infants in developed countries. Under these more favorable nutritional conditions, typically, the infant at birth is asymmetrically affected, with weight depressed but head circumference and length unaffected. The available data strongly support the hypothesis that this latter pattern results, as noted above, from retarded growth in the third trimester.

The differences between these two types of growth retardation are likely to be important if the hypothesis holds that neither their immediate nor their long-term effects are the same (Villar et al., 1984). With symmetrical growth retardation, infants are said not to experience a marked rise in perinatal mortality, but for the first year of life at least, the survivors remain stunted and track along the lower percentiles for height and weight. In some studies, stature has seemed to remain depressed through early childhood and into adolescence, and one study suggests that the same could be true for mental development. By contrast, infants with asymmetrical growth retardation undoubtedly experience increased perinatal mortality; those that survive this initial disadvantage quickly catch up in terms of weight and are not delayed in development. During the Dutch famine, maternal starvation in the third trimester produced asymmetrical growth retardation and raised mortality as noted, and the results conform with the hypothesis that these are effects of third trimester nutrient depletion, as we shall show below.

These observations and hypotheses emphasize that low birth weight is not the outcome of any single cause and that, even when it is a result of inadequate maternal nutrition, it might be the outcome of more than one pathogenetic mechanism. The existence of several causal paths could be one reason for the refractoriness of birth weight in the face of attempts to accelerate fetal growth by nutritional means. In rigorous experimental studies, supplementation of the maternal diet during pregnancy has at best produced a modest increment in birth weight (reviewed in Susser, 1980; Rush, 1982; Adair and Pollitt, 1985). In malnourished mothers in Latin America and elsewhere, the average increment in birth weight of the offspring of supplemented mothers had reached 60 or 70 g. (In one main study by Habicht et al. (1974), confounding of the relationship of supplementation with birth weight by length of gestation remains possible.) In the North American poor, the increment with supplementation has been nearer 40 g (Rush et al., 1980). These increments may be compared with the 200 g of birth weight that can be lost by maternal smoking during pregnancy.

A reanalysis of the major supplementation study carried out in rural Guatemala, however, suggests that for women who used dietary supplements during and between two successive pregnancies, the later-born infants have an advantage in birth weight over the earlier-born (Villar, 1985). Most controlled dietary experiments have tended to study supplementation of maternal diets through the last trimester of a single pregnancy. In the light of this latest analysis, the short duration of dietary supplementation would presumably account for the modest effects on birth weight observed in other studies. If confirmed, the substantial increment in birth weight after prolonged supplementation that extends well beyond a single pregnancy supports the view that low birth weight in less developed countries can be attributed in part to chronic undernutrition of the mother. Such a condition is unlikely to be remedied by short-term dietary supplementation. Observations on the effects of the Women, Infants and Children (WIC) food programs in the United States (Rush, 1986) are also compatible with the hypothesis that a moderate gain in the mean birth weight of infants born to poorly nourished mothers is to be expected from sustained supplementation of maternal diets.

On the other hand, certain results enjoin caution in the approach to supplementation. When prenatal supplements contain a high concentration of protein, there appears to be a risk of adverse effects. In the randomized controlled trial of prenatal supplementation in New York, such supplements significantly retarded fetal growth; there was also an excess of preterm infants with a high risk of neonatal death (Rush et al., 1980). With regard to fetal growth, it is now clear that other studies support this result. In eight instances (culled from all available sources), birth weight after high prenatal protein was compared with birthweight in a control group: in seven of the eight, birth weight was lower in the high protein group (Rush, 1982).

Neurological and Mental Deficit

When we turn to the second leg of the hypothetical sequence from nutrition to development, it has proved difficult to establish a causal connection between low birth weight following undernutrition of the mother

19-Year-Old Men After Prenatal Starvation (Dutch Famine)

Mental performance: no effect
Obesity: lowered frequency

Children After Prenatal Supplementation

Mental performance: no effect (Bogota, Guatemala, New York)

Habituation

At one year: New York high protein
Rhesus monkeys: high protein at 15 days: Bogota

Fig. 6.   Fetal stage (second leg).

and neurological and mental deficit. Several different causal models can account for many of the data observed (Fig. 6).

First, in one sequence, a common cause gives rise both to low birth weight and to mental impairment. Thus in some forms of mental retardation associated with low birth weight, a cause such as a chromosomal anomaly is the antecedent of intrauterine growth retardation on the one hand and mental retardation on the other.

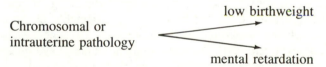

For purposes of elucidating the causal relationships of prenatal nutrition and subsequent development, this model has no salience.

In a second causal model, some factor (which might possibly be malnutrition among others) gives rise to marked prematurity and very low birth weight which, in turn, gives rise to neurological impairment and mental retardation.

Malnutrition→Preterm delivery→Neurological impairment and mental retardation
(very low birthweight)

Very low birth weight infants ($\leq$ 1,500 g) are undoubtedly at increased risk of cerebral palsy with mental retardation, and their prematurity, immaturity, and vulnerability may underlie that risk. Such infants comprise about 1% of births in New York City. In the 1960s, their risk for severe mental retardation was about 4–5%, that is, in the general population of births they could comprise up to 0.5/1,000. These infants almost invariably have had severe anoxia and accompanying neurological damage. Although the contribution of maternal diet to the incidence of preterm low birth weight offspring is not well understood, still, by most accounts it is not great. Therefore, this sequence too will not explain the association of preterm delivery with neurological damage.

A third causal sequence revolves around the central issue of the direct association of depressed birth weight with depressed mental performance (and/or mild mental retardation). This hypothesis stems in part from the association of both low birth weight and poor mental performance with poverty and poor dietary circumstances. This third model is of malnutrition leading to fetal growth retardation—a retardation that includes the brain and results in an irreversible depletion of brain cell number (Winick and Noble, 1966)—followed by the postnatal depression of mental function.

Malnutrition→fetal growth retardation→depressed mental performance

The animal experiments that support this model produced their effects through acute nutritional deprivation—usually of protein—applied during the period of maximum brain growth. This is precisely the model subjected to test—and rejected—by the Dutch Famine Study (Stein et al., 1975a). Records of infants born around the time of the famine confirm that, as in the animal experiments, fetal exposure to famine in the third trimester produced marked fetal growth retardation in all dimensions, including retarded growth of the head. In a complete national population of surviving 19-year-old men, however, such famine exposure produced no detectable effect on mental competence, whether measured by intelligence tests, special school attendance, or clinical evaluation. Some subsequent authors have questioned the experimental basis for the hypothesis: one challenger held that in primate experiments the depletion of brain cells did not occur (Cheek, 1985); another could not find histopathological or other evidence for the existence of irreversible depletion of cells in various organs (Sands et al., 1979; Dobbing and Sands, 1985).

Chronic malnutrition in the developing world is more relevant than famine in the developed world to the health of the world at large. The available evidence from the developing world does not support the idea that chronic maternal malnutrition during the fetal phase manifests effects on measures of cognition any more than does acute starvation, except in the one respect of attention. It remains to be seen whether persistent supplementation through more than one pregnancy or before a first pregnancy will improve mental performance as perhaps it improves birth weight. The exceptional finding relating to attention is that supplementation with high protein during the fetal phase has appeared to produce highly specific effects in infants, notably in augmenting the speed of habituation and dishabituation to visual or tactile stimuli. This result is one of the firmer in the literature on the mental effects of prenatal nutrition, having been found—not exactly in the same form—in two randomized trials of supplementation in human beings and in one trial in primates. The effect is apparently direct and not mediated by fetal growth or birth weight. Thus, in the New York study, all other psychometric measures of development but one correlated with each other and with physical size (both at birth and at 1 year of age) but not with the nutritional supplement. In contrast, the habituation measure correlated neither with the other psychometric measures nor with physical growth, but only with assignment to the high protein supplement.

POSTNATAL PHASE

Prenatal and early postnatal effects are difficult to separate. Histopathological studies (Dobbing and Sands, 1973) suggest that the phase of rapid brain growth which starts in mid-trimester slows, not after 3 or 6 months of postnatal life as was thought, but well into the second year. Thus, in one perspective, parturition may not mark a significant break in the biological development of the brain. A personal view is that the translation, at birth, of the gestating organism into a person with social roles has potential biological effects on central nervous system development, and that it is unwise to ignore them. However, some of the major experimental studies of prenatal supplementation considered below extend across the boundary of parturition and into the postnatal phase.

In diverse studies, using different designs and outcome measures, malnutrition alone during the postnatal phase has not been shown to produce permanent mental impairment (Lloyd-Still, 1976a). When combined with a lack of intellectual and social stimulation, however, such malnutrition does appear to depress mental performance. This conclusion rests on an array of observations from several studies. In some studies, the nutritional deprivation was caused by clinical conditions in children who did not lack social stimulation: for instance, cystic fibrosis (Lloyd-Still 1976b), celiac disease (Valman, 1974), ileal resection, and cyanotic congenital heart disease (Silbert et al., 1969). These impairments of nutrition under relatively good social conditions did not engender detectable mental impairment.

In other studies, episodes of acute nutritional failure in children reared in severely deprived environments gave rise to apparent deficits in mental performance in some well-controlled studies (Hertzig et al., 1972), although not in all (Hansen et al., 1971). These deficits have seemed to be recovered with food and/or mental stimulation, however (Richardson, 1976; Grantham-McGregor et al., 1980), and recovery could also explain the initially negative result in the study of Hansen et al. (1971). In further studies, the effect of food supplementation was tested experimentally among children exposed to chronic malnutrition. These experimental interventions have yielded equivocal responses (Freeman et al., 1980; Waber et al., 1981). One conclusion seems to apply throughout. In virtually all the experimental studies for which the necessary data are provided, the presence or absence of a response to supplementation can be seen to be mediated by the quality of the social environment.

One long-term and carefully conducted intervention study of the effect of early nutrition on cognition was conducted in four villages in Guatemala. The diet of the villagers is described as mild to moderately deficient in protein and calories. In each of the four villages, women and children were encouraged to partake twice daily and ad libitum of a supplementary beverage. In two of the villages the beverage was a protein-calorie mixture; in the other two, it contained no protein and fewer calories. At each visit, the amount consumed by each individual was recorded. At each birthday, from 3 to 7 years of age, the children were evaluated on psychosocial and anthropometric measures including family background and social interactions. Analyses of this study present problems; perhaps because there are many separate papers and even more authors, results and assertions from paper to paper are not entirely consistent. Exclusions of subjects are not all accounted for and could be confounding (Habicht et al., 1974); sometimes the longitudinal data are treated cross-sectionally with the same individuals appearing in several cells (Freeman et al., 1980); the amount of supplementation is confounded with duration of gestation because the shorter is gestation, the less the opportunity to consume the supplement, but also the lower the birth weight; home diet is measured but not analyzed, etc. One special problem, recognized by the investigators, is that in the analysis, the experimental design was abandoned in favor of a quasi-experimental one.

The relations of supplementation, physical growth, test scores and social indices were accounted for in a multivariate analysis. In the event, physical indices and social status indices both correlated significantly and independently with psychometric test scores, especially with language scores (Freeman et al., 1980). The total amount of supplementation of the mother during gestation and during lactation was considered separately from that of the child, and supplementation of both mother and child correlated wtih psychometric test scores and with growth. In the end, no significant postnatal effect solely owing to prenatal supplement consumption could be isolated. Consumption by the children themselves correlated most strongly with test scores and physical growth. Because the analysis abandoned the experimental design and left the way open for subjects as volunteers to select for themselves the use of supplements, this result immediately raises the question: was the child who took more supplement livelier because of the food or was the livelier child the one who took the most supplement? We note that language was the test measure associated most consistently with supplement, as well as with social indices and physical growth. The language tests are said by the researchers to relate meaningfully to behavior and social interaction outside the testing situation. This observation seems to point to initiative of the child, which might have led to self-selection in the consumption of supplement.

The Guatemalan findings show that children who make use of food supplements will grow taller and will do better on several cognitive tests than those who do not. What the causal sequence is among these changes is not established. For how long the advantage of supplemented children will last is also not known as yet, but it was observed over several years of development. Finally, both the use and the effect of the nutritional supplement is seen to be mediated by the sociofamilial environment.

In another carefully designed intervention study in Bogota, Colombia, (Waber et al., 1981), the effects of six blocked treatments could be compared: supplementation from the third trimester to 6 months postnatal; supplementation from the third trimester to 3 years, supplementation from 6 months postnatal to 3 years; no supplementation at all; and finally, maternal education from birth to 3 years given to two experimental groups, one without supplementation, and another supplemented from the third trimester to 3 years. In Bogota, prenatal diet supplementation in the third trimester had a modest effect on birth weight, significant (on a one-tail test, in our opinion unjustified) only in boys (Mora et al., 1979). We have already referred to the single postnatal mental or behavioral effect of prenatal supplements in the fetal phase; at 15 days of age, supplemented infants exhibited a more rapid response decrement on a test of auditory habituation.

In the postnatal period, diet supplementation influenced only motor measures, maternal education influenced only language, and there was no interaction between these effects. The advantage on motor measures of those supplemented through the third trimester and the first 6 months of postnatal life was short-lived. Thus, at 3 years of age, the children whose supplementation began postnatally at 6 months of age equalled the performance of those supplemented throughout the study period. In fact, the authors conclude that test scores reflect concurrent diet best. This study, like those in New York and Guatemala, offers no support for the concept of "critical period" during which a nutritrional insult results in irreversible damage that will be reflected in function (the results do not rule out cellular depletion that does not cause functional deficit detectable by the psychometric methods now in use).

In summary gains from supplementation in general were modest, affected mainly motor function, and were apparent only over the period that the supplement was used. We may conclude, with the investigators, that malnutrition probably decreased concurrent motivation and arousal, and that these effects may not be long-lasting. The long-term observational studies of Cravioto and Delicardie (1975) in a Mexican village provide a full examination of the connection between nutritional and social aspects of the environment and their combined effects on mental functioning. Poor mental function was indeed associated with poor nutrition, but always and only in the absence of social stimulation.

CONCLUSIONS

Specific dietary deficiencies and metabolic imbalances underlie a number of forms of mental retardation or depressed mental competence. As far as these are understood, they relate to periods before pregnancy—the periconceptional phase and the embryonic phase. With these disorders, the basis for prevention is much stronger than the basis for treatment. Apart from these effects of early pregnancy, neither acute nor chronic malnutrition in the prenatal, fetal, and early postnatal phases has been shown to be a lasting cause of depressed mental competence, still less of clinical mental retardation. When chronic nutritional deprivation is combined with social deprivation, however, cognitive performance in childhood is likely to be depressed. Whether such deficits persist into adulthood is not known, but examples of apparent rehabilitation (Hansen et al., 1971; Graham and Adrianzen, 1971; Hertzig et al., 1972; McLaren et al., 1973; Cravioto and DeLicardie, 1975; Richardson, 1976; Grantham-McGregor et al., 1978, 1980) make one reasonably optimistic that improvement can take place at older ages. The strongest hope for effective intervention, in our opinion, lies in the strong effect of social and educational stimulation coupled with good nutrition (Garber, 1975; McKay et al., 1978).

REFERENCES

Adair LS, Pollitt E (1985): Outcome of maternal nutritional supplementation: A comprehensive review of Bacon Chow study. Amer J Clin Nutrit 41:#5, 948–978.

Antonov AN (1947): Children born during the siege of Leningrad in 1942. J Pediat 30:250–259.

Cheek DB (1985): The control of cell mass and replication. The DNA unit—a personal 20-year study. Early Human Dev 12:211–239.

Cravioto J, DeLicardie E (1975): Environment and nutrition deprivation in children with learning disabilities. In Cruickshank W, Hallahan D (eds): "Perceptual and Learning Disabilities in Children." Vol. 2, "Research and Theory." New York: Syracuse University Press, pp 3–102.

Dobbing J, Sands J (1973): Quantitative growth and development of the human brain. Arch Dis Child 48:757–767.

Dobbing J, Sands J (1985): Cell size and cell number in tissue growth and development: An old hypothesis reconsidered. Arch Fr Pediatr 42:199–203.

Edwards JH (1958). Congenital malformations of the central nervous system in Scotland. Br J Prev Med 11:115–130.

Eichmann E, Gesenius H (1952): Die missgeburtenzunahme in Berlin und umberbung in den nachkriegs jahran. Arch Gynak 181:168–184.

Elwood JH (1972): Major central nervous system malformation notified in Northern Ireland 1964–1968. Dev Med Child Neurol 14:731–739.

Elwood JM, Elwood JH (1980): "Epidemiology of Anencephalies and Spina Bifida." London: Oxford University Press, p 234.

Freeman H, Klein R, Townsend J, Lechtig A (1980): Nutrition and cognitive development among rural Guatemalan children. Am J Public Health 70:1277–1286.

Garber HL (1975): Intervention in infancy: A developmental approach. In Begab MJ, Richardson SA (eds): The "Mentally Retarded and Society: A Social Science Prespective." Baltimore: University Park Press, pp 287–304.

Graham GG, Adrianzen B (1971): Growth, inheritance, and environment. Pediatr Res 5:691–697.

Grantham-McGregor SM, Stewart ME, Desai P (1978): A new look at the assessment of mental development in young children recovering from severe protein-energy malnutrition. Dev Med Child Neurol 20:773–778.

Grantham-McGregor SM, Steward ME, Schofeld WN (1980): Effect of long-term psychosocial stimulation on mental development of severely malnourished children. Lancet 2:785–789.

Habicht JP, Yarbrough C, Lechtig A, Klein R (1974): Relation of maternal supplementary feeding during pregnancy to birthweight and other sociological fators. In Winick M (ed): "Current Concepts in Nutrition." Vol. 2, "Nutrition and Fetal Development." New York: John Wiley and Sons, pp 127–146.

Hansen JD, Freesman C, Moodie AD (1971): What does nutritional growth retardation imply? Pediatrics 47:299–313.

Hertzig ME, Birch HG, Richardson SA, Tizard J (1972): Intellectual levels of school children severely malnourished during the first two years of life. Pediatrics 49:814–823.

Hetzel BS, Hay ID (1979): Thyroid function, iodine nutrition and fetal brain development. Clin Endocrinol 2:445–460.

Jones AP, Friedman MI (1982): Obesity and adipocyte abnormalities in offspring of rats undernourished during pregnancy. Science 215:1518–1519.

Laurence KM, James N, Miller M, Campbell H (1980): Inverse risk of pregnancies complicated by fetal neural tube defects in mothers receiving poor diets and possible benefit of dietary counselling. Br Med J 281:1592–1594.

Lenke RR, Levy HL (1980): Maternal phenylketonuria and hyperphenylalaninemia: An international survey of the outcome of untreated and treated pregnancies. N Engl J Med 202:1202–1208.

Lloyd-Still J (ed) (1976a): "Malnutrition and Intellectual Development." Lancaster: MTP Press Ltd.

Lloyd-Still J (1976b): Clinical studies on the effects of malnutrition during "Malnutrition and Intellectual Development." Lancaster: MTP Press Ltd, pp 103–159.

McKay H, Sinisterra L, McKay A, Gomez H, Lloreda P (1978): Improving cognitive ability in chronically deprived children. Science 270:278.

McLaren DS, Yaktin US, Kanawati AA, Sabbagh S, Kadi Z (1973): The subsequent mental and physical development of rehabilitated marasmic infants. J Ment Defic Res 17:273–281.

Miller E, Mare J, Cloherty J, Dunn P, Gleason R, Soeldner J, Kiutzmiller J (1981): Elevated maternal hemoglobin A in early pregnancy and major congenital anomalies in infants of diabetic mothers. N Engl J Med 304:1331–1333.

Mora JD, de Paredes B, Wagner M, de Navarro L, Suescun J, Christiansen N, Herrera MG (1979): Nutritional supplementation and the outcome of pregnancy. I. Birthweight Am J Clin Nutr 32:455–462.

Mulinaire J, Cordera JF, and Erickson JD (1981): Vitamin use and occurrence of neural tube defects. Am J Epidemial 114:428.

Ravelli GP, Stein Z, Susser M (1976): Obesity in young men after famine exposure in utero and early infancy. N Engl J Med 295:349–353.

Richardson SA (1976): The relation of severe malnutrition in infancy to the intelligence of school children having differing life histories. Pediatr Res 10:57–61.

Rush D (1982): Effects of changes in protein and caloric intake during pregnancy on the growth of the human fetus. In Enkin M, Chalmers I (eds): "Effectiveness and Satisfaction in Antenatal Care." Spastics International Medical Publications. London: Heinemann.

Rush D (1986): The National WIC Evaluation. VI. Summary. Office of Analyses and Evaluation, Food and Nutrition, SERV, Dept. of Agriculture, Washington, D.C.

Rush D, Stein Z, Susser M (1980): "Diet in Pregnancy: A Randomized Controlled Trial of Prenatal Nutritional Supplements." Birth Defects: Original Article Series, Vol. 16, No. 3. New York: Alan R. Liss.

Sands J, Dobbing J, Gratrix CA (1979): Cell number and cell size: organ growth and development and the control of catch-up growth in rats. Lancet ii:503–505.

Silbert A, Wolff PH, Mayer B, Rosenthal A, Nadas AS (1969): Cyanotic heart disease and psychological development. Pediatrics 43:192–200.

Smith CA (1947): Effect of wartime starvation in Holland on pregnancy and its products. Am J Obstet Gynecol 53:599–608.

Smithells RW, Sheppard S, Schorah CJ, Seller MJ, Nevin NC, Harris R, Read AO, Fielding DW (1980): Possible prevention of neural-tube defects by periconceptional vitamin supplementation. Lancet 1:339–340.

Stein ZA, Susser MW (1975): The Dutch famine, 1944/45 and the reproductive process. I. Effects on six indices at birth. Pediatr Res 9:70–76.

Stein ZA, Susser MW (1976): Maternal starvation and birth defects. In Hook EB (ed): "Birth Defects: Risks and Consequences." New York: Academic Press, pp 205–220.

Stein ZA, Susser MW, Saenger G, Marolla FA (1975a): "Famine and Human Development: The Dutch Hunger Winter of 1944/45." New York, Oxford University Press.

Stein ZA, Susser MW, Sturmans F (1975b): Famine and mortality. Tijdschr Soc Geneeskunde 53:134–141.

Valman HB (1974): Intelligence after malnutrition caused by neonatal resection of ileum. Lancet 1:425–429.

Villar J, Belizan JM (1982): The timing factor in the pathophysiology of the intrauterine growth retardation syndrome. Obst Gynecol Surv 37:499–506.

Villar J, Smeriglio V, Martorell R, Brown CH, Klein RE (1984): Heterogeneous growth and mental development of intrauterine growth-retarded infants during the first 3 years of life. Pediatrics 74:783–791.

Villar J (1985): Read at the American Public Health Association. Washington, D.C., 1985.

Waber DP, Vuori-Christiansen L, Ortiz N, Clement JR, Christiansen NE, Mora JO, Reed RB, Herrera MG (1981): Nutritional supplementation, maternal education, and cognitive development of infants at risk of malnutrition. Am J Clin Nutr 34:807–813.

Winick M, Noble A (1966): Cellular response in rats during malnutrition of various ages. J Nutr 89:300–306.

Yen S, MacMahon B (1968): Genetics of anencephaly and spina bifida? Lancet 2:623–626.

Current Topics in Nutrition and Disease, Volume 16
Basic and Clinical Aspects of Nutrition and Brain Development,
pages 339–357
© 1987 Alan R. Liss, Inc.

Maternal Nutrition and Fetal Growth: Implications for Subsequent Mental Competence

Pedro Rosso

Escuela de Medicina, Pontificia Universidad Católica de Chile, Santiago, Chile

INTRODUCTION

The possibility that mental competence may be permanently affected by prenatal exposure to malnutrition has been the subject of numerous studies since the early 1960s, when a link between postnatal malnutrition and subsequent mental development was first suggested (Stoch and Smythe, 1963). But these efforts, conducted in different populations throughout the world, have not provided definitive answers (Stein et al., 1975; Klein et al., 1977; Rush et al., 1980; Adair and Pollitt, 1985) because of the difficulty of extricating nutritional variables from the host of maternal and environmental factors known to influence mental competence (Stein et al., 1975) and because of inadequate knowledge on related aspects, such as maternal-fetal metabolic interactions during malnutrition, the consequences of maternal malnutrition on fetal brain growth, and the morphological and functional basis of mental competence. In addition, marked interspecies differences in reproductive biology, including the timing of fetal growth events in relation to analogous gestational times, have made the use of animal models to interpret the human stiuation of limited value (Holt et al., 1975; Dobbing and Sands, 1979).

Most investigators have approached the question of prenatal nutritional and mental competence by assuming that prenatal malnutrition affects fetal growth and, therefore, brain growth. Brain growth retardation at such a critical stage of development would determine lasting changes in brain structure which, in turn, would limit the capacity of the brain to perform some of the functions involved in mental competence (Dobbing, 1985). However, it is also theoretically possible that nutritional inadequacies may affect mental capacity or, at least, certain brain functions without affecting brain growth. To date this possiblity has not been directly investigated, although some of the available results discussed here suggest the existence of such an effect.

The present review will analyze the available information on prenatal nutrition and mental competence in humans while discussing the following key questions: Does maternal malnutrition affect fetal growth and, specifically, brain growth? Does a period of prenatal brain growth retardation permanently affect mental competence?

MATERNAL NUTRITION AND FETAL GROWTH

When considering the possible implications of maternal nutritional inadequacies on fetal growth, it is important to define certain terms. For the purpose of this review, only disorders of protein-energy intake will be considered. There is a general consensus that the most pervasive nutritional problem in the developing countries is a reduced intake of food, or "undernutrition," rather than "malnutrition," which implies an unbalanced intake of nutrients, generally reflecting a low protein diet.

During pregnancy, problems arising from a deficit in energy-protein intake can be observed in two situations: 1) women who were already undernourished when they became pregnant, as indicated by a low weight for height; and 2) women with a normal prepregnancy weight for height status who fail to meet the caloric needs of pregnancy, as indicated by a low weight gain. In the past, these two situations have not been properly recognized. The first type of undernutrition will be called "low prepregnancy weight" and the second type "gestational undernutrition."

In developing countries, undernutrition typically begins in early life, causing growth retardation, delayed skeletal ossification, delayed menarche, and a reduced adult stature (Chávez and Martínez, 1970). When these women become pregnant for the first time, they may have a normal body weight for their height; thus, they are not acutely undernourished. However, their reduced height determines a lower mean birth weight for their infants (Table I). The effect of maternal height on birth weight is well recognized (Love and Kinch, 1965; Niswander and Jackson, 1974; Lazar et al., 1975). By contrast, some women, besides being growth-stunted, also have a reduced body weight (weight for height less than 90% of standard weight). They constitute the classic type of chronic maternal undernutrition. Their combination of reduced maternal stature and low prepregnancy body mass has a strongly negative effect on fetal growth unless they can normalize their nutritional deficit during the course of pregnancy (Tompkins et al., 1955; Eastman and Jackson, 1968; Simpson et al., 1975; Niswander and Jackson, 1974; Bjerre and Bjerre, 1976; Edwards et al., 1979).

In more affluent populations, where food availability is not limited by either budgetary or climatic factors, it is common to find young women whose weight for height is less than 90% of standard weight. Most of these

TABLE I. Influence of Maternal Height on Birth Weight in
Low Income Chilean Women (mean ± SD)[a]

Maternal height (cm)	n	Birth weight (g)[b]
Less than 140	15	3,094 ± 361
140–144	103	3,231 ± 434
145–149	429	3,348 ± 384
150–154	716	3,377 ± 408
155–159	608	3,451 ± 409
160–164	232	3,535 ± 387
More than 165	60	3,495 ± 431

[a]Data from Rosso et al., 1987; unpublished.
[b]All births are singleton and full term.

young mothers are of average or above average height, consider themselves healthy, are physically active, and have been "thin" or "slim" all their lives. Clearly, the situation does not correspond to the chronic undernutrition described above, but their condition cannot be considered "normal" according to reference standards. These women with low weight/height also deliver infants whose mean birth weight is significantly below average (Tompkins et al., 1955; Edwards et al., 1979). Based on these considerations, we propose to classify them, together with the truly chronically undernourished mothers, as "low prepregnancy weight mothers." Thus, this clinical entity includes both women whose living conditions and diet history are consistent with "chronic undernutrition" and "underweight" mothers whose low weight/height may reflect a combination of genetic, cultural, and environmental factors.

During gestation, low prepregnancy weight women may either increase their food intake and meet pregnancy needs or maintain an inadequate food intake (Rosso, 1981b). In the first situation, weight gain can be normal and may help to improve maternal nutritional status. However, unless the initial maternal deficit of body nutrient stores is completely corrected, fetal growth will be less than average. In the second situation, when the mother fails to have normal food intake during pregnancy, she also becomes gestationally undernourished, and the newborn is usually considerably lighter than average (Rosso, 1981b; Eastman and Jackson, 1968; Abrams and Laros, 1986).

In both developing and industrialized countries, low prepregnancy weight mothers tend to gain more weight during pregnancy than either normal or obese women (Simpson et al., 1975; Eastman and Jackson, 1968). The available information indicates that the greater weight increments reflect a higher caloric intake (Beal, 1971), but it is unclear if this is an adaptive response or if it is due to the advice of health personnel. Unfortunately, as already mentioned, despite their greater gestational weight gains, the average

TABLE II. Influence of Maternal Weight Gain on Birth Weight in Low Income, Low Prepregnancy Weight-For-Height American and Chilean Women (mean ± SD)[a]

Weight gain (kg)	Birth weight (g)	
	American[b]	Chilean[c]
Less than 8.5	2,850 ± 321 (22)[d]	3,067 ± 367 (79)
8.5–13.5	2,980 ± 358 (42)	3,219 ± 377 (162)
More than 13.5	3,341 ± 361 (31)	3,351 ± 382 (182)

[a]Data from Rosso et al., 1987; unpublished.
[b]Racially mixed population from New York City approximately 50% black and approximately 50% white hispanics.
[c]White population with various proportions of Spanish and Indian ancestry.
[d]Number of subjects.

birth weight of neonates delivered by these mothers is generally lower than the birth weight of the newborns delivered by normal women, the difference ranging between 200–400 g (Simpson et al., 1975; Eastman and Jackson, 1968; Edwards et al., 1979; Gormican et al., 1980; Naeye et al., 1973; Niswander et al., 1969; Rosso, 1981b).

Low prepregnancy weight mothers can substantially increase the mean birth weight of their infants if they succeed in increasing their gestational body weight gains well above average values, i.e., 15–18 kg (Rosso, 1981b; Eastman and Jackson, 1968) (Table II). This applies only to those mothers of average height. In chronically undernourished mothers who suffered growth stunting, the mean birth weight of the infants is likely to remain somewhat depressed even when their gestational weight gains are above average (Lazar et al., 1975; McKeown and Record, 1954; Love and Kinch, 1965). This effect would be mediated by the reduced maternal height.

Contrary to chronic undernutrition, women who suffer from gestational undernutrition are "undernourished" only relative to what is considered normal nutritional status for a pregnant woman, including appropriate weight gain.

The fetal consequences of gestational undernutrition depend on the maternal nutritional status at conception and on the duration and intensity of the caloric deficit. An interesting study of acute gestational undernutrition is the report on the effects of a period of famine in the pregnant women living in northern Holland in 1944–1945 (Stein et al., 1975). The Dutch famine, a World War II-related event, lasted approximately 28 weeks and was well defined in terms of intensity and duration. A unique characteristic of this unfortunate event was that it affected a population which was among the most affluent, and presumably best fed, in the world. Because of the relatively short duration of the famine, pregnant women were affected at different gestational times. Some were affected during the last weeks only, some

TABLE III. Effect of Moderate Gestational Undernutrition (weight gain less than 8.5 kg) on Birth Weight in Low Income American and Chilean Women With Obese and Normal Prepregnancy Weight-For-Height (mean ± SD)[a,b]

	Birth weight (g)	
	American	Chilean[b]
Normal	3,072 ± 352 (32)[c]	3,253 ± 379 (272)
Obese	3,480 ± 381 (27)	3,471 ± 362 (146)

[a]Populations similar to those described in Table II.
[b]Data from Rosso et al., 1987; unpublished.
[c]Number of subjects.

during the entire second half, some during the first half only, and so on. The results of the study indicated that gestational undernutrition decreases mean birth weight if it occurs during the last half of pregnancy. If gestational undernutrition takes place during the first half of pregnancy, and it is subsequently corrected, mean birth weight is normal. In the most affected group (those women exposed during the entire second half of gestation), mean birth weight fell 327 g, or 9%, compared with the prefamine values.

A similar study was conducted with data collected during the siege of Leningrad (Antonov, 1947). This siege lasted nearly 16 months and caused a much more severe food shortage than the one suffered by the Dutch population. In addition, at the start of the siege, the average person may not have been as well fed as the Dutch and, furthermore, the population was subjected to much harsher living conditions. The contribution of each of these factors cannot be established, but a marked reduction in mean birth weight, more than 530 g at term, was observed. Nearly 50% of all term infants exposed to famine during the second half of gestation weighed less than 2,500 g.

Gestational undernutrition is common in any obstetric population and, similar to the wartime experience, it depresses mean birth weight in pregravid normal women (Rosso, 1981b; Eastman and Jackson, 1968; Simpson et al., 1975; Naeye et al., 1973). However, the effect of gestational undernutrition is unapparent in obese women. In massively obese mothers, even a weight loss during gestation may not decrease mean birth weight below average values (Rosso, 1981; Eastman and Jackson, 1968) (Table III). The observation of a normal mean birth weight in obese women who either gain little weight or even lose weight indicates that fetal growth is strongly influenced by the nutritional status of the mother at conception. If the mother is chronically undernourished and, in addition, she suffers from gestational undernutrition, the birthweight of her infant will be markedly below average (Table II). If she does not suffer gestational undernutrition, the infant's birthweight will be higher, but still below average. Only if the affected mother is able to recover from her chronic undernutrition and gains a normal weight will the infant weight reach average values. In this case, maternal recovery will be reflected by an above average weight gain during gestation (Eastman and Jackson, 1968; Rosso, 1981b).

The lack of recognition of the influence of prepregnancy weight and weight gain on birth weight has been the source of much confusion and controversy in the past. For example, many authors have misunderstood the role that maternal caloric intake has on fetal growth. They correctly assumed that caloric intake influences caloric weight gain and that weight gain should influence mean birth weight. However, in a healthy gravida population, maternal weight gain and birth weight have, at best, only a weak correlation (Darby et al., 1953; Thomson, 1959; Papoz et al., 1981). These results have generated considerable puzzlement and have contributed greatly to the misconception that in an affluent society, nutrition has little or no influence on fetal growth (Rosso, 1984). Most of these "negative" data can be easily explained. The lack of correlation between caloric intake and birth weight reflects the fact that underweight women with high caloric intakes will have infants of similar if not lower mean birth weight than obese women consuming an equal amount or even fewer calories. Similarly, normal women may have large differences in caloric intake for a similar weight gain and similar size infant. Further, the possibility of finding a significant correlation between caloric intake and birth weight also depends on sample size. With a very large sample size, i.e., 500 subjects or more, a large range of body sizes can be expected. The smaller women will have lower intakes, proportional to their smaller body size, and they will deliver smaller infants. On the contrary, larger women will be at the opposite end of the spectrum in both respects. Thus, a linear correlation will be established. By contrast a smaller sample, with predominantly normal weight women, will determine a cluster of points with no linear correlation.

The different mean birth weights associated with various maternal nutritional statuses reflect either positive or negative shifts in fetal skeletal growth and the accumulation of fat and lean dry mass in the fetal body.

In the past, the fetal consequences of prenatal exposure to either chronic or gestational undernutrition did not receive adequate consideration. Most studies on the effect of maternal nutrition on the fetus only report birth weight. Available data suggest that both chronic and gestational undernutrition cause similar types of fetal growth retardation. The affected newborns have a reduction in body length proportionally smaller than the reduction in body weight and, in the average case, a head circumference within the normal range (Tables IV and V). In more severe cases, for example, when birth weight is below 2,500 g, head circumference is also significantly reduced (Stein et al., 1975; Rosso et al., 1983).

TABLE IV. Effect of Chronic Maternal Undernutrition on Anthropometric Characteristics of the Newborn in a Low Income Chilean Population (mean ± SD)[a]

Group[b]	n	Birth weight (g)	Body length (cm)	Head circ. (cm)
Control	120	3,265 ± 367	49.9 ± 1.9	34.4 ± 1.2
Chronic maternal undernutrition	50	3,050 ± 352	48.6 ± 1.9	33.9 ± 1.2

[a]Data from Rosso et al., 1987; unpublished.
[b]All births are singleton and full term.

These anthropometric characteristics correspond to the so-called "disproportionate" type of growth retardation, in contrast with the "proportionate" type in which the different body segments are affected to the same degree (Rosso and Winick, 1974). The disproportionate type of prenatal growth retardation has been observed in fetuses of pre-eclampsia and chronically hypertensive mothers (Kurjak et al., 1978; Keirse, 1984). Since in this case fetal growth retardation is believed to be caused by reduced placental blood

TABLE V. Effect of Gestational Undernutrition Caused by Famine on the Anthropometric Characteristics of the Newborn in a Previously Well Nourished Dutch Population (1944–1945) (mean ± SD)[a]

Group	Birth weight (g)	Body length (cm)	Head circ. (cm)
Pre-famine	3,418 ± 516	50.3 ± 5.3	34.9 ± 1.7
Peak of famine	3,008 ± 556	48.9 ± 4.4	34.8 ± 1.6

[a]Adapted from Stein et al., 1975.

flow, the similarities with infants exposed to both chronic and gestational undernutrition support the idea that the main mechanisms determining fetal growth retardation in the undernourished gravida is a reduced placental blood flow (Rosso, 1981a).

FETAL GROWTH RETARDATION AND MENTAL CAPACITY

The human brain completes an important phase of its growth and development during prenatal life. Practically the entire neuronal cell population and approximately 50% of the glial cell population found in the adult brain are present at birth (Winick, 1968; Dobbing and Sands, 1973).

The growth of the brain is an orderly process in which a defined sequence of events of great complexity takes place. For example, in the cerebral cortex, neuroblast proliferation at the ventricular margin is followed by neuroblast migration to the cortical plate, differentiation of neuroblasts by the development of perikaryon, dendritic formation, axon growth, and synaptic connection. Parallel to these changes, biochemical maturation nd neuro-transmitter expression take place (Sidman and Rakic, 1973). Any situation capable of either interrupting or disorganizing this development may lead to permanent changes ranging from minimal neurological abnormalities to severe handicap.

Studies on the effect of early undernutrition conducted in the rat have shown that severe undernutrition imposed either prenatally or postnatally determines a permanent deficit in brain cell number (Winick, 1976). When the caloric restriction exists over both prenatal and early postnatal periods, the effect is even more pronounced.

Early postnatal undernutrition also determines reduced brain cell number (Winick and Rosso, 1969a). Since head circumference and brain cell number are highly correlated (Winick and Rosso, 1969b), the smaller head circum-ference of infants surviving early malnutrition supports the possibility of a permanent cell deficit in the human brain similar to that described in animals.

The consequences of early postnatal malnutrition on cognitive develop-ment and behavior have been the subject of numerous studies (Winick, 1976). These studies show that both experimental animals and children who have experienced early malnutrition have retarded psychomotor development and various behavioral abnormalities. The effect represents a combination of the biological impact of nutrition and the deprived environment in which the undernourished child grows and develops. Studies with adopted children have shown that an appropriate diet and a stimulating environment can largely reverse the negative effects attributed to malnutrition (Winick et al., 1975; Lien et al., 1977).

Acute gestational undernutrition of the type and severity observed during the Dutch famine does not affect intellectual development (Stein et al., 1975). This conclusion was reached after several tests of mental perfor-mance, applied to males prenatally exposed to famine, demonstrated no significant differences compared to a control group. However, it can be argued that this type of undernutrition was not severe enough to affect subsequent mental capacity because brain growth was not affected. As shown in Table V, during the peak of the famine period, mean head circumference in the newborn was similar to either pre-famine or post-famine periods.

Attempts have been made to modify the expected adverse outcome of prenatal exposure to undernutrition by providing the mothers with food supplements. The best known of these studies were conducted in markedly different environments: a low-income black population in New York City (Rush et al., 1980), a rural population in Taiwan (McDonald et al., 1981; Adair and Pollitt, 1985); and a rural population in Guatemala (Habicht et al., 1974; Lechtig et al., 1975; Klein et al., 1977).

The main purpose of the New York City study was to reduce the higher mortality rates among black infants by increasing mean birth weight with a nutritional supplement. This nutritional intervention is, undoubtedly, the most complex one, and a brief review of its strengths and weaknesses reveals many of the problems faced by those working in this field. The design, the control of compliance, and appropriate data analysis stand out as major strengths. The main problems are the selection of the study population and the type of supplement chosen. The main recruitment criteria, in addition to being healthy, black, and English-speaking, were a history of previous low weight gain for the duration of gestation, and low protein intake (less than 50 g) in the 24 hr preceding registration.

A low birth weight delivery may be caused by many factors besides undernutrition. In the prenatal study, there were no differences in caloric intake between mothers reporting at least one low birth weight delivery and other participants, excluding mothers recruited because of low protein intake.

Low weight at conception was perhaps the best of the main enrollment criteria, but by no means is nutritionally adequate. A small group of these women were probably normal but of small body size. These groups could have been defined using weight/height criteria.

A low weight gain in a woman with a normal nutritional status at conception indicates gestational undernutrition. However, as already mentioned, more often than not, low gestational weight gains are seen in obese women. Therefore, low weight gain alone does not indicate maternal undernutrition.

Protein intake of less than 50 g in the 24 hr prior to recruitment is an unreliable indicator of general dietary inadequacy. It can be argued that although a 24-hr protein intake may be an unreliable index when applied to a single individual, it may be helpful to identify an at-risk group. In fact, participants recruited because of their low protein intakes continued to report lower intakes than the rest of the subjects during the study, but their daily intakes (68.3 g/day) seem appropriate, especially if one considers the present RDAs, for protein to be unnecessarily high when compared with WHO recommendations.

The participants were randomly assigned to one of three treatment groups: 1) supplement, who received a high protein beverage containing 470 Kcal and 40 g protein daily; 2) complement, who received a balanced protein-calorie beverage containing 322 Kcal and 6 g protein; and 3) controls, who received only vitamin and minerals supplements routinely prescribed at prenatal clinics.

The results indicated no significant differences in mean birth weight between control and both supplemented groups despite the fact that these groups consumed a significantly greater amount of calories and protein.

TABLE VI. Psychological Measures at 1 Year of Age of Infants Delivered by Low Income Black Women Receiving Various Levels of Nutrient Supplementation During Pregnancy[a]

	Treatment group		
	Control	Complement	Supplement
Bayley mental score	99.39	98.65	98.97
Bayley motor score	45.81	45.79	45.78
Object permanence score	15.12	14.75	14.95
Play:			
Latency (sec)	108	129	125
Length of episode (sec)	71.7	59.7	87.3[*]
Sophistication (median score)	4.33	4.17	4.27
Habitation (slope)	-0.66	-0.57[*]	-0.84[**]
Dishabituation (sec)	1.33	2.2	4.6

[a]Adapted from Rush et al., 1980.
[*]$P < 0.05$ vs. other two groups combined.
[**]$P < 0.01$ vs. other two groups combined.

However, the differences in maternal weight gain between the control and either supplemented group were too small to cause any significant change, even if the women would have been undernourished. Moreover, there was a significant disproportion between the estimated cumulative caloric intake of the supplemented women and their weight gain. The supplemented women, as a group, consumed approximately 45,000 Kcal more than the control group, but they gained only 1.7 lb (0.77 kg) more than the controls. Based on a caloric cost of 3,500 Kcal per 1.0 lb of weight gained, the supplement group should have gained nearly 13 lb more than the control group. This finding strongly suggests an overestimation of the intake, but this explanation is not supported by the data on compliance, which seem rather convincing. The discrepancy has been attributed to undefined metabolic changes but, most likely, reflects methodological limitations.

Overall, the study seems to indicate that indiscriminate nutrient supplementation to women who, as a group, are not chronically undernourished has no beneficial influence on birth weight.

The infants were also studied at 12 months of age, and the different groups were compared on ten measures of psychological development adjusted for age and sex. Significant differences were found only in three of these measures: habituation, dishabituation, and length of play episodes. In each instance, the infants from the mother who received the largest quantity of nutritional supplementation (supplement group) were significantly different from the other two groups (Table VI). These changes were not correlated with somatic measures of growth, and thus, they were attributed to the maternal consumption of the supplement. The meaning of the findings is tentative. Since the effects were unrelated to a significant change in fetal somatic growth, they must reflect a more subtle change in either brain morphology or cell function. The visual habituation test would reflect "a more efficient central nervous system function" (Lewis, 1971), indicating that the supplemented infant may have better I.Q. scores later in life, but this possibility remains to be investigated. Overall, the importance of these findings is that they support the possibility of fetal effects mediated by the quality of the maternal diet, a fact of great potential relevance.

The Taiwan study (Adair and Pollitt, 1985) was conducted in a group of rural villages considered to be economically distressed when the study began in 1967. The local diet contained little meat, consisting mainly of rice, sweet potatoes, and peanuts. A dietary survey of the female population indicated a mean daily intake of about 1,200 Kcal and 36–37 g protein.

The study was a longitudinal, double blind, nutrition intervention. Women were recruited in the last trimester of pregnancy if they were married with at least one male child, planned to have one additional child, and were judged to be of low socio-economic status. A total of 294 women, ages 19–30 years, were enrolled in the study. The subjects were randomly assigned to a supplement group A or B. Group A received a chocolate-flavored nutrient-rich liquid supplement, expected to provide, if consumed, an additional daily intake of 20 g of protein, 13.3 g of fat, and 50 g of carbodydrate. Mothers in group B received a placebo providing only 10 g of carbohydrates. In addition, both groups received a multivitamin-mineral tablet daily and were provided with medical care. The supplements were distributed twice daily at a village field station or, if required, were delivered directly to the mother, either at home or in the fields.

The women were followed continuously from the final trimester of one pregnancy and subsequent lactation period through a second pregnancy and lactation period, but supplemented only after the birth of the first study infant. Comparison of the supplemented and unsupplemented groups showed no differences in any of the anthropometric measurements, including weight, length, Rohrer's index (wt/length^3), head circumference, and subscapular skinfold. Intragroup comparisons of the first and second sibling in group A revealed a statistically significant difference in male infants, who weighed 162 g more than the previous infant. Anthropometric covariations between siblings were significantly reduced for Rohrer's index in the females of group A, indicating an effect of maternal supplementation.

Infant motor and mental development was assessed using a research version of the Bayley Scales of Infant Development. The test was administered to 8-month-old infants and intergroup comparison revealed no significant differences, except for motor scores when male and female infants were analyzed together.

The Stanford Binet Intelligence Scale was administered when the infants were 5 years of age and, again, none of the inter- or intragroup comparisons indicated significant differences.

This study, which was well designed in terms of the intervention and the control of confounding variables, suffers from many of the problems which have been previously discussed. The mothers were a heterogeneous group, with only a minority being really underweight before pregnancy. The mean weight for height corresponds to 93% of standard weight, therefore, within normal limits. More important, the supplement failed to cause a significant increase in maternal weight gain compared with the placebo group. Finally, given the expected individual variability in some of the key measures, for example birth weight, sample size is too small to detect a moderate change.

The Guatemalan study was conducted in four small villages. The initial experiment was designed to compare the effect of protein supplementation in a diet providing approximately 1,500 Kcal/day and about 40 g protein. Two types of supplements were provided: atole (a gruel) and fresco (a refreshing cool drink). Two villages received one type of supplement and two the other. Women were encouraged to come daily to a supplementation center, and this resulted in a wide range of supplemented intake. Comparisons of protein and non-protein-supplemented villages revealed no apparent effects on the main variables. On the supposition that both supplementation terms were equally effective, the investigators decided to organize cohorts according to the level of cumulative caloric intake provided by supplementation. Thus, two groups were finally organized: women who consumed more than 20,000 Kcal and women who consumed less than 20,000 Kcal.

The main finding was a higher mean birth weight in the high consumption group of approximately 110 g and a lower percentage of low birth weight infants (9 vs. 28%, approximately). Children were tested at 36, 48 and 60 months of age. The sample of 671 infants born during the 4 years of maternal supplementation and 412 who were already born, but under 3 years of age when the study began. At each examination the supplemented children performed better than the unsupplemented ones on the composite measure of cognitive tests and other individual tests. Socio-economic status did not account for the differences and within-families comparison revealed sibling differences associated with the intervention.

Although the results reflect in most cases the influence of combined pre- and postnatal supplementation, regression analysis suggests that the gestational period and the first 2 years of life are the most important in determining subsequent mental developmental.

This study provides the strongest support presented so far for the possibility that maternal diet and nutritional status during pregnancy influence psychological outcome, but it has some limitations. The most serious difficulty derives from the self-selection present in the type of data analysis performed. Since in each village the mothers themselves chose whether to visit the supplementation centers and also the quantity of beverage to be consumed, it is reasonable to assume that those who consumed more supplement could have been "different" than the low consumers. The investigators examined this possibility by analyzing maternal height, weight, age, morbidity, parity, birth interval, and home diet and concluded that none of these factors could account for the effect on birth weight. Another possibility investigated was that the growth potential of the fetus could influence maternal appetite, thus causing mothers bearing larger fetuses to consume more supplements. This highly theoretical possibility can be ruled out based on the similarities in caloric consumption of women carrying male and females infants despite the heavier birth weight of the males. Perhaps the greatest problem for the interpretation of the psychological outcome is to separate the prenatal from the postnatal effects caused by supplementation. In this respect the data cannot be considered conclusive.

Similar to the Taiwan data, the initial nutritional status of the Guatemalan mothers was considerably less dramatic than suggested by the caloric intake data. The mean maternal height of only 149 cm suggests chronic exposure to a nutritionally deprived environment. The mean weight at the end of the first trimester was 49 kg. This indicates a mean weight for height equivalent to 98% of standard weight, therefore, within normal limits. Perhaps the main problem in these women was inadequate caloric intake during pregnancy, as reflected by an average weight gain of only 7 kg. Thus, the results would be more representative of the effects of gestational undernutrition than low maternal prepregnancy weight. However, a group of mothers probably experienced both types of problems. The consequences of either type of undernutrition on the fetus could be substantially different. For example, the prenatal growth of infants of mothers with low prepregnancy weight who also suffer from gestational undernutrition may be more depressed than those suffering from gestational undernutrition alone. The postnatal consequences of either situation, in terms of postnatal physical growth and mental development, could be important.

A followup study (Villar et al., 1984) of intrauterine-growth-retarded and normal infants included in the Guatemalan supplementation study compared their growth and development. The growth-retarded infants were divided in two groups: those with normal ponderal index [PI = (wt/length^3) $\times$ 100], and those with low ponderal index. Both groups had a similar mean birth weight. Overall, at 3 years of age, the infants with low ponderal index were lighter, shorter, and had smaller head circumferences than those with normal ponderal index. The low ponderal index infants also had the lowest values in seven of eight developmental measures and in the composite score. This study indicates the urgent need to better define the maternal situation as well as the characteristics of the newborn to begin to clear up some of the present confusion. In this respect, most of the data now available is of little help.

Another approach to the problem of establishing the postnatal consequences of growth retardation caused by maternal undernutrition is to observe the growth and development of infants prenatally growth-retarded for other causes. The basis for this approach is the evidence indicating that maternal diet has little influence on subsequent outcome compared with the effect of growth retardation. If this assumption is correct, an infant who is growth-retarded because of maternal undernutrition would be comparable to a child who is growth-retarded because the mother has been chronically hypertensive. As previously mentioned, these infants may have similar anthropometric characteristics and may be the product of a placenta with reduced maternal blood perfusion. There are numerous studies on the postnatal growth of infants who suffered growth retardation in utero. The data pose many questions derived from the fact that until recently, the infants have been considered a homogeneous group. Despite this serious problem, the overall impression is that these infants have a greater risk of developmental problems, ranging from minor neurological abnormalities to severe handicap, than the normal size newborns (Taylor, 1984).

When considering the postnatal consequences of fetal growth retardation it is important to remember that most of these infants have suffered the effect of a reduced maternal placental blood flow and, therefore, in addition to growth retardation, they may suffer the effect of intrapartum asphyxia. During the newborn period they may also have hypothermia, hyperbilirubinemia, and hypoglycemia, especially those born before term (Oh, 1977). These problems are reflected in considerably higher mortality rates in intrauterine-growth-retarded infants than in those fully grown (Starfield et al., 1982).

The best-known followup study of infants who suffered intrauterine growth retardation was conducted in 96 full-term growth-retarded infants by Fitzhardinge and Steven (1972) in Montreal, Canada. All infants had a birth weight 2 standard deviations below mean birth weight for gestation and, approximately, one-third were more than 3 standard deviations below the mean. The infants were followed for a minimum of 6 years. Most of these infants suffered from a disproportionate type of growth retardation, as indicated by higher mean values for head circumference than body weight in comparison with the general population means. Incremental growth patterns were compared with a control group of 24 normal newborn infants born at the same time as the test children. The incremental growth pattern was significantly greater for the study children during the first 6 months of life but remained the same as the normal birth weight for the rest of the study period.

As a result of the intrauterine and immediate postnatal failure, these children tended to remain small. At the age of 2 years, their average weight and length was just above the 3rd percentile, while head circumference was at the 10th percentile. Neurological and psychological assessment revealed various problems. One of the children developed cerebral palsy, while six others were subject to repeated convulsions. These abnormalities were associated with neonatal asphyxia. The remaining 89 children were free of any major sequelae, but 16 had problems in coordination and fine motor ability. The average I.Q. at school was 95 for boys and 101 for girls. The curve was skewed to the left for the males, with 25% of the children scoring 80 or less. No significant correlation was found between birth weight and subsequent intelligence scores. A number of children (50% of the males and 36% of the females) had poor school performance which required special care. The patients followed into adolescence (Westwood et al., 1983) did not include those with neonatal asphyxia. This subgroup of children was similar to controls in terms of motor function, coordination, gait, and stretch reflexes. The mean IQ scores continued to be lower in the test children than controls, but this difference was attributed to socio-economic differences. There were no differences in the number of school years successfully completed and in post high school education.

A study in a British population (Neligan et al., 1976) measured performance at 5, 6, and 7 years of age in children who had suffered fetal growth retardation. Measurements were adjusted for maternal age and care of the child, sex, birth order, antepartum hemorrhage, and mode of delivery. The results indicate stunted growth, retarded language, and increased incidence of neurological abnormalities compared with a control group of children who had a normal size at birth either full term or preterm. Verbal IQ (Wechsler) was also significantly lower at 6 years of age in the intrauterine growth retardation group. In contrast with the Canadian study (Fitzhardinge and Steven, 1972), a significant positive correlation was found between the degree of impairement and the severity of growth retardation at birth. A similar correlation between fetal growth retardation and low IQ scores has been reported by others (Francis-Williams and Davis, 1974).

Studies conducted in twins of unequal size have provided additional information regarding postnatal development of children who have suffered intrauterine growth retardation while controlling for intervening factors such as birth order and family environment. Four studies of intelligence in like-sex twins have been reported (Babson et al., 1964; Churchill, 1965; Kaelberg and Pugh, 1969; Hohenauer, 1971). Except for Babson et al. (1964) who used a 25% difference in birth weight, the rest of the authors have used a 300-g difference in birth weight as criterion for inclusion in the study. The number of twin pairs in each study ranged from 12 to 17. The results show a consistant difference of 5.8–7.7 points in IQ scores, with values lower in the smaller twin.

Thus, the available data indicate that infants exposed to prenatal growth retardation have a high risk of important sequelae. It remains undetermined if the observed abnormalities are largely determined by intrapartum insults or early postnatal complications. Therefore, it is still unknown to what extent better prenatal and postnatal care could reduce the possibility of later handicap. It is also important to better define the influence of time of onset and severity of the prenatal growth retardation on subsequent physical growth and mental capacity. Clinical studies suggest that growth retardation must begin before week 26 of gestation for significant deficits to appear later in life (Fancourt et al., 1976; Harvey et al., 1982). However, the possibility remains that a later onset fetal growth retardation including brain growth retardation, such as that associated with severe gestational undernutrition in a previously well nourished mother, may also affect subsequent development. Future studies may provide an answer to that question.

REFERENCES

Abrams BF, Laros RK (1986): Prepregnancy weight gain and birth weight. Am J Obstet Gynecol 154:503–509.

Adair LS, Pollitt E (1985): Outcome of maternal nutritional supplementation: A comprehensive review of the Bacon Chow study. Am J Clin Nutr 41:948–978.

Antonov A (1947): Children born during the siege of Leningrad in 1942. J Pediatr 30:250–259.

Babson SG, Kangas J, Young N, Bramhall JL (1964): Growth and development of twins of dissimilar size at birth. Pediatrics 33:327–333.

Beal VA (1971): Nutrition studies during pregnancy. II. Dietary intake, maternal weight gain, and size of infant. J Am Diet Assoc 58:321–326.

Bjerre B, Bjerre I (1976): Significance of obstetric factors in prognosis of low birth weight children. Acta Paediatr Scand 65:577–583.

Chávez A, Martínez C (1970): "Nutrición y Desarrollo Infantil". México DF: Interamericana, pp 52–64.

Churchill JA (1965): Relationship between intelligence and birth weight in twins. Neurology 15:341–347.

Darby WJ, McGanity WJ, Martin MP, Bridgeforth E, Densen PM, Kaser MM, Ogle PJ, Newbill JS, Stockwell A, Ferguson ME, Touster W, McClellen GS, Williams C, Cannon RO (1953): The Vanderbilt cooperative study of maternal and iron nutrition. IV. Dietary, laboratory and physical findings in 2129 delivered pregnancies. J Nutr 51:565–597.

Dobbing J 1985): Maternal nutrition in pregnancy and later achievment of the offspring: A personal interpretation. Early Hum Dev 12:1–8.

Dobbing J, Sands J (1973): Quantitative growth and development of human brain. Arch Dis Child 48:757–763

Dobbing J, Sands J (1979): Comparative aspects of the brain growth spurt. Early Hum Dev 3:79–83.

Eastman NJ, Jackson EC (1968): Weight relationships in pregnancy. I. The bearing of maternal weight gain and prepregnancy weight in full term pregnancies. Obstet Gynecol Surv 21:1003–1025.

Edwards LE, Alton IR, Barrada MI, Hakanson EY (1979): Pregnancy in the underweight woman. Am J Obstet Gynecol 135:297–302.

Fancourt R, Campbell S, Harvey D, Norman AP (1976): Follow-up study of small-for-dates babies. Br Med J 1:1435–1437.

Fitzhardinge PM, Steven EM (1972): The small for date infant. II. Neurological and intellectual sequelae. Pediatrics 50:50–57.

Francis-Williams J, Davies PA (1974): Very low birthweight and later intelligence. Dev Med Child Neurol 16:709–728.

Gormican A, Valentine J, Satter E (1980): Relationships of maternal weight gain, prepregnancy weight and infant birthweight. J Am Diet Assoc 77:662–667.

Habicht JP, Lechtig A, Yarbrough C, Klein R (1974): Maternal nutrition, birth weight and infant mortality. In: "Size at Birth." Ciba Foundation Symposium 27 (new series). Amsterdam: Elsevier-Excerpta Medica-North Holland pp 353–377.

Harvey C, Prince J, Bunton J (1982): Abilities of children who were small-for-gestational age babies. Pediatrics 69:296–300.

Hohenauer L (1971): Prenatal nutrition and subsequent development. Lancet I: 644–645.

Holt AB, Cheek DB, Mellits ED, Hill DE (1975): Brain size and the relation of the primate to the nonprimate. In Cheek DB (ed): "Fetal and Postnatal Cellular Growth." New York: John Wiley and Sons, pp 23–44.

Kaelberg CT, Pugh TF (1969): Influence of intrauterine relations on the intelligence of twins. N Engl J Med 19:1030–1034.

Keirse MJNC (1984): Epidemiology and aetiology of the growth retarded baby. Clin Obstet Gynaecol 11:415–436.

Klein RE, Irwin M, Engle PL, Towned J, Lechtig A, Martorell R, Delgado H (1977): Malnutrition, child health and behavioural development. Data from an intervention study. In Mitter P (ed): "Research to Practice in Mental Retardation." Vol. 3, "Biomedical Aspects". Baltimore: University Park Press, pp 299–310.

Kurjac A, Latin V, Polak J (1978): Ultrasonic recognition of two types of fetal growth retardation by measurement of four fetal dimensions. J Perinat Med 6:102–108.

Lazar P, Dreyfus J, Papiernik O, Berkauer E (1975): Individual correction of birthweight for parental stature with special reference to small-for-date and large-for-date infants. J Perinat Med 3:242–247.

Lechtig A, Martorell R, Delgado H, Yarbrough C, Klein RE (1975): Food supplementation during pregnancy and birthweight. Pediatrics 56:508–520.

Lewis M (1971): Individual differences in the measurement of early cognitive growth. In Hellmuth J (ed): "Exceptional Infant, Studies in Abnormalities," Vol. 2. New York: Brunner-Mazel, pp 172–210.

Lien NM, Meyer KK, Winick M (1977): Early malnutrition and "late" adoption: A study of their effects on the development of Korean orphans adopted into American families. Am J Clin Nutr 30:1734–1739.

Love EJ, Kinch RAH (1965): Factors influencing the birth weight in normal pregnancy. Am J Obstet Gynecol 91:342–349.

McDonald EC, Pollitt E, Mueller W, Hsueh AM, Sherwin R (1981): The Bacon Chow study: Maternal nutritional supplementation and birthweight of offspring. Am J Clin Nutr 34:2133–2144.

McKeoun T, Record RG (1954): Influence of prenatal environment on correlation between birthweight and parental height. Am J Hum Genet 6:457–463.

Naeye RL, Blanc W, Paul C (1973): Effects of maternal nutrition on the human fetus. Pediatrics 52:494–503.

Neligan GA, Kolvin I, Scott DM, Garside RF (1976): Born too soon or born too small. A follow-up study to seven years of age. Spastic International Medical Publications. London: William Heinemann Medical Books, Philadelphia: J. B. Lippincott, pp 66–79.

Niswander K, Jackson EC (1974): Physical characteristics of the gravida and their association with birthweight and perinatal death. Am J Obstet Gynecol 119:306–313.

Niswander KR, Singer J, Westphal M Jr, Weiss W (1969): Weight gain during pregnancy and prepregnancy weight. Obstet Gynecol 33:482–491.

Oh W (1977): Considerations in neonates with intrauterine growth retardation. Clin Obstet Gynecol 20:991–1003.

Papoz L, Eschwege E, Pequignot G, Barrat J (1981): Dietary behavior during pregnancy: The St. Antoine Maternity Hospital study in Paris. In Dobbing J (ed): "Maternal Nutrition in Pregnancy. Eating for Two?" New York: Academic Press, pp 71–80.

Rosso P (1981a): Nutrition and maternal-fetal exchange. Am J Clin Nutr 34:744–755.

Rosso P (1981b): Prenatal nutrition and fetal growth. Pediatr Ann 10:430–439.

Rosso P (1984): Nutrition during pregnancy: Myths and realities. In Winick M (ed): "Concurrent Concepts in Nutrition. Vol 13, "Nutrition in the 20th Century," New York: John Wiley and Sons, pp 47–70.

Rosso P, Arteaga A, Foradori A, Grebe G, Lira P, Torres J, Vela P (1983): Physiological adjustments and pregnancy outcome in low-income Chilean women. Fed Proc 17:138A.

Rosso P, Winick M (1974): Intrauterine growth retardation. A new systematic approach based on the clinical and biochemical characteristics of this condition. J Perinat Med 2:147–160.

Rush D, Stein Z, Susser M (1980): Diet in pregnancy: A randomized controlled trial of nutritional supplements. Birth Defects 26(3), pp 87–104.

Sidman RL, Rakic P (1973): Neuronal migration with special reference to developing human brain: A review. Brain Res 62:1–35.

Simpson JW, Lawless RW, Mitchell AC (1975): Responsibility of the obstetrician to the fetus. II. Influence of prepregnancy weight and pregnancy weight gain on birthweight. Am J Obstet Gynecol 45:481–487.

Starfield B, Shapiro S, McCormick M, Bross D (1982): Mortality and morbidity in infants with intrauterine growth retardation. J Pediatr 101:978–983.

Stein Z, Susser M, Saenger G, Marolla F (1975): "Famine and Human Development." New York: Oxford University Press.

Stoch MB, Smythe PM (1963): Does undernutrition during infancy inhibit brain growth and subsequent metnal development? Arch Dis Child 38:546–552.

Taylor DJ (1984): Low birthweight and neurodevelopmental handicap. Clin Obstet Gynaecol 11:525–542.

Thomson Am (1959): Diet in pregnancy. 3. Diet in relation to the course and outcome of pregnancy. Br J Nutr 13:509–525.

Tompkins MT, Mitchell RM, Wiehl DG (1955): Maternal nutrition studies at Philadelphia Lying-in Hospital. 2. Prematurity and maternal nutrition. In "The Promotion of Newborn and Maternal Health." New York: Milkbank Memorial Fund, pp 25–50.

Villar J, Smeriglio V, Martorell R, Brown CH, Klein R (1984): Heterogeneous growth and mental development of intrauterine growth retarded infants during the first three years of life. Pediatrics 74:783–791.

Westwood M, Kramer MS, Munz D, Lovett JM, Watters GV (1983): Growth and development of non-asphyxiated small-for-gestational age newborns: Follow-up through adolescence. Pediatrics 71:376–382.

Winick M (1968): Changes in nucleic acid and protein content of the human brain during growth. Pediatr Res 2:352–355.

Winick M (1976): "Malnutrition and Brain Development." New York: Oxford University Press.

Winick M, Meyer KK, Harris RC (1975): Malnutrition and environmental enrichment by early adoption. Science 190:1173–1175.

Winick M, Rosso P (1969a): The effect of severe early malnutrition on cellular growth of the human brain. Pediatr Res 3:181–184.

Winick M, Rosso P (1969b): Head circumference and cellular growth of the brain in normal and marasmic children. J Pediatr 74:774–778.

Index